TEXTS AND
TRANSFORMATIONS

For Anne,
Victor H. Mair
25/III/18

TEXTS AND
TRANSFORMATIONS

Essays in Honor of
the 75th Birthday of
VICTOR H. MAIR

EDITED BY

Haun Saussy

CAMBRIA
PRESS

Amherst, New York

Requests for permission should be directed to
permissions@cambriapress.com, or mailed to:
Cambria Press
100 Corporate Parkway, Suite 128
Amherst, New York 14226, USA.

Library of Congress Cataloging-in-Publication Data on file.

ISBN: 978-1-60497-956-5

Table of Contents

Chapter 10: Fotudeng's Spell Practice and the Dhāraṇī Recitation Ritual
Koichi Shinohara 271

Chapter 11: The Not-So-Long Arm of the Law
Phyllis Granoff 289

Chapter 12: Who Guards the Buddha-Word?
Tanya Storch 311

Chapter 13: Yijing and the Buddhist Cosmopolis of the Seventh Century
Tansen Sen 345

Chapter 14: Countdown to 1051
Mimi Yiengpruksawan 369

About the Contributors 435

Cambria Sinophone World Series 441

Index 445

LIST OF FIGURES

Tabula Gratulatoria

The following individuals have entered their names in this tabula gratulatoria to express their gratitude for what Victor Mair has done and as a tribute to his impact on Asian studies throughout the world. While we did our best to reach all who might have wanted to add their names, we did not reach everyone and know that this list represents only a fraction of those whose lives and work have been greatly enriched by Victor Mair.

* * *

Susan R. Anderson

Center for Buddhist Studies, University of Arizona

East Asian Studies Department, University of Arizona

Kathlene Baldanza

Anthony Barbieri-Low

T. H. Barrett

Wolfgang Behr

Mark Bender

James A. Benn

Rostislav Berezkin

Michael Berry

Susan D. Blum

Gayle Foster Bodorff

Stephen R. Bokenkamp

Daniel Boucher

Jim Breen

Katharine P. Burnett

Cambria Press

Linda H. Chance

Kang-i Sun Chang

Huaiyu Chen

Chen Jinhua

Kaijun Chen

Xiaomei Chen

Cheng Fangyi

Eva Shan Chou

John Colarusso

Jennifer Crewe

Wiebke Denecke

Nicola Di Cosmo

June Teufel Dreyer

Ronald Egan

Gina Elia

Lothar von Falkenhausen

Geraldine Fiss

Erika Forte

Charlotte Furth

Liangyan Ge

Levi Gibbs

Erika H Gilson

Peter B. Golden

Phyllis Granoff

Linda Greene

Alison Groppe

Guinsr Peggy Guinsr

Chris Hamm

Valerie Hansen

Hartley Lauran R. Hartley

Hartman Charles Hartman

Rowena He

Anne Henochowicz

Jane Hickman

Gene Hill

Michel Hockx

Laura Hostetler

H. M. Agnes Hsu-Tang

Minghui Hu

Hu Ying

Wilt L. Idema

Lionel Jensen

Jiang Chenxin

Nicholas A. Kaldis

Paize Keulemans

Ross King

Jeffrey C. Kinkley

Cornelius C. Kubler

Wendy Larson

Charles A. Laughlin

Mabel Lee

Dore J. Levy

Melody Yunzi Li

Qiancheng Li

Perry Link

Jonathan Lipman

Liu Jianmei

Zhenzhen Lu

Liang Luo

Christopher Lupke

Richard John Lynn

In memory of Joseph C. and Esther F.L. Mair

David M. Mair

Denis C. Mair

Joseph R. Mair

Thomas Krishna Mair

Thomas L. Mair

Jim Mallory

Paul Manfredi

Justin McDaniel

Joseph P. McDermott

Tsu-Lin Mei

Xiuyuan Mi

Arina Mikhalevskaya

James Millward

Diane Moderski

Thomas Moran

David Moser

Brendan O'Kane

EALC, University of Pennsylvania

Peter Perdue

Martin Powers

Nanxiu Qian

Bob Ramsey

Evelyn S. Rawski

Jeffrey Rice

John S. Rohsenow

Carlos Rojas

Haun Saussy

Neil Schmid

David K. Schneider

Leander Seah

Cecilia Segawa Seigle

Tansen Sen

Kelsey Seymour

Ed Shaughnessy

Shu-mei Shih

Koichi Shinohara

Jerome Silbergeld

Jonathan Stalling

Tanya Storch

E. K. Tan

Toni Tan

Ori Tavor

Emma J. Teng

Jing Tsu

J. Marshall Unger

Rudolph Wagner

David Der-wei Wang

Jiajia Wang

Yuanfei Wang

Sophie Ling-chia Wei

Stephen H. West

Ellen Widmer

Carrie E. Wiebe

Endymion Wilkinson

Dorothy C. Wong

Chia-rong Wu

I-Hsien Wu

Jiang Wu

Kunbing Xiao

Xie Bo

Xu Wenkan

Xiaowen Xu

Mimi Yiengpruksawan

Leqi Yu

Li Yu

Zhansui Yu

Zhang Xing

TEXTS AND TRANSFORMATIONS

INTRODUCTION

FROM THE CAVE OF
A THOUSAND BOOKS

AN APPRECIATION OF VICTOR MAIR

Haun Saussy

A story must begin somewhere. To start this one in Ohio or at Harvard would yield too short a run-up; more momentum is needed to stage the leap that has been Victor Mair's scholarly career.[1] Not a leap of faith, incidentally, but a leap or series of flights outside the area that is familiar to China scholars.

Let the story begin, rather, with a day around the year 1000 CE, when (we conjecture) a group of monks under threat of invasion hid their abbey's library holdings in a cave near Mogao, Dunhuang County, in northwest China. In "a small cave, a little bigger than ten feet" they arranged "countless numbers of white packets... In each packet were ten scrolls. In addition, Buddhist flags embroidered with figures were spread out underneath the white packets."[2] Alongside the carefully prepared bundles of Buddhist scrolls were "mixed bundles" of Sanskrit, Tibetan, Uyghur, Sogdian, Khotanese, Turkish, and Kuchean manuscripts, as well as paintings, textiles, and what we might call library supplies (silk wrappers, wooden rollers, snippets of fabric, wooden strainers and the like). The door to the cave was sealed and the library experienced almost nine hundred years of quiet. Then in 1900 a local Daoist priest and freelance abbot, Wang Yuanlu, looking to restore the paintings and furnishings of the long-abandoned temple caves, broke through the mud-brick wall and discovered the treasures within. Unable to read the materials in languages other than Chinese, Daoist Wang took samples of painting and calligraphy to present to provincial officials and sold a few items for restoration expenses. In 1907–1908, Aurel Stein and Paul Pelliot successively convinced Wang to part with thousands of scrolls for the collections of the British Museum and the Bibliothèque Nationale. (The International Dunhuang Project now seeks to reconstitute the dispersed collection through digital means.[3])

Whatever moved the people of a thousand years ago to wall up a roomful of documents, one consequence, unknowable at the time, of their action was to create the conditions for the emergence of the scholarly species we know as Victor Mair. Victor Mair's mind is Dunhuangian, if the expression may be permitted: polyglot, heteroclite, multimedia, syncretic, vernacular, with strong currents flowing from presumed margins to presumed center and back again. It contains a well-organized Indo-Chinese compartment and holds items from many other linguistic areas arranged in singular ways. It is a Silk Road kind of mind, a place of interaction, exchange, and overlay.[4] It is a mind that loves lists:

> These men wrote about such topics as wars, temples, belvederes, gazebos, huts, scholars, maids, courtesans, actors, storytellers, ventriloquists, dogs, calligraphy, stationery, bamboo, canes, trips to the countryside, attendants, fools, paintings, portraits, poetry, retirement, old age, death, dreams, the mind of a child, peach blossoms, flowers, excursions, brooks, lakes, ponds, mountains, drinking, and all manner of books.[5]

> [...]The spectrum of Chinese intellectual orientations can by no means be limited to Buddhism, Taoism, and Confucianism. Also

to be taken into account are Magianism, shamanism, legalism, hedonism, eremitism, utilitarianism, naturalism, technocracy, rationalism, Nestorian Christianity, Manicheism, Zoroastrianism, Judaism, Islam, Hinduism, Catholicism, Protestantism, and many other assorted teachings and practices.... Traditional Chinese culture, like contemporary Chinese culture, consisted of a virtually infinite number of separate strands and fibers...[6]

This multifarious, raucous, come-all-ye, never-finished conception of culture contrasts markedly with the generally received paradigm of a benevolent "assimilation" of foreignness into a lasting Chinese cultural "mainstream" the beginnings of which go back to the Neolithic villages of the Yellow River Valley. "Whether in real life or at the level of thought and the emotions, it is the tradition of Confucius and Mencius that has proved the mainstay of generations of intellectuals in China," says the assimilationist paradigm; "it was the Confucian-educated scholar-intellectuals who produced almost all of Chinese philosophy, aesthetics, art, and literature," in a tradition whose "basic character remained unchanged" from beginning to end.[7] In that view of Chinese literary and intellectual history, the flower and fruit can be discerned from the seed; but in the perspective of a Dunhuang cave-dweller, nothing can be predicted because the path of culture can at any moment be turned this way or that by reckoning with new inputs. Unauthorized writers compose in unrecognizable genres; forgotten tombs yield mummies that were not on anyone's ancestor list. Transformation can be sudden and total, since perduring identity is not assumed.[8] The vernacular, in Victor Mair's histories, operates rather as in Erich Auerbach's history of European realism: as a force dissolving classical hierarchies of genre and style, a channel whereby unmastered "antagonisms" enter literary representation.[9]

This attention to what breaks with precedent is not a mere matter of taste. Scholarly works have, no less than works of fiction or poetry, their plots and genres. Although fluent in such genres as translation, annotation, didactic expansion, stylistic appreciation, ingenious allegory,

identification of common threads, life and works, intercultural comparison, and reframing, Victor Mair has always been drawn to the mystery
genre. In even the best-settled accounts of literature and culture, something requires explanation. The *bianwen* 變文 of Dunhuang are "texts of
extraordinary significance for the subsequent development of popular
literature in China," everyone agrees, and yet "no one knew with any
degree of certainty where they came from or how they arose. Nor was
there any agreement on the size of the *bianwen* corpus or the formal
nature of the genre."[10] The key to the mystery is not to be sought in genre
theory or indeed in literature generally: it comes down to properties of
the material artifact, which brings us back to the Mogao caves.

One of the manuscripts kept in Paris, Pelliot chinois 4524, bears on one
side a painted account of Śāriputra's conjuring contest with Raudrākṣa,
chief of the Heretical Masters, in six scenes, and on the other side the six
verse sections of the *bianwen*, "Transformation Text on the Subjugation
of Demons."[11] There is nothing inherently surprising about a scroll with
words and pictures. Such objects readily lend themselves to description as
illustrated narration, a familiar type of object with many variants: labels,
legends, cartouches, speech bubbles, comments. But the fact that only
the verse segments of an originally prosimetric narrative are recorded,
added to the fact that in C 4524 they are copied onto the reverse of the
illustration (where they would be of little use as captions or legends),
leads Mair to deduce that the artifact is not made for individual reading,
as an illustrated book would be. It is, rather, a tool used in picture-
aided, story-telling performances. The form of the material object (lost in
transcription) indicates the function: while the front of the scroll with its
painted scenes was unwound and shown to the public in six successive
stages, a storyteller, positioned behind the scroll, would have offered
a relatively free prose narration of the events, punctuated by exactly
worded verse sections read from the paper. For "it is the verses that are the
central, stable core of a prosimetric folk narrative in the Indian tradition
and in other Asian traditions influenced by it"; the verses are the reciter's
"fixed capital."[12] As Mair documents the practice of picture-narration

throughout Europe and Asia, he supplies abundant iconography and calls attention to the recurrent deictic exclamations in the Chinese texts: "Please look for a moment at the place where X occurs. How should I present it?"[13] The "place" (*chu* 處) is a spot on the picture; other *bianwen* repeatedly refer to "the time when..." (*shi* 時). These deictics can only refer to the specifics of this mixed-media performance, an act of artistic enchantment whereby audiences were led to visualize and temporarily dwell in sublime alternate worlds of the religious imagination. And from this arises vernacular theater in China, a composite art that drew from many sources but whose catalyst is Indic.[14]

Thus, the Mystery begins with a Clue, a puzzling object that falls between the expected categories of literary studies and art history. Solving the Mystery involves reconstructing the original function of the Clue, placing it in a history of diffusion, and establishing parallels. The Clue, once understood, clarifies a whole series of phenomena, often far surpassing the scope of the original problem that called for solution. Thus: why does Xie He put forth just "six laws" of painting? Is that number, if not an organic development from prior Chinese painting theory, indicative of an unstated methodological orientation?[15] Why is tonal prosody unknown in Chinese before Xu Shen, and why must it have eight and only eight defects?[16] The numbered list stands out as seemingly extrinsic and thus points to an origin outside the immediate context —in both cases, that means an Indian origin for a motif incompletely adapted to the Chinese milieu which it irreversibly affected. Such puzzles, typically, can be solved only be reaching for combinations of knowledge fields, languages, and cultures that the existing disciplines were not anticipating.

Sometimes, as in the best classical precedents, the Clue is a dead body. Gainsaying the common beliefs that dead men both wear no plaid and tell no tales, the dessicated mummies of the Tarim Basin speak to us, through their physiognomies and clothing, of Bronze Age and Iron Age populations residing in what is now China but whose cultural ties seem to be with civilizations to the west (with the steppe cultures, the Middle East and even central Europe).[17] A mystery indeed, to be resolved only by retracing long-obliterated footprints! These Missing Persons call for new accounts of personal and cultural traffic across Central Asia in the centuries preceding our earliest Chinese records (that is, around three thousand years prior to the Dunhuang document trove).

Victor Mair takes seriously his responsibilities as a teacher. Courses in Chinese language, literature, and history have been transformed by the anthologies of translated primary sources that he has edited: not only the aforementioned *Columbia Anthology of Traditional Chinese Literature* (1996) and its shorter version (2001), but the coedited *Hawai'i Reader in Traditional Chinese Culture* (2005, with Nancy Steinhardt and Paul Goldin), and the *Columbia Anthology of Chinese Folk and Popular Literature* (2011, with Mark Bender).[18] Through such works as *The True History of Tea* (2009, with Erling Hoh), *Sacred Display: Divine and Magical Female Figures of Eurasia* (2010, with Miriam Robbins Dexter), *Traditional China in Asian and World History* (2012, with Tansen Sen), *Chinese Lives: The People Who Made a Civilization* (2013, with Sanping Chen and Frances Wood), and his exhibition catalogues, Victor Mair has informed and intrigued a broader public.[19] His translations of Laozi, Zhuangzi, and Sunzi are steadily reprinted.[20] Scholarly homages such as the volume assembled in memory of Antonino Forte, *Buddhist Transformations and Interactions: Essays in Honor of Antonino Forte* (2017) show another facet of Victor Mair's generosity.[21] And let us not forget the ongoing adventure of *Sino-Platonic Papers* (273 numbers and counting), his contributions to "Language Log," or the Cambria Sinophone Series.[22] With such roving attention and boundless curiosity, Victor Mair keeps Chinese studies on the move.

> Master Chuang said, "If a man is capable of wandering, what's to keep him from wandering? If a man is incapable of wandering, will he ever get to wander? ... Only the ultimate man can wander through the world without deviation, accommodating others

without losing himself. Though he doesn't study their doctrines, he can accept ideas without being dismissive."[23]

No one is actually "the ultimate man," any more than reading Nietzsche turns one into the *Übermensch*, but it is good to "wander" and to take risks, for as another chapter of that work maintains, a fearless spirit "might pass over a great mountain without impediment, enter a deep spring without getting wet, dwell in humble circumstances without feeling wretched." Such a person is "filled with heaven and earth, so that he more he gave to others, the more he had for himself."[24]

The contributors to this volume join Victor Mair's many friends, students and colleagues in greeting his seventy-fifth birthday and wishing him undiminished energy for many years to come.

The combination of Victor Mair's scholarly distinction and his legendary generosity toward students and younger scholars has already resulted in several congratulatory publications, such as the 2006 double number of *Asia Major* entitled "China at the Crossroads: A Festschrift for Victor Mair" and the retrospective volume *China and Beyond by Victor H. Mair: A Collection of Essays.* By way of continuing the celebration, we offer here a group of essays by friends, former students, associates, and beneficiaries of Victor Mair. In countless ways, not just by footnote references, they bespeak his influence on us.

The volume opens with a chapter by Perry Link on one of Victor Mair's favorite topics—the eternally controversial conundrums of translation. Link notes that "What good translators actually do, and Victor's translations of Lao-Zhuang texts could be exhibit A for this, might better be called 'live re-creation.'" What this means, Link illuminates by taking us through the fascinating step-by-step example of a *shunkouliu* 順口 溜 or doggerel ditty. Through the process, he demonstrates how each translation is "only one of a family of possible translations, none intrinsically more 'correct' than the others," underscoring how "we can narrow things down, but we can never pin them down in a way that eradicates every possible ambiguity."

Translation figures largely in Mabel Lee's chapter on Gao Xingjian as well. For at the same time as he was writing *Bus Stop* and *Soul Mountain*, Gao was translating Prévert and Ionesco and writing critically on Sartre, Camus, Beckett, Brecht, and Artaud. Gao's "absurdist aesthetics," however, is an original formulation sprung from the contact, in a restless and searching mind, of Chan Buddhism with the Theatre of the Absurd. The failure to give this Chan element its due weight often leads critics to misunderstand Gao Xingjian's drama, fiction, and essay writing as derivative. Lee shows the continuity of themes and attitudes in Gao's work across many genres and media, despite isolation, political opprobrium and exile.

The heavy hand of politics on Chinese twentieth-century writing gives the background to David Der-wei Wang's essay on Sinophone literature. The Sinophone, originally proposed as a label for literature written in Chinese outside of the People's Republic of China, reveals a difference in the relation to political struggles and the nation: just as Sinophone writers in countries such as Malaysia or Indonesia have often been suspected of insufficient local patriotism, so too the availability of other political and cultural frameworks gives these authors opportunities to define Chineseness differently. Wang suggests that the full potential of the Sinophone is realized when these discourses, no longer viewed as the productions of "overseas Chinese," enter the Chinese national conversation and break down hierarchical binaries that have long been indispensable to Chinese cultural identity. In what he calls "postloyalism," "the politics of anachrony and displacement," Wang sees a project of cultural reclamation, an "intervention with China" from several places of "heterotemporality."

Mice occupy a "heterotopia" at the edges of human habitation—an alternate world structured, according to the New Year's prints and ballads examined by Wilt Idema, exactly like the human one. Mice hold wedding processions, always looking over their little shoulders for the cat; in the underworld, they are even so bold as to take the cat to court for murder—

an unwise move, as King Yama finds for the cat and condemns the mouse tribe to eternal persecution by cats. This folk tale with its many variants in China links up with motifs from Europe, ancient Egypt, Persia and Turkey, indeed from wherever settled agricultural societies are found. King Yama expresses the majority human point of view: of course, mice steal grain and it is the job of cats to stop them. But the mouse's plight must have had particular resonance for Chinese villagers, accustomed to visits from the tax collector and the yamen runners, and this double sympathy accounts for much of the tale's charm.

The interplay of agriculture, climate, settlement, and technology forms the basis of the two following essays. Nicola di Cosmo explores the alliance between the Tang and Uyghur empires at the moment of Manichaeism's widest spread. Undergirding the alliance was a system of exchange: silk for horses; and we have many documents from the Chinese side complaining that the horses received were too feeble. Climate data shows that the reason for the complaints was not Uyghur dishonesty but a drop in average temperatures and desertification, resulting in poorly nourished horses. The exchanges ended in 830, weakening the Uyghur state and sapping the Tang defenses.

Mark Bender writes on the significance of hunting equipment in "origin stories, creation myth-epics, ritual and folk songs, bridal capture tales, migration and colonization narratives, legendary accounts of wars, personal narratives/hunting tales, folk dramas, festival, crafting narratives," and the like from minority regions of China. Though self-evidently out of date, these attributes refer, like the Homeric chariots and boar's-tusk helmets, to the heroic period of the poems' setting. The weapons also intersect—without redoubling them—the myths of cosmic foundation integrated into Chinese quasi-historical legends, suggesting a "pool" of epic and mythological material from which different neighboring countries selected their leading motifs. The tools used by hunters and warriors also provide indices of cultural interchange, sometimes permitting inferences about the dates of creation of epic narratives or their links to outside cultures.

Ties to outside cultures are foregrounded in the cultural conversion narrative described by Emma Teng, whose essay examines a nineteenth-century story about an Englishwoman who adopts Chinese language, dress, and deportment. It has long been said that the criterion of Chinese identity is cultural, not ethnic, with Mencius's statement "Shun was a *dongyi* 東夷 [Eastern barbarian]" often called to attest that Chinese civilization assimilates foreigners rather than putting them beyond the pale.[25] Wang Tao's "The Story of Mary" from 1887 or thereabouts puts this assertion to the test. Both a reflection on debates of the time and a "what if?" work of narrative speculation, the story provokes reflection on the category of Chineseness and looks forward to the Sinophone interrogations of our time.

Boundary-crossing women are at the center of Ellen Widmer's study, both thematic and bibliographical, of the late-Qing romance *Nü yuhua*. Combining the urgencies of national salvation and feminist rebellion, Wang Miaoru, the novel's author, died young and was commemorated as a modern Bodhisattva by her grieving husband, in language that echoes that used to describe one of her heroines. Her novel, full of superhuman exploits and defiance of then-current law and morals, must have been extremely provocative for the readership of 1904, and Widmer sees in its illustrations some attempt to soften it. The illustrator's "informed diminution" of the story demonstrates the degree to which the novel's implications were inadmissible in its time.

From jail cells to gardens is a large step in the semiotics of space. Jerome Silbergeld takes us, in spirit, through several masterpieces of the Chinese art of garden design in order to reveal the thought that went into planning each turn, contrast, or vista. The art is so demanding that even the coloration of a background wall can throw off the whole effect. Gardens are not merely places for entertaining "a green thought in a green shade"; they "tease us into thought," memory, and comparison.

The arrival of Buddhist teaching expanded the Chinese universe in many dimensions—in time, in space, and in ontological possibility.[26] The group of five essays that concludes the book retraces the consequences of the expansion, indeed explosion, that resulted from the shoehorning of the Buddhist *shijie* 世界 into the traditional Chinese *tianxia* 天下.[27]

One aspect of early Chinese Buddhism that has come increasingly into view in recent years is the attention paid to wonder-working personages and magical language. Seemingly far from the philosophical concerns of such Six Dynasties gentry Buddhists as Dao'an, Huiyuan, or Zhi Mindu, these prodigies seem to have captured the popular imagination and to have conferred extraordinary prestige on the language(s) of India. The *Gaoseng zhuan* (Lives of Eminent Monks) reflects these exotic views of early Buddhist practitioners in China. Koichi Shinohara's study of Fotudeng (232–348), a foreign monk who found a succession of patrons partly through his ability to overcome natural and human disasters, present him as exemplary of many similar cases, evincing "a common culture of spell practice" that Shinohara then further relates to questions of ritual, the use of images, and the invocation of deities in this phase of Esoteric Buddhism.

The legal status of monks and nuns—their relative, absolute or nonexistent exemption from corvée labor, taxation, and other requirements—was a matter of intense dispute between members of the samgha and Chinese officials ever since the first monastic establishments were created, at a moment of disorder and fragmentation in the Chinese state. Phyllis Granoff retraces the uneasy relation between monastics and the legal system in Indic texts. Although "both philosophical debates and law cases take place in the court of the king" and the Buddha is often likened to an examining judge called to determine the truth of a dispute, recourse to actual law was seen as disreputable and virtually polluting. Lay support, far more important for Buddhist and Jain communities living from alms, and moral standing are preferable to legal victory.

If the Buddhist samgha had any inalienable privilege, one reasons, surely it should have been that of managing its internal doctrinal affairs: of deciding which texts were to be maintained in the canon, how those texts were to be interpreted, and which versions or translations were to be adopted in doubtful cases. But as Tanya Storch shows in her essay, successive Chinese dynasties sought opportunistically to intervene in the processes of canon formation, and traces of this manipulation subsist in the catalogues and histories usually considered internal to the Buddhist establishment. From Han to the verge of the Tang, the balance of forces shifted, now this way, now that. We should read these bibliographies as the outcomes of complex processes of negotiation in which the imperial dynasties most often had the advantage.

Tansen Sen's essay looks at medieval world history through the travel writings of the Tang monk Yijing, who traveled to India and Sumatra in search of Buddhist monuments, learning, and texts. (A translation by Yijing is the basis of the *Sutra of the Wise and the Foolish* that eventually gave rise to the Dunhuang scroll that plays such a large part in Mair's *T'ang Transformation Texts*.) Yijing's interest in monastic rules differentiates his travel goals from those of the better-known Xuanzang and Faxian, and this in part explains his itinerary. His travel report demonstrates how the Buddhist cosmopolis of his time was stitched together, though "collaborations between itinerant monks, mercantile networks, and the state sponsorship of Buddhist activities." For monastic rules and for the organization of this cosmopolis, the Nālandā monastery and university complex apparently served Yijing as a model.

A cosmopolis, however vast, must be bounded in space and in time; whoever proposes an account of the world must conceive of its beginning, end, and change. The imaginative construction of "the last days of the Dharma" in Heian Japan and Liao-dynasty China is the subject of Mimi Yiengpruksawan's essay. Mahāyāna commentators plotted the extinction of the Dharma onto calendrical time and registered unforeseeable events such as smallpox epidemics as evidence for it. In both China and

Japan, the expectation of end times underwrote such preparations as making a stone copy of the Buddhist canon or restoring pagodas, on an astonishingly precise shared schedule—the temporal equivalent of the spatial realm of exchanges and communications among Buddhists. Like two clocks synchronized in the past and left to run, the Heian and Liao prognostications testified to both a common origin and to a reliable continuity of operation.

I see in the essays of this book—with their breadth of concern, their carefully documented scholarship, and the boldness of some of their conclusions—a fitting homage to Victor Mair, whose readers, students, and colleagues have long recognized the same qualities in him.

Notes

1. For a comprehensive view of Mair's career up to *Contact and Exchange in the Ancient World* (2006), see Daniel Boucher, Neil Schmid, and Tansen Sen, "The Scholarly Contributions of Professor Victor H. Mair: A Retrospective Survey," *Asia Major* third series, 19 (2006): 1–11. The pace of Mair's activity has, if anything, increased since that stock taking: see below for a partial list of new titles.

2. Xie Zhiliu, "Dunhuang shishi ji," cited in Rong Xinjiang, "The Nature of the Dunhuang Library Cave and the Reasons for its Sealing," trans. Valerie Hansen, *Cahiers d'Extrême-Asie* 11 (1999): 247–275, at 248–249. See also Sir Aurel Stein, *On Ancient Central-Asian Tracks* (London: Macmillan, 1933), 201–216, and Wang Jiqing, "Aurel Stein's Dealings with Wang Yuanlu and Chinese Officials in Dunhuang in 1907," in Helen Wang, ed., *Sir Aurel Stein: Colleagues and Collections* (London: British Museum, 2012), 1–6.

3. See the Dunhuang Project's website, http://idp.bl.uk.

4. As the "Silk Road" has recently become the object of vast imaginative and financial investment ("one belt, one road") in the People's Republic of China under Core Leader Xi Jinping, it is necessary to disavow the image of an international highway channeling trade and culture between East and West. Multilateral trade was, rather, conducted in a series of linked marketplaces across the Central Asian region and beyond, with no end-to-end communication. The "road" was rather a set of co-occurring conditions than a structure. For a description of these conditions, see Lothar von Falkenhausen, "Notes on the History of the 'Silk Routes': From the Rise of the Xiongnu to the Mongol Conquest (250 BC–AD 1283)," in Victor H. Mair, ed., *Secrets of the Silk Road* (Santa Ana, CA: Bowers Museum, 2010), 58–68. But the fact of encounter among languages, religions, peoples and forms of political organization in the region over millennia is certain. On the "mirages," see Peter Brown, "The Silk Road in Late Antiquity," in Victor H. Mair and Jane Hickman, eds., *Reconfiguring the Silk Road: New Research on East-West Exchange in Antiquity* (Philadelphia: University of Pennsylvania Museum of Archaeology and Anthropology, 2014), 15–22.

5. Victor H. Mair, "Introduction," in Victor H. Mair, ed., *The Columbia History of Chinese Literature* (New York: Columbia University Press, 2001), 7.

6. Mair, "Introduction," 9.
7. Li Zehou, *The Chinese Aesthetic Tradition*, trans. Maija Bell Samei (Honolulu: University of Hawai'i Press, 2010), 90, 219, 194.
8. On the Buddhist concept of "transformational manifestation" and its effects on Chinese fiction, see Victor H. Mair, "Transformation as Imagination in Medieval Popular Buddhist Literature," in John Kieschnick and Meir Shahar, eds., *India in the Chinese Imagination: Myth, Religion, and Thought* (Philadelphia: University of Pennsylvania Press, 2014), 13–20.
9. Erich Auerbach, *Mimesis: The Representation of Reality in Western Literature*, tr. Willard R. Trask (Princeton: Princeton University Press, 1953), 49, 72, 248.
10. Victor H. Mair, *T'ang Transformation Texts: A Study of the Buddhist Contribution to the Rise of Vernacular Fiction and Drama in China* (Cambridge, Mass.: Harvard University Press, 1989), ix; transliteration altered.
11. See the digitized scroll at http://idp.bl.uk, under Pelliot chinois 4524, or Nicole Vandier-Nicolas, ed., *Śāriputra et les six maîtres d'erreur: fac-similé du manuscrit chinois 4524 de la Bibliothèque nationale, avec traduction et commentaire du texte* (Paris: Imprimerie nationale, 1954). This facsimile includes both sides of the scroll, showing the placement and orientation of the verse passages.
12. Victor H. Mair, *T'ang Transformation Texts*, 97–98.
13. Ibid., 73. For the broader account of picture recitation ranging from Japan to Tunisia, see *Tun-Huang Popular Narratives* (Cambridge, Eng.: Cambridge University Press, 1983); *Painting and Performance: Chinese Picture Recitation and its Indian Genesis* (Honolulu: University of Hawai'i Press, 1988).
14. Victor H. Mair, "The Contributions of T'ang and Five Dynasties Transformation Texts (*pien-wen*) to Later Chinese Popular Literature," *Sino-Platonic Papers* 12 (1989). Cf. Vandier-Nicolas, *Śāriputra et les six maîtres d'erreur*, 9–11.
15. Victor H. Mair, "Xie He's 'Six Laws' of Painting and Their Indian Parallels," in Zong-qi Cai, ed., *Chinese Aesthetics: The Ordering of Literature, the Arts, and the Universe in the Six Dynasties* (Honolulu: University of Hawaii Press, 2004), 81–122.
16. Victor H. Mair and Tsu-Lin Mei, "The Sanskrit Origins of Recent-Style Prosody," *Harvard Journal of Asiatic Studies* 51 (1991): 375–470.
17. J. P. Mallory and Victor H. Mair, *The Tarim Mummies: Ancient China and the Mystery of the Earliest Peoples from the West* (London: Thames & Hudson, 2000); Elizabeth Wayland Barber, *The Mummies of Ürümchi*

(New York: Norton, 1999); Victor H. Mair, ed., *Contact and Exchange in the Ancient World* (Honolulu: University of Hawai'i Press, 2006); Mair and Hickman, eds., *Reconfiguring the Silk Road.* For a genetic perspective on population changes and migrations, see Christopher P. Thornton and Theodore G. Schurr, "Genes, Language, and Culture: An Example from the Tarim Basin," *Oxford Journal of Archaeology* 23 (2004): 83-106. Cf. Carl Reiner, dir., *Dead Men Don't Wear Plaid* (Universal Pictures, 1982).

18. *The Columbia Anthology of Traditional Chinese Literature* (New York: Columbia University Press, 1996); *The Shorter Columbia Anthology of Traditional Chinese Literature* (New York: Columbia University Press, 2001); *The Hawai'i Reader in Traditional Chinese Culture* (Honolulu: University of Hawai'i Press, 2005); *The Columbia Anthology of Chinese Folk and Popular Literature* (New York: Columbia University Press, 2011).

19. *The True History of Tea* (London: Thames & Hudson, 2009); *Sacred Display: Divine and Magical Female Figures of Eurasia* (Amherst, NY: Cambria Press, 2010); *Traditional China in Asian and World History* (Ann Arbor: Association for Asian Studies, 2012); *Chinese Lives: The People Who Made a Civilization* (London: Thames & Hudson, 2013).

20. Victor H. Mair, tr., *Tao Te Ching: The Classic Book of Integrity and the Way* (New York: Bantam, 1990); *Wandering on the Way: Early Taoist Tales and Parables of Chuang Tzu* (New York: Bantam, 1994); *The Art of War: Sun Zi's Military Methods* (New York: Columbia University Press, 2007).

21. *Buddhist Transformations and Interactions: Essays in Honor of Antonino Forte* (Amherst, NY: Cambria Press, 2017).

22. See http://www.sino-platonic.org for the complete catalogue of SPP's occasional publications. For "Language Log," see http://languagelog. ldc.upenn.edu. The Sinophone Series catalogue may be consulted at www.cambriapress.com/sinophone-series.

23. *Zhuangzi,* chapter 26; Mair, tr., *Wandering on the Way,* 274–275.

24. *Zhuangzi,* chapter 21; Mair, tr., *Wandering on the Way,* 208.

25. *Mencius* 4b: 1, in Zhu Xi 朱熹, comm., *Si shu zhangju jizhu* 四書章句集注 (Beijing: Zhonghua shuju, 1983), 289.

26. Once again, see Victor H. Mair, "Transformation as Imagination."

27. For an intellectual history of this process, see Wang Yongping 王永平, *Cong 'tianxia' dao 'shijie': Han-Tang shiqi de zhongguo yu shijie* 從天下到世界：漢、唐時期的中國與世界 (Beijing: Shehui kexue chubanshe, 2015).

Chapter 1

On Translation

How and Why Can Something Less than a Mirror Be Useful?

Perry Link

When a physicist tells a non-physicist that the solid surface of a table is, in fact, mostly empty space between the components of atoms, the non-physicist might be surprised, and temporarily fascinated, but afterwards will likely revert to thinking of solid tables in the normal way. Similarly a language maven like Victor Mair can tell non-specialists, quite correctly, that what they think of as "translation" (roughly, the substitution of one code for another) simply does not exist. The non-specialists might or might not understand, but in either case they will likely move forward with life, relying on their wrong but serviceable notions.

Most people think a translation is an *equivalent* in a second language of something in a first, but equivalence is rarely, if ever, possible. A person who has mastered French and English can easily find untranslatable subtleties between examples of the two. For someone who works with languages as different as Chinese and English, subtle examples are hardly necessary. Nonequivalences abound and the question turns around, as it were, into one where the truly subtle challenge is to find any two phrases that do exactly match. What good translators actually do, and Victor's translations of Lao-Zhuang texts could be exhibit A for this, might better be called "live re-creation."

In Chinese and English, *shu* and "book" are far from equivalent, even when each is restricted to its use as a noun (both can also be verbs, and as verbs are very obviously not "equivalent"). This is because "book" is concrete and can be made plural whereas *shu* is abstract and neither singular nor plural. *Shu* is more like "bookness," if we may invent an English word. To talk about a concrete book you may, of course, add a "measure word" and say *yi ben shu* 一本书 in three nifty syllables, but, if you were to aim for "equivalence," you would have to say something in English like "one volume of bookness," which is six syllables and sounds ridiculous from several points of view. So right away a dilemma arises between fidelity to grammar and fidelity to style, and there is no perfect answer to it. Value judgments by the translator are necessary.

For years, my students of beginning Chinese at Princeton—who on the whole were at least as bright as ordinary people—irritated me, without meaning to, by asking questions like, "What is the Chinese word for X?" The question reflected the language-as-code approach that I wanted them to stop using as soon as possible. I used to fight back by showing two or three ways in which words like *shu* and "book" might differ and then giving a mini-lecture on what the word "translation" does not mean. I told them that even "one, two, three, and four" are not "the same" as *yi* 一, *er* 二, *san* 三, and *si* 四, because, for example, *yi* can mean something like "as soon as" when paired with *jiu* 就 in adjacent clauses, but "one" cannot; and "two" can mean *er* 二 or *liang* 两 or *lia* 俩; and you can say that somebody is *bu san bu si* 不三不四 but not that he is "neither three nor four"; and so on. I told them that the only exact equivalents between the two languages might be high numbers or, perhaps, modern words like *tansuangai* 碳酸钙 "calcium carbonate"—words, that is, that are invented in one language precisely in order to serve as the equivalent in another. I told them they were better off not looking for equivalents but just trying to start thinking in Chinese. Sooner or later, I told them, they would have the experience of thinking something in Chinese and not knowing exactly how to put it into English. This happens to almost everyone who gets very far into learning Chinese as a second language.

I always felt vaguely guilty when handing vocabulary lists to students. You can use these to cram when you're short of time, I told them. But whatever you do, don't imagine that X "means" Y. My departed colleague Fritz Mote made the point very well in the 1970s during a faculty discussion of whether graduate students should be required to submit English translations of the key texts they are working on. "Yes," said a colleague, "because making them translate is the only way to tell whether they really understand correctly." Fritz took the point but raised the bar. "The best test of how well they *understand*," he said, "is not how well they translate but how dissatisfied they are with even the best of translations."

But if the lay conception of translation as equivalence is an illusion, what are we to conclude? That we should abandon translation? Of course not. It is too useful in too many ways, both scholarly and otherwise. We just need a more sophisticated concept of what it is.

We might begin by recognizing that there are, broadly speaking, two ways in which translations of a text can differ. One way is through mistakes: a translator might misunderstand an original text in some relatively gross way, a way that cannot be attributed to different interpretations of nuance. (What if, for example, someone read "The Road Not Taken" by Robert Frost too quickly and thought he meant "two toads diverged in a yellow wood..."?) Alternatively a translator might understand well enough, but then miswrite a translation with incorrect spelling, bad grammar, wrong usage, or the like ("two roads submerged in a yellow wood," for example). But setting aside these kinds of gross error, there remains a very large area within which pretty good translations can vary. By "pretty good" translations I mean translations that come from people who have not misread the original and who, if they were to sit down in a room and talk about the original, would agree fairly well about what it is saying. Each, though, in deciding on which particular words to choose, would need to make judgments on many kinds of trade-off. Results would inevitably be affected by the values of the translator and, perhaps, by the translator's judgment of the backgrounds and needs of the imagined readership. The results of course would vary. Final decisions would be arbitrary, and everyone would realize that translation in the end is an art, not a science.

Eliot Weinberger has a little book called *Nineteen Ways of Looking at Wang Wei*, which was originally published in 1987 and was updated "with more ways" in 2016.[1] In it he offers thirty-four different translations into English, French, Spanish, or German of Wang Wei's famous poem *Lu Zhai* 鹿柴. Weinberger criticizes nearly all the translations for their imperfections—some large, some fine—but wisely adds that "quite a few possible readings" can all be "equally 'correct'." Or—to put the point another way—all are equally doomed to one or another kind of imperfection. Perfect translation is a useful ideal, but in the end a mirage. But Weinberger argues that several of the translations of Wang Wei, whatever else one says about them, are good poems in their own rights. They are not mirrors of the original, but its offspring.

Let's push this inquiry further with a contemporary example. In 2002 Kate Zhou and I published an essay on *shunkouliu* 顺口溜, the satiric rhythmical sayings that Chinese people pass around on their oral grapevines.[2] *Shunkouliu* are not easy to translate, but we had to try. Here's one that comments on how China's new state-capitalist economy has brought back old social ills and created a new kind of class society:

辛辛苦苦四十年
一朝回到解放前
既然回到解放前
当年革命又为谁

How should one try to translate it? Although no one, I think, would want to be so super-literal as to go character by character, let's start there anyway, just in order to stake out one extreme position. The Chinese-English dictionary that I most often use is the *Han-Ying Cidian* edited by the English Department of the Beijing Foreign Languages University and first published in 1995. Using that source, a character-by-character rendition (using hyphens to link two English words that correspond to a single Chinese character) would be:

> Hard hard bitter bitter four ten years
> One morning return to untie release before
> Already thus return to untie release before
> Just-at year change fate in-fact for whom?

Now let us take the very minimal steps of recognizing standard compounds (like *jiefang* "Liberation") and standard grammatical conventions (like "before X" for X *yiqian*), but still stick word-for-word to the *Han-Ying Cidian*. The result is still extremely "literal":

> Strenuous, strenuous forty years
> One morning return to before Liberation
> Given that return to before Liberation
> In those days revolution in fact for whom?

Despite its literal faithfulness, this rendition conveys misimpressions to the native speaker of English. "Strenuous, strenuous" sounds quaint, and maybe a bit childlike; but there is nothing quaint or childlike in the original. In the last line "revolution in fact for whom?" might also seem, in its broken grammar, "cute Chinesey," while the line in the original is neither broken nor cute but quite the opposite. We need to weigh fidelity to the whole against fidelity to parts. We need to let ourselves import un-quaint English grammar and supply words like "an," "we" and others so that the resulting English matches the original Chinese in tone. Some call this "taking liberties," but I do not. I think of it as balancing one kind of fidelity against another, given that full fidelity in all respects is impossible. If inserting some words and tenses in order to get rid of quaintness is "taking liberties," then, in my view, *not* inserting them and letting the misimpression of quaintness remain could equally well be called the "taking of a liberty."

Anyway, to supply our *shunkouliu* with trappings that make the English more natural (if still not graceful), we might get:

> An extremely strenuous forty years
> And one morning we [find ourselves having]
>   returned to before Liberation
> And given that we've returned to before Liberation
> [We might ask] whom, in fact, the revolution
>   back in those days was for

Academic translations sometimes read like this, but I don't like them, especially when something terse and sprightly like a *shunkouliu* is at stake. We should worry about fidelity to form and spirit as well as content. As a rule of thumb, I try to devise translations that will, as much as possible, *give to the native-speaking reader of English the same overall reading experience that the native-speaking reader of Chinese gets in reading the original.* I admit that this rule can bring us uncomfortably close to metaphysics, because who is to say, for any reader of any text, what an "overall experience" is, let alone how to average that experience over many possible readers? Still, I believe that it is better to aim at this standard than not to. We should at least try, for a start, to put the lines of our example into less awkwardly different lengths. So perhaps:

> An extremely strenuous forty years
> And suddenly we're back to before Liberation
> And given our return to before Liberation
> Whom, in fact, was the revolution for?

This is not too bad, in my view. It may be fair enough as a balance among different kinds of "liberties taken." One of the remaining problems, though, is that the rhythm is awkward. "Before Liberation" in line two is a poor syllabic match for "forty years" in the first line; lines three and four also mismatch rhythmically. But in the original the rhythm is fine. What can we do? Maybe something like:

> An extremely strenuous forty years
> And suddenly we're back to 'forty-nine,
> And since we've gone back to 'forty-nine
> Whom, in fact, was it all for?

This version has the advantage, in terms of rhythm, that it can be read in four-beat lines:

> An exTREMEly STRENuous FORty YEARS
> And SUDdenly we're BACK to 'FORty-NINE,
> And SINCE we've gone BACK to 'FORty-NINE
> WHOM, in FACT, was it all FOR? (...REST)

But this version makes the lexical compromise of trading "forty-nine" for "Liberation," and, for the sake of rhythm, completely omits *dangnian* "in those days" and *geming* "revolution" from the last line. Moreover, it does not match the rhyme of the original, in which the final syllables of lines one through three rhyme. Can we somehow restore *dangnian* and *geming*, and add rhyme? Probably, but again only at the cost of other fidelities. How about:

> For forty long years ever more perspiration
> And we just circle back to before Liberation
> And speaking again of that big revolution
> Whom, after all, was it for?

Here "perspiration" goes in for "strenuous," a lexical and syntactic liberty taken in exchange for a rhyme with "Liberation." "Speaking again" in line three can do partial justice to *dangnian* that appears in line four. "Revolution" is restored, even though it appears now in line three, not line four where the original has it, and even though "-ution" is not the best rhyme-match for "-ation" in lines one and two. "Circle back" for "return" helps to preserve the rhythm, which on the whole survives. The stunted rhythm of line four does not match the original but the abrupt effect that it provides, in my view, creates an effect that is similar to the abrupt non-rhyme of line four in the original.

One could set a higher standard in the matter of rhythm. The original can be read in four-beat lines, like 4/4 time in music, and so, except for its last line, can our translation. But the original is in traditional Chinese *qiyan* 七言 form, which invites a reading in the more sedate and more elegant 2-2-3 rhythm. What if we wanted to do that with this *shunkouliu* (even though, in practice, it would be a bit unusual to pronounce a *shunkouliu* sedately). Then even more attention to rhythm, at the cost of even more compromises of other kinds, would be necessary. We might have something like:

> Forty long years crack our spine
> Back we go to forty-nine
> Since we go to forty-nine
> Back then whom was it all for?

Here each line in the English, as in the Chinese, is exactly seven syllables, and the grammar allows a reading in 2-2-3 rhythm to make sense. But, I would argue, formal fidelity has now begun to go too far. Just as when literal fidelity went too far, the result is to produce a misleading quaintness.

But formal fidelity could, if one chose, go even further. What about rectangularity, for example? Although Chinese *qiyan* verse does not have to be written to form a rectangle, it always can be so written, and I have printed our example that way earlier (see page 20). Can we do it in English? Something like:

> Forty years we bend our spine
> And just go back to forty-nine
> And having gone to forty-nine
> Whom back then was this for?

When David Bellos, a professor of French at Princeton and an expert on translation, saw this, he devised a version whose lines are even more exactly of the same length. Each uses twenty-one digits (where spaces and punctuation marks also count as digits) per line. Moreover, rhyme is supplied:

> Blood sweat and tears
> Over forty long years
> Now it's utterly over
> Who stole the clover?

These last two curious results should be enough to show definitively that the translator at some point has to make an arbitrary choice about balance, and to settle for one or another kind of imperfection. Anyone who still wants to pursue perfection should remember that classical Chinese poetry also pays attention to the tone patterns of parallelism and mirroring that the categories *ping* 平 and *ze* 仄 make possible. *Shunkouliu* rarely observe *ping* and *ze*, but for poems that do, how could one possibly translate? Considerable ingenuity would be needed even to conceive a way to try to begin. If Y.R. Chao had not translated Lewis Carroll's "Jabberwocky," we might simply say such a project is unthinkable.

Given that 1) perfection is impossible, 2) a range of imperfect possibilities are plausible, and 3) the choice among them is ultimately artistic, what is the best policy for a translator? Here I can only give my personal view, which is to try to imagine who the readers of a translation will be, and then use, as well as one can, the principle I have stated earlier: try to give native-speaking readers of language two the same overall reading experience that native-speaking readers of language one get in reading the original. Kate Zhou and I, in our article on *shunkouliu*, chose the sixth of the eight aforementioned versions (the one that begins, "For forty long years ever more perspiration..."). I feel that this rendition gets across most of the lexical meaning as well as the basic rhythm and rhyme without creating a quaint or exotic sense by going too far in any one direction. But in the end it is only one of a family of possible translations, none intrinsically more "correct" than the others.

I want to underscore the danger of producing artificial quaintness. Very often, in my view, East and West cultures find the other side to be strange more because of problems in perception processes (including translations) than because of original differences in how human beings on the two sides live life. The sense of exoticism that Western readers get when they read translations of Chinese literature are often rooted less in the original Chinese than they are in the awkwardness that overly literal translations produce. In time, if a person reads too much literal translation, the strangeness that it generates can come to seem authentic. It is almost as though a third culture grows up: on one side we have Chinese, on the other we have English, and in between we have a Chinglish that people who don't know Chinese take to be authentic Chinese.

Let me offer an example. When I was working on an English edition of *The Tiananmen Papers*,[3] a friend of mine, a political scientist, was led to question the authenticity of the *Papers* because, in his view, the documents "just don't sound right". He had read thousands of translated Chinese Communist documents in his career, and the *Papers* did not strike his ear as the real McCoy.

He had not seen the original Chinese texts, but this, he said, was not the problem that he was talking about. His sense of inauthenticity came from the fact that the English translations in *Papers* did not sound like the English translations of documents that he had read before. He was accustomed to a kind of document translatese that the US and other Western governments produce in large quantity and from which he habitually worked. The style of these translations is overly literal, roughly equivalent to the third *shunkouliu* rendition listed above (the one that begins, "An extremely strenuous forty years..."). Because this style has appeared in such volume, for my friend it had come to be a kind of authentic Chinese. He was so deeply accustomed to it that, for him, it could even be the standard by which to measure the authenticity of other texts.

I relate this anecdote not to show that China-field political scientists are naïve about language, although that observation, far too often, is fair enough; I relate it because I see it as an extreme example of a much broader problem. Even good translators with wonderful sensitivity to language must struggle to avoid producing inadvertent quaintness or exoticism. When Lu Xun's mendicant scholar Kong Yiji eats *huixiangdou* 茴香豆, for example, is that "aniseed peas" (Gladys Yang)[4] or "fennel-flavored beans" (William Lyell)?[5] Or should the translator just leave it in romanization as *huixiangdou*? Any of these alternatives will strike the English reader as somewhat exotic, yet the original *douzi* 豆子, to the Chinese reader, are utterly ordinary, and the art of the story is better when the ordinariness is preserved.

My maxim of "try to create the same overall experience...(etc.)" rests not only on a conception of what translation is but on an underlying conception of what language itself is. As noted earlier, I am often troubled by assertions that "X means Y" where X and Y are words in Chinese and English. The popular tendency to speak in this way is rooted, I think, in the conception that words are labels for things. "Book," people think, is the English label for that stack of paper between covers that lies on a desk, and *shu* 书 is the Chinese label for the same thing: therefore "book" equals *shu*. But not only are "book" and *shu* hardly equivalent; even "book" and that stack of paper between covers do match up neatly as "thing" plus "label for thing." "Book," for example, can be a transitive verb when I book a room. Is it now still a label, in some sense? A label for what? And even if we speak only of noun-labels for concrete things, it is ultimately impossible, as W. V. Quine famously showed in his example of "rabbit," to make a reference that is unambiguous.[6] If you and I see a rabbit running across a field and I say "rabbit," how do you know what I mean? I could mean rabbit fur or rabbit ears or undisaggregated rabbit parts or running rabbit or running animal or any number of things.

You can ask what I mean, and I can answer, and we can narrow things down, but we can never pin them down in a way that eradicates every possible ambiguity.

So how should we think of words, if not as labels? Postmodernism has gone to town on this question. On the whole, postmodernists share a premise that words are things in the world, existing in the same plane, as it were, as other things in the world, rather than as labels that exist on a separate but corresponding plane. Insofar as this thought can be made clear, it seems to me a sound position. The thick jargon that tends to infect postmodernist writing (aiming at ostentation and obfuscation simultaneously, it seems) makes it a difficult place to go in search of clarity in the matter. To my mind, no postmodernist has made intellectual progress beyond what Ludwig Wittgenstein made when he renounced his rigorous *Tractatus Logico-Philosophicus* (1921) in favor of his sketchy *Blue and Brown Books* (1933–1935) and *Philosophical Investigations* (1953) —that is, when he moved from the confident view that words are labels for things to a vaguer but sounder understanding that words and things are all things, and have their various uses. An anecdote from *Philosophical Investigations*, about a mason and his assistant, sticks in my mind. "Brick!" says the mason. The assistant brings him a brick. "Brick," the mason repeats. Another brick. What is happening? How do language and life interact? The bricklayer gives the assistant a word, and the assistant gives the bricklayer a brick. They are passing things back and forth as they do the living of life. That way of thinking about language, according to "the later" Wittgenstein, works better than the item-and-label model.

If the later Wittgenstein is roughly right, and I think he is, then it follows that words in different languages cannot be equivalent labels and further follows that translation can never be a project of replacing one set of labels with another. *Pace* most people, most of the time, in most of the world. A translation turns out to be a separate creation, inspired by an original but never, even possibly, its clone, its mirror image, its copy in another code, or "the" translation. Original and translation exist side by side. Both can be passed around, like bricks and other things, and can be useful to readers in various ways. Depending on the skill of the translator, and on the backgrounds of readers, what I have called "overall experiences" of reading a text and a translation of it can be closer or further apart, but we must not expect them ever to be "the same."

NOTES

1. Eliot Weinberger and Octavio Paz, *Nineteen Ways of Looking at Wang Wei (with More Ways)* (New York: New Directions, 2016).
2. Perry Link and Kate Zhou, "*Shunkouliu*: Popular Satirical Sayings and Popular Thought" in Perry Link, Richard Madsen, and Paul Pickowicz, ed. *Popular China: Unofficial Culture in a Globalizing Society* (Lanham MD: Rowman and Littlefield, 2002), 89–110.
3. *The Tiananmen Papers: The Chinese Leadership's Decision to Use Force Against Their Own People—in Their Own Words,* compiled by Zhang Liang and edited by Andrew J. Nathan and Perry Link (New York: Public Affairs, 2001).
4. *Selected Stories of Lu Xun* (Beijing: Foreign Languages Press, 1960), 42.
5. *Diary of a Madman and Other Stories* (Hawaii, 1990), 45.
6. "On the Reasons for Indeterminacy of Translation" *Journal of Philosophy* LXVII, 178–183 (1970).

Chapter 2

Gao Xingjian's Chan-Inspired Absurdist Aesthetics

Mabel Lee

Gao Xingjian (b. 4 January 1940, China) was proclaimed Nobel Laureate of Literature in 2000, the first time the honor had been bestowed on a body of works originally created in Chinese. After the repressive regime of the Cultural Revolution (1966–1976) had ended in China, intellectuals and overseas "China experts" began an annual ritual of naming potential Chinese Nobel laureates. As the year 2000 approached, there was a general sense of anxiety because it would mean that in the 100-year history of the Nobel Prize, no Chinese writings had been able to match the standard of literature achieved in other languages. However, that year the Swedish Academy announced that "Chinese writer Gao Xingjian" had won the Nobel Prize for Literature, finally signaling a clear victory for Chinese writings in the global context.[1]

Unfortunately, there were no grounds for national jubilation in China because Gao had taken French citizenship in 1997. In fact, he had relocated to Paris in late 1987 precisely because his play *The Other Shore*[2] had been banned after a few rehearsals, and the authorities were also using various insidious means to block his advancement as a writer. Furthermore, when the military crackdown on Tiananmen Square protesters in Beijing shocked the world on June 4, 1989, Gao had condemned the Chinese authorities on radio and television in France and Italy, and at the same time renounced his membership in the Chinese Communist Party (CPC) and the Chinese Writers' Association:[3] these had been prerequisites for his writing and publishing in China. Before the end of the year, he had written a play titled *Escape* about those events.[4] His instructions for staging the play suggest that the performance "should be imbued with the declamatory style of ancient Greek tragedy and the ritualized solemnity of ancient Chinese theatre. The play is political, philosophical, and psychological, and should not be performed as a social-realist play reflecting only a single political event of the present."[5]

In May of 1991, Gao's play *Escape* was reprinted in *On the Diaspora "Elite": Who They Are and What They Are Doing*, published in Beijing by Chinese Youth Publishing House. It would be the last time any of his works was published in China. The play was preceded by a three-page diatribe attacking Gao for alleging that thousands of students had been killed in Tiananmen Square when he had not been present; it also condemned the three characters of the play for their sexual promiscuity and moral depravity. Soon after, Zeng Huiyan's essay "Publication of the Amazing Book *On the Diaspora 'Elite': Who They Are and What They Are Doing*" published in the Hong Kong bimonthly magazine, *Baixing*, no. 244 (1991) indicated "absurd theatre" was actually unfolding on a national scale. The authorities had approved a print run of 25,000 copies of the book that sold out in two months and was reprinted. The aim of the book was to provide examples of "reactionary" writings by "unpatriotic" Chinese elites living abroad; and while eagerly read, the book failed to achieve its intended "educational" effect. Nonetheless, over the next decade, Gao's *Escape* premiered at Kungliga Dramatiska Teatern (Stockholm, 1992), and was followed with performances at Nürnberg Theater (Nürnberg, 1992) and Teatr Polski (Poznan, 1994); and the following theatre groups took the play to Africa and Asia: RA Theater Company (Tours, 1994), Ryunokai Gekidan (Osaka, Kobe, Tokyo, 1997), Atelier Nomade (Benin, 1998), and Haiyuza Gekidan (Tokyo, 1998).[6]

It was also in 1991 that Gao was formally expelled from the Chinese Writers' Association and CPC, and his Beijing apartment seized.[7] His works have been banned in China ever since, although they can be collected by libraries in the form of gifts. While the banning of his works has stymied research or impact prospects stemming from his creative genius in China, Gao enjoys celebrity status in the literary, theatrical and art worlds of Taiwan, Hong Kong, Singapore, and South Korea, and certainly in the rest of the world, particularly in the Francophone and Anglophone spheres.

The ban on Gao's works meant that he was airbrushed out of existence during the 1990s in China, as well as from overseas studies of contemporary Chinese literature because the discipline was influenced by what was happening in China. During that decade in China, the subject matter of literature tended to focus on incidences of grotesque inhumanity in remote areas of the hinterland; and literary studies required the application of various strands of postmodern, postcolonial, gender, and feminist analysis, and the citing of cult Western thinkers such as Michel Foucault and Jacques Derrida. These avant-garde developments had occurred while China was cut off from the rest of the world, and while they were introduced over decades in the West, they were introduced together within that decade. In any case, Gao was not considered a contender for the Nobel Prize in 2000, and in fact less than a handful of academics had kept up with reading his prolific publications, and even fewer were engaged in Gao Xingjian research.

Henry Y.H. Zhao was an exception. The English edition of his *Towards a Modern Zen Theatre: Gao Xingjian and Chinese Theatre Experimentalism* was published on the eve of Gao Xingjian's receiving the Nobel award on December 10, 2000, in Stockholm.[8] Zhao was familiar with the entire corpus of Gao Xingjian's writings. In addition, he was equally erudite in Chinese and Western literature and philosophy, as well as comparative theatre studies. His knowledge of Chan (Zen) texts, allowed him to intuit immediately the unique wit, irony, satire and humor of Chan *gong'an* (Japanese kōan) in Gao's writings. While the Japanese terms Zen and kōan are familiar in the West, these are adaptations of the Chinese words "Chan" and "gong'an." My preference is to use the Chinese terms because they were in common use in China prior to their transmission to Japan, and because Chan and Zen subsequently evolved differently in their respective sociocultural milieus.

It is worth noting the role of translation in Gao Xingjian's Nobel success. From 1990–2000, academics from various parts of the world worked independently to translate Gao Xingjian's major works, and moreover succeeded in placing them with commercial publishers. Göran Malmqvist of Stockholm University worked on Swedish editions; and Noël and Liliane Dutrait, husband and wife team of the University of Provence (now known as Aix Marseille University), worked together on French editions.[9] English-language publications were by comparison slow. Nonetheless, Gilbert C.F. Fong, for many years at the Chinese University of Hong Kong and now Provost of Hang Seng Management College, worked on Gao's book of five plays in English, titled *The Other Shore: Plays by Gao Xingjian*, which was published in 1999[10]; and I worked on Gao's novel *Soul Mountain*, which was published by HarperCollins in 2000, four months before the Nobel announcement.[11]

Gao Xingjian's own absurdist reality in China is outlined in the following paragraphs to provide a context for appreciating various facets of his absurdist aesthetics later in this essay. He was appointed resident playwright in 1981 to the Beijing People's Art Theatre, and in 1982 on the staging of his play *Absolute Signal* the French newspaper *Le Monde* announced that avant-garde theatre had arrived in Beijing. The narrative tells how a planned train robbery is aborted because one of the robbers changes his mind. Unlike the propaganda plays of the past forty years, the audience had to form their own opinion about the characters, and this was a new experience for anyone born after the founding of the People's Republic of China (PRC) on October 1, 1949. Gao's interest is focused on the psychology of the characters, and modern European dramaturgical techniques such as flashbacks and change of perspective are introduced for the first time to audiences in China. The play displeased the custodians of Mao Zedong's guidelines for cultural production although no action was taken, and the play was staged a hundred times before being taken by theatre groups for performances in other cities.

The Cultural Revolution had ended, and while most older writers remained paralyzed by those times, younger writers were loudly clamoring for greater expressive freedom. Already aged forty, Gao Xingjian had been waiting more than twenty years just to be able to submit his works to an editor. At the beginning of the Cultural Revolution he had burned a suitcase of unpublished manuscripts—ten plays, numerous short stories, as well as poems and a novella—rather than risk having them found and be branded a counterrevolutionary. Afterwards, by devising strategies to effectively hide what he wrote, he wrote in secret to affirm the existence of his self, and to console himself in those bleak times when absolute conformity of thought was demanded and self-expression forbidden.

The end of the Cultural Revolution opened China to foreign influences after decades of isolation, and Gao soon found that his French major at the Foreign Languages Institute was a wonderful asset. A prolific reader since childhood, he had read through the Institute library holdings a shelf at a time during his five-year degree course (1957–1962). While literature and philosophy sections in libraries everywhere were systematically sealed off by censors, the Institute miraculously escaped such visits by zealous censors. In addition to reading French writings, Gao also read widely in Chinese writings that had been sealed off in libraries elsewhere. Through French publications he kept abreast of developments in the world that were not available to the rest of the population, a situation that continued when on graduating he was assigned work as a translator and editor at the Foreign Languages Press. In 1979, Gao travelled as official translator of the first PRC delegation of writers to France led by veteran writer Ba Jin (1904–2005), and as new literary publications proliferated, manuscripts that Gao Xingjian had been incubating for years began to assume concrete form and were welcomed by editors. In 1980, he traveled to Italy and France as a new member of the Chinese Writers' Association.

In a two-year period (1980–1981), his publications included two novellas, *Stars on a Cold Night* (1980) and *A Pigeon Called Red Beak* (1981); two scholarly critiques, "The French Modernist People's Poet Prévert and his *Paroles*" (1980) and "The Agony of Modern French Literature" (1980); two prose essays, "Ba Jin in Paris" (1980) and "Italian Caprice" (1981); and two short stories "Friends" (1981) and "Rain, Snow and Other" (1981). His *Preliminary Explorations into the Art of Modern Fiction*, serialized during 1980–1981 in the Guangzhou monthly, *Suibi*, was published as a book in 1981, and argues that the rise of cinema and technological developments requires that writers give greater attention to literary techniques and language use in the narration of fiction. In the West, fiction as a genre had been given new life through the introduction of flashbacks and stream of consciousness, but such strategies were virtually unknown in China. He explained how these strategies worked, and why they were effective, then followed by detailing the techniques used by the great novelists of premodern China and Russia. He spoke with the authority of erudition and concluded with the powerful assertion that fiction is ineffectual if its aim is to preach: it can only succeed when it is based on the freedom of the author, the characters, and the reader.

What Gao Xingjian advocated was audaciously subversive, and diametrically opposed the guidelines Mao Zedong had formulated for cultural production in Yan'an (1942) that were later enshrined as cultural policy after the founding of the PRC. Gao's *Preliminary Explorations* was widely read and reprinted in 1982, but it went unnoticed by the custodians of cultural production until it was praised by some veteran writers. In early 1983, a power shift in the upper echelons of the CPC allowed the Chinese Writers' Association to organize mass meetings to attack a "minor writer" who was challenging the social-realist traditions of the nation, and having a harmful effect on young writers. Being that "minor writer," Gao Xingjian was summoned to attend separate meetings at three different locations, but each time established writers came forward to speak in defense of both the author and the book, so none of the meetings turned into mass criticism sessions.[12]

Buoyed by such an outcome, in July of 1983, without securing the required approval, Gao proceeded to stage his play *Bus Stop* to wildly enthusiastic audiences. After the tenth staging, he was served notice that further performances were banned. The play tells of a motley crowd waiting for a bus to town at what seems to be a defunct stop. Beijing audiences encountered some common Western stage practices for the first time, such as the polyphony of conversations at the bus stop, and the actors going amongst the members of the audience to engage in conversation. At the time, securing permission for the most basic of things inevitably involved interminable waiting, and usually with no guarantee of success, so the theme resonated with audiences. However, the absurd and futile act of waiting, as well as the absurd and comic conversations between the characters, was a new and highly entertaining experience for audiences.

Geremie Barmé of the Australian National University wrote the first detailed study of Gao Xingjian in any language about this play. Barmé's "A Touch of the Absurd: Introducing Gao Xingjian, and His Play *The Bus-stop*" includes an abridged translation of the play, and was published in the Hong Kong translation magazine *Renditions* in 1983.[13] Gao's play was without precedent in China, but the obvious theme of waiting, and Gao's special interest in Samuel Beckett and Theatre of the Absurd in general, had commentators suggesting connections with Beckett's *Waiting for Godot*. Barmé's study correctly dismisses the notion that the play is Theatre of the Absurd and genealogically linked to Beckett. The Chinese authorities opposed the transmission of ambiguous messages to theatre audiences, and it was unlikely they understood absurdist aesthetics of any genealogical lineage. For them cultural production was serious business aimed specifically at educating the masses. However, having heard he was to be sent for "re-education" to the notorious prison farms of Qinghai from which one in ten was likely to return, Gao had no time to engage in debate on absurdist matters. It was certainly not his intention to wait around to be sent, so promptly reporting to his workplace that he was going to the mountain forests in the Southwest to carry out research on the lives of the woodcutters for a novel, he immediately boarded a train headed south out of Beijing.

During Gao's absence from Beijing, the Anti-Spiritual-Pollution Campaign escalated and he was publicly denounced for promoting the modernism of the decadent capitalist West. Wandering alone for five months on the fringes of Han civilization, he had much time to reflect on his own life, human relationships, history, and society. His solitary journey forms the backbone of his novel *Soul Mountain*, which he began in Beijing in 1982 and concluded in Paris in September 1989.[14] The campaign lost traction towards the end of 1983, and Gao returned to Beijing. His manuscripts that had been shelved for almost a year were released for publication in 1984, and his new play *Wild Man*[15] was staged in the main theatre of the Beijing People's Art Theatre in 1985. For the duration of the staging of *Wild Man*, in the theatre foyer he held the first solo exhibition of his Chinese ink paintings. He had been painting with Western oils since he was a young teenager, but after his second visit to Europe in 1980, he abandoned oils and turned to painting with Chinese inks. For five years, he had been exploring the potential of Chinese inks to gratify his need to express himself in visual images.[16]

The play *Wild Man* identifies poor management and corrupt bureaucratic practices as the cause of deforestation and serious destruction of the ecology, but the focus of the narrative is male-female relationships in the ancient past and in present times. He travelled to Germany for the first time on a D.A.A.D fellowship in 1985, and in Berlin at the Künstlerhaus Bethanien held a solo exhibition of his ink paintings as well as reading from his works and presenting seminars. He travelled from Berlin on invitation to various German universities, and to the UK and Denmark. After returning to China, in 1986 his play *The Other Shore* was stopped after a few rehearsals. He travelled to Germany on a second D.A.A.D fellowship in 1987, and by the end of the year had taken up residence in Paris where he has since lived.

Gao Xingjian's first three plays had made him a celebrity in literary and art circles in China and internationally, and during the 1980s he was arguably the most "notorious" writer in the land, best known for his three plays *Absolute Signal, Bus Stop*, and *Wild Man* that had been staged. He wrote plays for actualization on the stage, yet his close attention to the musicality—or auditory sensuousness—meant his plays could also be appreciated as audio texts, or as poetry. Of course, to watch his plays performed in the theatre space, directed by him or other talented directors, is an unforgettable experience. He no longer directs his own plays, but theatre groups all over the world are becoming increasingly sophisticated in documenting their productions and are now forwarding excellent archival copies to the Gao Xingjian Library Collections located at The Chinese University of Hong Kong and at Aix Marseille University in France.

* * *

Gao Xingjian has developed a unique Chan-inspired absurdist aesthetics that has a conspicuous presence in his plays, his first novel *Soul Mountain*, and especially in his second novel *One Man's Bible*. The following section seeks to substantiate this assertion, even though this may not count as high-level Chan intellectual enquiry. Nonetheless, by surveying Gao's repertoire of plays that focus on different dramaturgical, philosophical, historical, anthropological, psychological or social issues, folk religions and practices, male-female relationships, and includes mega-scale works such as *Snow in August* (2000), *City of the Dead* (1991), and *Of Mountains and Seas: A Tragicomedy of the Gods in Three Acts* (1989), it becomes clear that there is invariably a striking presence of absurdist aesthetics. With Gao's meticulous understanding of the theory and practice of performance arts in Eastern and Western traditions, he knew that the staging of his play *Bus Stop* in 1983, with its theme of waiting and dependency on absurdist dialogues, would remind foreigners of Beckett and Theatre of the Absurd. Western critics often saw the "late-modernizing" cultural efforts of Eastern writers as "derivative" or having been "influenced by" certain Western authors, but such insinuations with Gao Xingjian or *Bus Stop* did not emerge. When his works were first published, Gao's harshest critics were the Chinese authorities, although they had never succeeded in forcing him to change whatever he had written. Gao had uncompromising confidence in his own aesthetic judgments.[17]

Playwrights, theatre scholars, and critics in China had for decades been denied knowledge of literary developments in the outside world, and catching up would take time. A few years after the appearance of Barmé's 1983 essay, English-language research again dominated the field in analyzing the lively theatre scene of Beijing, Shanghai, and other cities, as well as examining Gao Xingjian's early plays in the context of Western playwrights, which he made no secret of having read. The following essays by Western-trained theatre experts were published between 1989–1992: Kwok-kan Tam, "Drama of Paradox: Waiting as Form and Motif in *The Bus-Stop* and *Waiting for Godot*" (1990); William Tay, "Avant-Garde Theatre in Post-Mao China: *The Bus-Stop* by Gao Xingjian" (1990); Ma Sen, "The Theatre of the Absurd in China: Gao Xingjian's *The Bus-Stop*" (1989); Xiaomei Chen, "*Wild Man* Between Two

Cultures" (1992); Jo Riley and Michael Gissenwehrer, "The Myth of Gao Xingjian" (1989).[18] These essays mainly consider Western playwrights who may have informed certain aspects of Gao's *Bus Stop*, or aspects of *Bus Stop* with similarities to *Waiting for Godot*. While Gao's knowledge of traditional Chinese theatre is sometimes mentioned, it was never the focus of research.

In the 1980s Gao wrote essays on Jean-Paul Sartre, Albert Camus, Beckett, Eugène Ionesco, Bertolt Brecht, Antonin Artaud, Jerzy Grotowski, and Tadeusz Kantor, translated Jacques Prévert's *Paroles* (1984) and Ionesco's *La Cantatrice Chauve* (1985). Gao also published exploratory essays on various theoretical aspects of traditional Chinese drama, and the year after his relocation to Paris a collection of these essays was published as *Searching for a New Kind of Modern Theatre* (Beijing: Theatre Publishing House, 1988). The decade of the 1990s was one of intense creation for Gao Xingjian as a highly innovative artist, playwright, novelist, as well as a highly perceptive literary and cultural critic. Living in France, he treasured the creative freedom of not having to exercise self-censorship as he subconsciously did during his short career, lasting less than a decade, as a writer publishing in China. In his second autobiographical novel *One Man's Bible* (1999), the word "freedom" is used twenty-three times over two consecutive pages, clearly defining the significance of freedom both for the individual and the creative self.

> Freedom is not conferred, nor can it be bought, it is your own awareness of life...Freedom castigates others. To take account of the approval or appreciation of others, and worse still to pander to the masses, is to live according to the dictates of others. Thus, it is they who are happy, but not you yourself, and that would be the end of this freedom of yours.[19]

His clearest statements on theatre are contained in his essay "The Potential of Theatre" (October 1, 2007), in which he demonstrates superb erudition in performance as an art form in Eastern and Western traditions. By careful study, he had isolated the "neutral actor" status found in traditional Eastern (Chinese and Japanese) performance. The actor consciously sheds his everyday self at the instant of mounting the stage to acknowledge the audience, and he is transformed into a "neutral actor" who is aware that he is to act a specific role or several roles. In other words, the actor does not try to merge with the role he plays, as is the case with modern Western theatrical practice. Both actor and audience know that the actor is playing a role. This important discovery led to Gao spending time to train actors before the staging of performances, and he began this practice with rehearsals for *The Other Shore* which was written with actor training in mind.[20]

In "The Potential of Theatre," Gao notes that Theatre of the Absurd emerged in the aftermath of World War II Europe, and flaunted as "anti-theatre," aimed at subverting traditional theatre.

> The story and plot essential in plays of the past were completely discarded, the characters were divested of any individuality and became mere ciphers, and theatrical conflicts constructed between characters also vanished. All that remained were words that were spoken on the stage—that is, a whole lot of talking.[21]

However, that was not what Gao Xingjian sought to achieve in theatre. He also argued against theatre replicating real life: authenticity is unnecessary on the stage. Audiences go to the theatre to see actors presenting a performance, and performance is not reality. He adds matter-of-factly: "naturalist performances are not particularly interesting but are in fact usually dull and boring."[22]

Having returned to the origins of theatre, Gao Xingjian wanted to restore in his plays the carnival atmosphere of "omnipotent theatre"—with its singing, dancing, acrobatics, walking on stilts, local folk stunts, music, punning, innuendo and asides—that is inherent in performance art. Within that context, as playwright he can freely interrogate serious human issues in a dedicated theatre space before his audience. Five of his works have large casts, and are written as "omnipotent theatre": *Wild Man* (1985), *The Other Shore* (1986), *City of the Dead* (1989), *Of*

Mountains and Seas: A Tragicomedy in Three Acts (1993), and *Snow in August* (2000). These five works included, between 1982 and 2007, he had written a total of seventeen works for the stage, and a large proportion of these explore the psychology of men and women regarding male-female sexual relationships, which have traditionally formed the stuff of theatre, whether in the East or the West.

The theatre is ideally suited for exploring such relationships because either men or women can be recruited to play the required "gendered" role. However, because in traditional Chinese theatre, women were banned from the stage, male performers were trained to perform female roles to perfection, even as tantalizing seductresses. Crossdressing is a feature of theatre in many countries, including China. The practice was severely punished during the Cultural Revolution and for many years temporarily went underground. Gao had grown up in the theatre world, and it is likely he would psychologically "cross-dress" to write the female roles for his plays. As a male playwright in contemporary times, he had the added advantage of being able to recruit female actors to perform the female roles of his plays.

A survey of the full range of Gao's plays that explore male-female sexual relationships reveals that he promotes the notion that men and women alike are biologically endowed with sexual instincts, as well as a sex drive. In the past, society regarded promiscuous women as sluts, but Gao consistently argues through his female characters that a woman's sex drive can be as strong as any man's, and just like men, women can and do propose and initiate sexual liaisons. What also emerges is that women who fall in love with men or have sexual liaisons with men demonstrate great courage, but are bound to suffer, whether in the remote past or in present times. Men are invariably depicted as emotional retards. For example, in his play *Wild Man*, the ecologist's wife tells her husband she is divorcing him just as he is setting off on a field trip into the mountains. She will not tolerate his long absences from home any longer. His impending divorce preys on his mind, but before long he finds himself flirting with a young village woman who falls in love with him. The woman is to be married off by her family to a local man with good prospects. Desperately in love with the ecologist, she has the courage to propose marriage but is cruelly rejected.

The gravity of male-female sex-related relationships is punctuated with Gao's unique absurdist aesthetics that intrudes as counterpoints to heighten the dramatic impact as events unfold. Gao invariably stands firmly on the side of the female characters in such relationships. His absurdist aesthetics is used to full extent in the play *City of the Dead*[23] that is based on the tale of how Zhuang Zhou (the philosopher Zhuangzi) plays a cruel trick on his wife, leading to her suicide and subsequent endless suffering in Hell. This play is Gao Xingjian's strongest indictment of the flippant attitude of men towards women who love them. Zhuang Zhou, his male accomplices who act in the charade of carrying his coffin home after he has died, as well as the male tormenters of Zhuang Zhou's wife in Hell are all knavish and cowardly.

Zhuang Zhou had been living in the mountains away from home to observe natural phenomena in his search to understand the Heavenly Way. However, missing the embrace of his young and beautiful wife, he pretends to have died of illness and arranges to be carried home in a coffin. His hapless wife, who had been yearning for her husband day and night, is distraught with grief and furthermore faces the grim prospect of not having a livelihood. Disguised as a Chu prince, Zhuang Zhou suddenly appears and announces that the King of Chu had sent him to invite Zhuang Zhou to serve at the Chu court. However, as Zhuang Zhou was apparently dead, the imposter proceeds to seduce the young widow and manages to steal a kiss. She flirts in response and makes a coquettish show of pushing him away. He falls and cannot get up, and tells her he has a fatal disease that can only be cured if he is fed the brain of a fresh corpse. Infatuated by the imposter, she goes off to find an axe to break open her husband's coffin. When she returns to the scene, Zhuang Zhou is dressed in his philosopher's clothes and steps out of the coffin. He laughs at her, mocks her, calls her a slut, then cowers in fear as she approaches him holding high the axe that she uses on herself and not on him.

The second part of the play shows Zhuang Zhou's wife mercilessly tormented by the obnoxious keepers of the various levels of Hell: both her morality and suicide are deemed reprehensible. There is a carnival-like atmosphere as performances of traditional Chinese theatrical stunts are presented by the tormentors of Zhuang Zhou's wife, all of whom are presented as "tyrannical, cruel, bullying, mendacious, foolish, ridiculous and knavish males, and they can also be seen as theatrical exaggerations of male behavior towards females in real life."[24] Witnessing these events in Hell unfolding, female singers lining the stage condemn the despicable joke Zhuang Zhou has played on his wife. The play insists several times that these events took place a long time ago, implying that this is no longer the case. However, a strong subliminal message is conveyed at the same time: women will always suffer because of their sexual liaisons with men. First drafted in 1987 in Beijing, *City of the Dead* defines Gao Xingjian's stance that men have a cavalier attitude towards their female sexual partners and that women in such relationships are "doomed to suffer."[25]

Gao Xingjian's modern Peking Opera *Snow in August* (2000) is the high point of his achievements in theatre, and his absurdist aesthetics has a strong presence throughout. The 2002 production of the play at The National Theatre in Taipei was directed by Gao Xingjian, and according to Gilbert C.F. Fong's description, featured fifty actors, a chorus of fifty, four percussionists, a symphony orchestra of ninety musicians, hence totaling 200-odd performers. *Snow in August* recounts the life of Huineng (633–713), Sixth Patriarch of Chan and the founder of the Sudden Enlightenment School. "He was an outsider to the religious order —he did not belong to any temple, and he was not even an ordained monk when he became Sixth Patriarch."[26] The brilliant music for the opera, composed by Xu Shuya (b. 1961, Changchun, Jilin province, China),[27] lingers tenaciously long after one has viewed the production,[28] and the absurdist aesthetics permeating the beginning of the work indicates that for Gao Xingjian the dimensions of male-female sexual relationships are endlessly intriguing in the ways they affect human behavior.

In *Snow in August* the youthful woodcutter Huineng has delivered a load of firewood to the temple, and introducing himself approaches the nun Boundless Treasure who is beating a wooden fish and chanting a sutra with her back to the audience. Mesmerized by her chanting, Huineng refuses to leave. She offers him a copy of the sutra to take with him, but he says he is illiterate and would not be able to read the words. Boundless Treasure is alarmed, and thinks to herself:

> What should I do now? I'm a nun, and I should not get caught in any romantic entanglement. That was the reason I decided to seek refuge here at the Mountain Stream Temple! But now... Deep autumn, early chill, the raindrops hit the banana leaves. The night is long, and this young woodcutter insists on staying by my side. He refuses to leave the temple. What should I do? Amitabha, what should I do?[29]

Being pure of mind, Huineng fails to understand why Boundless Treasure is troubled by his presence. The two engage in dialogue through song. She sings a haunting song of perpetual loneliness with a solitary lamp as her only company, and of long and endless nights. Life for her is "Endless regrets, / Boundless remorse; / Endless and boundless sorrow."[30] While Huineng remains unmoved and uncomprehending, it is clear to the audience why the nun is frustrated. The whole scene is flush with the absurd, yet the snatches of Boundless Treasure's singing tell of her loneliness and her desire for companionship during the long and endless nights, even if that loneliness is self-imposed by her choosing to become a nun.

Absurdist aesthetics is inevitably present in any of his plays that discuss male-female sex-based relationships, whether they concern short-term encounters as in *Escape* (1989) and *Dialogue and Rebuttal* (1992), or a long-term relationship as in *Between Life and Death* (1991). Discussions of male-female sex encounters, liaisons, or relationships in Gao Xingjian's plays are always narrated by a female performer, and she will invariably present a woman's point of view. A man's point of view on the subject is never presented, even though Gao Xingjian is a male playwright. It is exploring the female psychology regarding male-female sexual relationships that is fascinating for him.

As mentioned earlier, in the mid-1980s after isolating the "neutral actor" status in traditional Chinese performance, he began training actors in this technique when they began rehearsals for his plays. The actor would discard his/her everyday persona on mounting the stage as a "neutral actor," acknowledge the audience, and proceed to perform a specific role or roles. Moreover, because the male playwright Gao Xingjian is adept in achieving "neutral actor" status in performing a role, it is not a quantum leap for him to assume the psychology of a female character or any character in the writing of his plays. For example, in *Between Life and Death*, the female performer narrates how third-person "she" is a nervous wreck because of her man's profligate lifestyle, and she releases a barrage of complaints about the man who does not speak throughout, and responds only with a grimace, a pout, a shake of the head, or raises an arm trying to explain. The female performer complains that "she" and her man cannot communicate, but she admits she still loves him and will forgive him, even if he continues to have his flings. Eventually, she goes to grab him because he makes no response and finds he has transformed into a jacket on a clothes hanger, a pair of empty trousers, a pair of shoes, and a hat. "She" thinks she has killed her man, and proceeds to talk about her loneliness, her fear of growing old, her memories, her sexual longing, as well as about how her mother's boyfriend had been allowed to rape her with her mother's consent.

In 1999 Gao Xingjian drafted a theatre piece in French titled *Ballade Nocturne*. Claire Conceison's English translation of his 2007 revised French version was published in 2010 and retains the French title *Ballade Nocturne*.[31] In 2009 Gao wrote a Chinese version that was published in his poetry collection *Wandering Spirit and Metaphysical Thoughts.*[32] My translation from the Chinese version is titled *Song of the Night.*[33] A female actor performs the role of "She," and is accompanied by two female dancers, one melancholy and the other vivacious, and together they form a composite image of contemporary woman. A male musician plays a saxophone or some instrument but does not speak. Appraising male behavior towards women, "She" maintains that sex leaves a woman like a butterfly pinned alive to the wall. If men could be women for a while, they would be more intelligent and deserving of a woman's love. Men think they own a woman but have no inkling of her loneliness. "She" calls on women to wage war against men. It is men who cause wars and destroy lives, while women offer love and become pregnant again. In the final analysis, "She" concedes that the desire for sex between men and women in nature's grand plan for procreation of the species will prevail.[34]

Gao's absurdist aesthetics is a definite presence in his autobiographical novels *Soul Mountain* and *One Man's Bible.* In fact, these works encapsulate elements of poetry, theatre, art, photography, and film, and may be considered simultaneously trans-genre and transmedia. In *One Man's Bible,* the author/narrator of the present (i.e., "you") distances himself from "he" of the past (i.e., during the Cultural Revolution). This psychological distancing by the author/narrator allows the thoughts and actions of "he" of those times to be subjected to rigorous scrutiny. So "distanced," the author/narrator stands at a position identical to that of reader, and there is no reason to create excuses for his "distanced" self or to treat him as a victim of those times. The unfortunate "he" is subjected to strong lashings of Gao's absurdist aesthetics that are scattered throughout the novel.

> You then stand at the window and watch snowflakes falling soundlessly outside. Snow covers the whole city like a huge white shroud wrapping corpses, and you, by the window, mourn his loss of self...
>
> Or, for a different perspective, it is you in the audience, watching him crawl onto the stage, a deserted stage. He is standing naked

in the bright light, and it will take a little time for him to get used to it, to see past the stage lights, and to see you sitting in the red velvet seat in the last row of the empty theater.[35]

Having imputed a definite absurdist aesthetics to Gao Xingjian's plays and novels, some facts are worth noting. His extensive study of French authors or French translations of writings in other languages during his studies at the Beijing Foreign Languages Institute had inflamed his lust to write, and he began interrogating Western narrative and dramaturgical theories and practices to inform his writings. Whereas a tradition of Western literary criticism had evolved over recent centuries, a similar process did not occur in China. Gao Xingjian applied the critical skills he had developed in his study of Western writings and used these to scrutinize Chinese narratology and theatre in their various forms, including storytelling, local theatre, and shamanistic and religious practices. He was intent on learning about the dynamics involved so that he would be able to create writings that would satisfy himself as the reader. Because he totally rejected the idea of writing according to the national guidelines for cultural production, he wrote in secret. This meant that he alone had enjoyed and critiqued his own works for more than three decades. It was as if he were sitting in a theatre, watching a play that he had written and directed. This was in fact the situation he describes in Chapter 60 of *One Man's Bible*. "He" the protagonist of the Cultural Revolution era protests.

> He says enough, put an end to him!
> Who are you talking about?
> Who is to put an end to whom?
> Him, the character you're writing about, put an end to him.
> You say you are not the author.
> Then who is?
> Surely, it's clear, himself, of course!
> You are only his conscious mind.
> Then what will happen to you?
> If he is finished off, will you also be finished off?
> You say you can be a reader,

You will be just like the audience watching a play...[36]

Chapter 58 of *One Man's Bible* demonstrates the powerful impact of Gao's absurdist aesthetics.

"Run, run, run!" the crowd shouted.

He said he was busy, he had personal matters to deal with.

"Personal matters? No matters are as important as this! Run, run with us, run with all of us!"

"Why are you running?" he asked.

"We're going to greet the good times, the good times will be here soon, we're going to greet the good times! How can your piffling personal matters be as important?"[37]

"He" was caught in a crowd that was loudly singing uplifting good-time songs. He had to sing loudly or be called a deaf-mute, and he also had to keep in step. If he were half a step slower, the heel of his shoe would be trodden on, and he would lose his shoe. If he tried to pick up his shoe, people's feet would trample his head. He would just have to stumble along with one shoe and continue singing loudly in praise of the good times.[38] This absurdist episode continues and approximates some of the descriptions of crowd behavior portrayed in his play *Escape*.

None of Gao Xingjian's works confront a single issue; instead they deal with several at the same time: controversial themes and issues, and technical or linguistic innovations within genres or across genres to satisfy his curiosity as a writer. It is therefore easy not to register the unique absurdist aesthetics pervading most of his literary works. His absurdist aesthetics is partly due to his innate fun-loving nature, but equally due to his deliberate strategy to provide release to readers who have been subjected to prolonged tension in the narration: it is a release that functions like counterpoint in musical composition. Although he does not claim to compose music, he is highly sensitive to music, and movements, harmonies, variations, symphonic connections are often used to structure his writings. Gao's absurdist aesthetics is prevalent yet subtle, adding considerable dramatic force to his creative endeavors. It is present in his recent cine-poem *Requiem for Beauty* (2016)[39] that he had written in 2011 as a poem with the same title.[40] An accomplished novelist, playwright, artist, photographer, filmmaker, and director, he is the embodiment of creative genius in multiple disciplines, genres and media, so he does not balk at ignoring what are manifestly "borders": for him such borders have been created over the ages by humans. In his cine-poem *Requiem for Beauty*, paintings, performance, music, and poetry replace the narrative episodes of film, and the cine-poem grieves the death of beauty in contemporary urban life that has been eroded by material lust.

In the "Postscript" to his poetry collection *Wandering Spirit and Metaphysical Thoughts* he writes that in preparing for his cine-poem *Requiem for Beauty*, he wanted to express his condolences to beauty, and to shout out: "Return to human nature, return to the investigation of beauty, and in what is meaningless seek after what has meaning; through observation and scrutiny, awaken the conscience so that hopefully some traces of the poetic may be captured." He notes also that the series of poems titled *Wandering Spirit and Metaphysical Thoughts* is the only work without links to plays or films.[41] Amongst his writings, the thirty-six poems of *Wandering Spirit and Metaphysical Thoughts* contain the highest concentration of his absurdist aesthetics. A few poems show definite traces of Chan or perhaps even Daoist thinking, but overwhelmingly it is Gao Xingjian's own unique absurdist aesthetics that is the driving force. "Poem 26" states that poetry is just a language game, but that poetry expressing a person's ambitions "is boring." His suggestion instead is to use poetry to "tease humanity" and in the process not to "forget first to amuse yourself."[42]

In "Poem 1" we learn that the poet was to have been dispatched by Death, but God had given him a reprieve because "the reprobate still had things to say," and God "being the epitome of kindness" gives him a horse, and treats him as his favorite son.[43] The poems concerning God, the Devil, and the poet are honest, extremely funny, and resonate loudly with truth. "Poem 15" notes that compared with the poet's experiences as a human being, to have an association with the Devil is carefree and relaxing. In conversations with the Devil, nothing is taboo and talk turns from scandals involving chairmen and presidents to women's skirts and panties. The latter is the Devil's specialty, so he talks with great gusto and laughs so much that he ends up rolling about on the ground. However, God is solemn. He wields the scepter of supreme power, and having an odd temperament sends forth diseases and natural disasters that virtually wipe out the human species. In contrasdistinction, the Devil only engages in a bit of debauchery from time to time.[44]

The absurd aesthetics of "Poem 12"[45] below is a none-too-subtle reminder of human insignificance in the grand order of the universe.

> How this began
> You've forgotten
> Anyway
> God and the Devil
> Are sitting with you
> Although to say sitting is strictly not accurate
> Because in Heaven which lacks gravity
> Sitting, standing or standing upside-down
> Are all meaningless
> Also, meaning is beyond language
> So, speaking or not is the same as being silent
> And the discussion proceeded like that
>
> God, the Devil and humankind are in three-way conference
> You represent humankind
> Even if no one has elected you
> Democracy and majority rule
> That scrap of human rationale
> Is totally absent in Heaven
> As for reasoning and logic

Pay attention!
What I am saying is
Grand and glorious principles
Amount to less than a rag for wiping feet
And bear in mind
Shoes aren't worn in the Garden of Eden
The Devil has hoofs
And God is floating in the clouds
So, you're the only one who is barefoot

* * *

After a second trip to Europe in 1980, realizing he would never be capable of painting like the European masters, Gao Xingjian abandoned oils and turned to Chinese inks to give concrete form to the ephemeral and tantalizing images that surged endlessly from the depths of his mind.[46] By the end of 1987, after relocating to Paris, it was by selling his Chinese ink paintings that he covered his living expenses. During the period 1985–2012 he held sixty-eight solo exhibitions worldwide, including exhibitions such as "La Fin du Monde" at Ludwig Museum, Germany (2007) and "Depois do dilúvio" at Sintra Musem of Modern Art, Portugal (2009). Detailed analytical studies on his art are now being published, the most recent being Daniel Bergez, *Gao Xingjian: Painter of the Soul.*[47] Belgium has conferred an extraordinary honor on Gao Xingjian as an artist. On February 25, 2015, in Brussels his *The Awakening of Consciousness* went on permanent display in a large dedicated hall of the Royal Museums of Fine Arts of Belgium. Comprising six large-scale works, *The Awakening of Consciousness* explores the psychological states he has designated *Subconscious, Illusion, Impulse, Introspection, Somewhere Else,* and *Bewilderment.* On the following day, the "Gao Xingjian Retrospective" was launched at Musée Ixelles (February 26– May 31, 2015).[48]

Gao uses traditional calligraphy and ink-wash techniques in his painting, but his art does not accord with traditional Chinese aesthetics that emphasizes the one-dimensionality of the flat painting surface.

Instead, his works demonstrate his fascination for the texture and tactile sensuousness of Western oil painting, and for black-and-white photography.[49] He rejects the use of language in his art and focuses purely on the visual: his visual aesthetic is anti-intellectual and anti-analytical, perhaps a reflection on his career as a writer from a perspective distinct from that of literature.

Notes

1. See detailed discussions in Kwok-kan Tam, "Gao Xingjian, the Nobel Prize and the Politics of Recognition," in Kwok-kan Tam, ed., *Soul of Chaos: Critical Perspectives on Gao Xingjian* (Hong Kong: The Chinese University Press, 2001), 1–20; and Julia Lovell, "Gao Xingjian, the Nobel Prize, and the Chinese Intellectuals: Notes on the Aftermath of the Nobel Prize 2000," *Modern Chinese Literature and Culture*, 14.2 (Fall 2002), 1–50.
2. In Gao Xingjian, *The Other Shore: Plays by Gao Xingjian*, tr. Gilbert C.F. Fong (Hong Kong: The Chinese University Press, 1999).
3. See Gao Xingjian, "Wilted Chrysanthemums" (1991), in Gao, *The Case for Literature*, tr. Mabel Lee (New Haven and London: Yale University Press, 2007; first published in Sydney: HarperCollins, 2006), 140–155.
4. In Gao Xingjian, *Escape & The Man Who Questions Death*, tr. Gilbert C. F. Fong (Hong Kong: The Chinese University Press, 2007).
5. See Mabel Lee, Introduction: "Two Autobiographical Plays by Gao Xingjian," in Gao, *Escape & The Man Who Questions Death*, xiv–xvi.
6. Ibid.
7. See Gao, "Wilted Chrysanthemums."
8. London: School of Oriental and African Studies, 2000. The Chinese edition was published in Taipei in 1999.
9. Liliane died an untimely death of illness in 2010, but Noël Dutrait continues to translate and write on Gao's works.
10. Gilbert Fong continues to translate and write on Gao's works.
11. For five years, 1995–1999, I included Gao Xingjian's works in my Chinese literature courses at the University of Sydney, and it is possible these were the only Gao Xingjian courses in the world at the time. I continue to engage in Gao Xingjian research projects—my latest book is a forthcoming volume coedited with Liu Jianmei and titled *Gao Xingjian and Transmedia Aesthetics* (Amherst, NY: Cambria Press, 2018), which demonstrates the extensive reach of Gao Xingjian's transcultural, transdisciplinary and transmedia explorations—and to translate his writings.
12. See Gao, "Wilted Chrysanthemums."
13. *Renditions: A Chinese-English Translation Magazine*, 19–20 (1983): 373–386.

14. The Chinese edition was published in Taipei by Lianjing in 1990. See Gao, *Soul Mountain*, tr. Mabel Lee (Sydney and New York: HarperCollins, 2000; London: HarperCollins, 2001).
15. Gao's play *Wild Man*, tr. Bruno Roubicek, is attached to Roubicek's essay, "*Wild Man*: A Contemporary Chinese Spoken Drama," *Asian Theatre Journal*, 7. 2 (1990): 184–191.
16. As a young teenager, Gao Xingjian read widely about Western art history and he studied painting with Western oils under an instructor. He also developed a keen interest in black-and-white photography, and the textures of oil painting and photography can be discerned in his Chinese ink paintings. A departure from traditional themes, the female nude is a presence in his Chinese inks, but they are calligraphic representations, sensuous forms that radiate energy. Kinesthetic sensation is also represented in his works: the wind blowing through the branches of trees is motivated by the Chan notion that the wind can be represented.
17. Following the June 4, 1989, military crackdown on students in Tiananmen Square, Gao was approached to write a play about the events for an American theatre company. In September, he completed the play *Escape*, but having read the English translation the theatre company requested revisions. Gao sent word that the Chinese authorities could not make him change his manuscripts, nor could the American theatre company. See Gao, "About *Escape*," tr. Shelby K.Y. Chan in Gao, *Escape & The Man Who Questions Death*, 69–71.
18. All of these essays have been reprinted with full citations in Kwok-kan Tam, ed., *Soul of Chaos*.
19. Gao Xingjian, *One Man's Bible*, tr. Mabel Lee (New York, Sydney, London: HarperCollins, 2002), 358–359. For a detailed discussion, see Mabel Lee, "Gao Xingjian's Transcultural Aesthetics in Fiction, Theater, Art, and Film," in Michael Lackner and Nikola Chardonnens, eds, *Polyphony Embodied: Freedom and Fate in Gao Xingjian's Writings* (Berlin and Boston: de Gruyter, 2014), 20–42, esp. 26–27.
20. Discussed at length by Gao in "Dramaturgical Method and the Neutral Actor" (July 4, 1995). See Gao, *Aesthetics and Creation*, tr. Mabel Lee (Amherst, NY: Cambria Press, 2012), 159–177.
21. Gao, "The Potential of Theatre," in Gao, *Aesthetics and Creation*, 42.
22. Ibid., 44.
23. Gao completed the first draft of *City of the Dead* in 1987 before leaving Beijing and completed the final draft in Paris in late 1991.

24. See Mabel Lee, Introduction: "Gao Xingjian: Autobiography and the Portrayal of the Female Psyche," in Gao Xingjian, *City of the Dead* and *Song of the Night*, tr. Gilbert C. F. Fong and Mabel Lee (respectively) (Hong Kong: The Chinese University Press, 2015), xv.
25. See Mabel Lee, Introduction: "Gao Xingjian: Autobiography and the Portrayal of the Female Psyche," xiv–xv.
26. See Gilbert C.F. Fong, Introduction: "Marginality, Zen, and Omnipotent Theatre," in Gao, *Snow in August* (Hong Kong: The Chinese University Press, 2003), vii–x.
27. Xu Shuya had been living in Paris since 1988 and is now professor of composition and director of the Academic Committee of the Shanghai Conservatory of Music (his alma mater).
28. Gao Xingjian, *August Snow* (DVD) (Taipei: Council for Cultural Affairs, Executive Yuan, 19–22 December 2002).
29. Gao, *Snow in August*, 5.
30. Ibid., 6–7.
31. Lewes, UK: Sylph Editions and the American University of Paris, 2010.
32. Gao Xingjian, *Wandering Spirit and Metaphysical Thoughts* (Taipei: Lianjing, 2014).
33. See Gao, *City of the Dead* and *Song of the Night*, 64–84.
34. For further discussion, see Lee, "Gao Xingjian: Autobiography and the Portrayal of the Female Psyche," xxi–xxiii.
35. Gao, *One Man's Bible*, 251.
36. Ibid., 441.
37. Ibid., 432
38. Ibid., 433.
39. Gao Xingjian, *Requiem for Beauty*, tr. Yang Xiling, Sherry Buchanan, Gilbert C.F. Fong, Wu Jia-Shan, Noël Dutrait, Hsu Chia-Yu (Taipei: National Taiwan Normal University, 2016). The book includes a CD of the cine-poem.
40. First published in Gao Xingjian, *Wandering Spirit and Metaphysical Thoughts: Collected Poems by Gao Xingjian* (Taipei: Lianjing, 2012), 139–199. Of this series, Mabel Lee has translated Poems 10–12, in *Contrappasso: Special Issue: Long Distance*, edited by Theodore Ell (November 2015): 21–23; and Poems 1–9 in *Portal: Journal of Multidisciplinary International Studies*, 14.1 (April 2017).
41. See Gao, *Wandering Spirit*, 252–254.
42. Ibid., 122.
43. Ibid., 89–90.

44. Ibid., 107–111.

45. Ibid., 99–101.

46. See Mabel Lee, "Aesthetic Dimensions of Gao Xingjian's Painting." In Gao Xingjian, *Between Figurative and Abstract: Paintings by Gao Xingjian* (West Bend IN: Notre Dame University, Snite Museum of Art, 2007), 127–145.

47. Published in French as *Gao Xingjian: Peintre de l'âme* (Paris, Seuil, 2013), and followed in the same year by the English edition tr. Sherry Buchanan, *Gao Xingjian: Painter of the Soul* (London: Asia Ink, 2013).

48. See Michel Draguet, *Gao Xingjian: Le Goût de l'encre* (Brussels: Musée d'Ixelles, 2015.

49. See Lee, "Aesthetic Dimensions of Gao Xingjian's Painting," 127–145.

CHAPTER 3

SINOPHONE INTERVENTION WITH CHINA

BETWEEN NATIONAL AND WORLD LITERATURE

David Der-wei Wang

"Sinophone" is arguably the most provocative keyword of Chinese literary studies since the turn of the new millennium. Although the term has been used since the 1990s in select contexts, it was not made popular until 2007 when Professor Shu-mei Shih published *Visuality and Identity: Sinophone Articulations across the Pacific*.[1] In her book, Shih invokes the "Sinophone" as a language-based critical perspective from which to engage the linguistic, cultural, ethnic, and political dynamics in China, as well as Chinese-speaking communities worldwide.[2] In opposition to conventional reference to "China" as a homogenized entity, she argues that the dispersal of the Chinese people across the world needs to be reconceptualized in terms of vibrant or vanishing communities of Sinitic-language cultures rather than of ethnicity and nationality. With the Sinophone paradigm, Shih seeks to intervene in both Sinology and Chinese Area Studies, in the hope of unleashing (or dispelling) the contested forces in the discourse about China.

In the wake of Shu-mei Shih's groundbreaking work, there have been waves of attempts to rethink the conditions of Sinophone literature, its spatiotemporal boundaries, its methodological feasibility, and above all, its geopolitical and geopoetic implications. Meanwhile, questions have been raised as to the relationship between Sinophone literature and the extant paradigm of Chinese literary studies: Is Sinophone merely a nomenclature in place of the familiar term "overseas Chinese literature"? If not, what is the new theoretical ground and critical goal at stake? Is it a Sinitic brand of popular theories in North America, such as postcolonialism, multiculturalism, diaspora studies, and empire studies? How can it be brought to bear on the literary productions in Chinese speaking communities? Most important, what is its relevance to Chinese national literature produced in China?

In this essay I engage with Sinophone Chinese literary studies by examining the strengths and limitations of the extant models, which are largely predicated on postcolonialism. Instead of the postcolonial model, which stresses the politics of spatiality, I introduce postloyalism as a way to tease out the historical bearings of Sinophone discourse, thereby calling forth its inherent politics of temporalities. Moreover, I ponder the dialogic of "Sinophone obsession with China" versus "Sinophone intervention with China," and propose that a Sinophone imaginary provides a critical interface through which to rethink the configuration of (Chinese) national literature vis à vis world literature. With fictional examples drawn from Taiwan, Hong Kong, Malaysia, and Mainland China, I highlight the textual and spatial loci where postcolonial and postloyalist inscriptions are intertwined with each other, and contend that these loci generate some of the most perplexing Sinophone conditions for further deliberation.

I.

To begin with, Sinophone literature represents a most recent intervention with the mapping of Chinese literary modernity based on national boundaries. For decades, the writing and reading of modern Chinese literary history has been couched in the national discourse, as part of the world circulation of nationalism and literary representation. By way of contrast, Chinese language literature produced outside the territory of sovereignty (of either the Republic of China or the People's Republic of China; hereafter ROC and PRC) has been treated as that which is subordinate to, or derivative of, the corpus of Chinese national literature. As a result, it is not difficult to discern in overseas Chinese-language literature a geopolitical subtext of center versus periphery, authenticity versus mimicry, homeland versus diaspora.

Sinophone literature seeks to reconsider such a dichotomized view of Chinese literature, by projecting a sphere where multiple Chinese language literatures are being produced, circulated, and contested. Shu-mei Shih derives her definition of "Sinophone" from the Sinitic-language family, an immense network comprising more than four hundred toplects, dialects and ethnic languages.[3] Such a Sinophone vision opens up a new terrain for studying Chinese literature. At its most dynamic, "Sinophone" amounts to nothing less than a realm of Bakhtinian "heterglossia," in which the centripetal and centrifugal sources and forces of languages interact with each other. But beyond this shared recognition of plural soundings of the Chinese language, critics of Sinophone Studies are taking different approaches to the questions raised above. For instance, Shih emphasizes the oppositional potential of the Sinophone vis-à-vis the imperialist hegemony of China, thus echoing the tenor of postcolonialism and empire studies. Jing Tsu contends that "Sinophone governance" is a nebulous process of negotiation through which Chinese speaking regions and cultures form a communicative network. Between these positions, one observes a spectrum of proposals addressing the affective, cultural, semiotic, and political terms of Sinophone articulations. These stances compel us to understand modern Chinese literature not as a fixed field but a flux of practices and imaginaries.

The invocation of "Sinophone" is ineluctably related to the geopolitics of modern China since the Cold War era and its literary representation in the global circuit. Before Sinophone discourse drew our attention, there had existed a trend to rethink China "beyond" China. The Tiananmen Incident in 1989 served as an impetus for overseas intellectuals to confront the issue of political crisis and cultural sustainability. Wei-ming Tu, for instance, famously proclaimed in 1989 that on top of China as a political entity, there has existed a cultural lineage that outlasts dynastic changes and modern power struggles.[4] The turn of the new millennium witnessed another wave of engagements with Chinese identity and culture in a more polemical manner. Whereas Rey Chow argues vehemently against the "consanguinity of Chineseness," a concept that links ethnic heritage with patriotic solidarity,[5] Ien Ang goes one step further, tackling the irony of one's being "unable to speak Chinese" despite one's Chinese ancestral roots.[6] Kim-chew Ng, a Chinese Malaysian writer based in Taiwan, critiques Chinese Malaysians' predicament as resulting from both their fetishizing everything about China and their disempowerment under Malaysian government's hegemonic rule.[7]

It was amid these inquiries into "China" as a *problematique* that Shih Shu-mei's Sinophone discourse surfaced on the horizon. For Shih, "Sinophone studies takes as its objects of study the Sinitic-language communities and cultures outside China as well as ethnic minority communities and cultures within China where Mandarin is adopted or imposed."[8] She contends that, just as is the case of Anglophone, Francophone, or Hispanophone articulations, Sinophone brings to mind the colonizing and colonized conditions in greater China in military, economic, and cultural terms. Shih's research concludes with the claim that the Sinophone subjectivity is predicated on the disavowal of diaspora. If diaspora studies focuses on issues such as the loss of roots and the yearning for homecoming, Sinophone studies, according to Shih, seeks to pin down the "expiration date" of diaspora.

Shih's reflection leads one to Jing Tsu's theory of "governance," which she defines as an "implicit coordination between linguistic antagonisms and the notion of the 'native speaker' that makes something like a 'national literature' both possible but conceptually fraught."[9] Tsu is vigilantly aware of the temptation of phonocentrism in the Sinophone agenda, therefore directing her study to the interactive relationship between the sound and script systems. For her, the script system of the Han language is a textual assemblage, one that requires a genealogical investigation of its ideological and technological interactions. Thus, in contrast with Shih who insists on the politics of resistance, Tsu explores the diplomatic dispersal and coalition of Sinophone communication.

I would suggest that, despite their interventional efforts, neither Shih nor Tsu goes far enough to confront the most polemical dimension of Sinophone studies. In my view, for a Sinophone project to exert its critical potential, one must not engage merely with the domain of conventional overseas Chinese literature plus ethnic literature on the Mainland. Rather, one should test its power *within* the nation-state of China. In light of the translingual dynamics on the global scale, we need to reimagine the cartography of the Chinese center versus the periphery so as to enact a new linguistic and literary arena of contestations. As a matter of fact, to truly subvert the foundation of Chinese national literature, we should no longer consider it apart from the Sinophone literary system.

My proposal may sound self-contradictory because, as defined by Shih and Tsu respectively, the Sinophone is invoked in the first place to deal with the literary and cultural production outside China proper. Nevertheless, I argue that while Sinophone scholars can avert their attention from Chinese national literature for various reasons in praxis, they must reject the temptation of a dichotomized logic of the Chinese versus the Sinophone. My argument actually derives from Shih's and Tsu's logic. If "Chinese" is not a homogenized entity but a constellation of

Sinitic utterances amid the flux of historical changes, a Sinophone scholar can conclude that even the official Han language, however standardized by the state, comprises complex soundings and transformations, therefore subject to the rhizomic tapestry of Sinoglossia. Coming to mind are the variations of the *putonghua* articulation, in discursive format as in tonality, from the revolutionary era to the post-revolutionary era, and from one area of China to another. By corollary, Chinese national literature, just like overseas Chinese literature, is always a proliferating *process* of expressions and experimentations in both script and sound.

More importantly, despite her assertion of Chinese "continental colonialism" over the minorities on the Chinese mainland, Shih falls short in explaining the spread of the Chinese language overseas in the modern period. It had less to do with China's (and Chinese settlers') "colonial expansion" and coercion, as claimed by Shih, than with the overdetermined motivations inherent in the waves of Chinese people's travel, emigration, and diaspora. That is, when Chinese travelers, emigrants, and refugees relocated to the new places of settlement for economic and political reasons, they kept the Chinese language—often in terms of dialects and topolects—and script system as the linkage to their homeland (but not necessarily the home country). Chinese served as less a political vehicle overpowering indigenous languages and cultures than a linguistic register—and an affective index—sustaining the cultural legacy and ethnic bonding among Chinese themselves. The result is a hybrid linguistic culture fraught with both naturalized foreignness and alienated nativity, both Sinophone utterance and cacophonous reverberations.

It is in this context that postloyalism becomes a notable phenomenon. Postloyalism is a coinage derived from a critical reflection on loyalism, or *yimin* 遺民, a unique political and cultural discourse in Chinese history. The term *yimin* originally meant "one who remains loyal to a former dynasty and is ashamed to serve a new dynasty when a change in state power occurs."[10] Loyalism is a discourse premised on the politics of anachronism and displacement. When a political subject of the ancient times insists on retaining his bereavement for a fallen dynasty or a lost culture against all odds, loyalist sentiment abounds. There underlies a paradox in loyalism, however, as it derives its claim to legitimacy, be it political, cultural, emotional, ethnic, or ethical, from a reluctant awareness of the loss of that legitimacy. In other words, loyalism gestures toward the belatedness of time and yet gains an unlikely agency in the hope of restoring that which is (forever) lost. Caught between the desire for the past to be realized in the future and the future to be restored to the past, loyalist plays out a unique politics of time "in fold."

The etymological root of *yi* already contains a sematic ambiguity. *Yi* suggests losing something (*yishi* 遺失) while at the same time it means the leaving of something (*canyi* 殘遺); the former points to a total loss, the latter a leftover or a remnant. But *yi* also means giving or bequeathing (*yiliu* 遺留), implying leaving someone a thing or a gift. The three meanings of *yi* speak to the complex historical and affective syndrome that is loyalism: thrown into the abysmal condition of dynastic cataclysm, a political subject feels entrenched in a irrecoverable loss of his affiliations while cherishing all the more his identity as a survivor, a remnant of the loss; more engagingly, he is compelled to preserve the loss as a legacy, a gift, from the past into the future despite the historical fact that suggests otherwise.[11]

When one comes to postloyalism, something more complex arises. The prefix "post" as I am using here partakes of a postmodernist undertone. Literally, postloyalism refers to that which happens, in conceptual, affective, and political terms, *after* loyalism. But insofar as loyalism already implies temporal posteriority, and a resultant sense of mourning and nostalgia, the "post" of postloyalism doubles the temporal and psychological complexity inherent in loyalism. It could mean either that which is over with, or that which is subsequent to, loyalism. More intriguingly, in line with the postmodern subversion of the causal sequence of time, "post" loyalism could point to an anticipatory re-visioning of the past on behalf of the future, therefore implying a reopening of the pastness of the past. As such, the "post" of postloyalism refers to a desire for a timeline that comes prior, rather than posterior, to the extant historical closure: it implies the (renewed) beginning rather than the ending of a desired history.

Politically, loyalism engages itself with the polemics of (dynastic and cultural) legitimacy; it generates the force of its platform from that which has already been overthrown. That is to say, if loyalism is a thought or act predicated on anachronistic desire, to turn back the clock so as to return to the primal state of nationhood and selfhood, postloyalism is an exercise that "anachornizes" anachronism. It is aimed to alter or displace a timeline that is already irrecoverably altered or displaced. As such, postloyalism intensifies the precarious nature of loyalism as it seeks to upset—delegitimize— what has already been delegitimized. The result is the opening of Pandora's box, unleashing multiple demons with regard to the politics of recognition and loyalty. Postloyalism plays with the double bind underlying the art and politics of loyalty and betrayal.

Here, Derrida's notion of "hauntology" finds its complex Eastern parallel. With "hauntology," Derrida intended to draw attention to the haunting influence of the "specters of Marx" after the decline of Marxist thought in the West. He criticizes the ontological style of dialectics perpetuated by theorists and philosophers who evade discussion of the shadowy origins of these theories. He writes that "haunting is historical, to be sure, but it is not dated, it is never docilely given a date in the chain of presents, day after day, according to the instituted order of a calendar."[12] In other words, the specter not only comes from the past but also foretells its continuous, lingering presence in the future. Based on Derrida's argument, we can speak of the postloyalist's "refusal to comprehend the mandate." On the one hand, this act ultimately dislodges the loyalist memory from the neat order of time, while on the other hand it extends and exaggerates the postloyalist ego's *a priori* attachments to the loyalist consciousness. Time's continuum becomes disjointed and forms of remembering become unrestricted. The postloyalist's sense of loss and his inability to let go of his love and resentment are no longer bound by systematic thinking. These feelings rather become endlessly evolving burdens and quagmires—or ghostly seductions. In the meantime, they may also serve as an unlikely source of imagination or agency for a community to reorient—and invent—its political or cultural legacy.

To conclude this section, let me reiterate that I have no intention to promote postloyalism as the sole critical vehicle through which to engage the extant Sinophone paradigm based on postcolonialism. Nor do I intend to treat postloyalism as a normative tenet, prescribing the direction of Sinophone studies. I do, however, intend to point out that postcolonialism cannot fully address the mapping of the Sinitic world. It is too much grounded in the geopolitical dialectics of the modern times and cannot address the historical intricacies of Chinese/Sinitic world. By introducing postloyalism, I call attention to the legacy of "China," both its assets and liabilities, inherent in Sinophone Studies, which project a long, sprawling historical perspective onto both Chinese and Sinophone studies otherwise constrained by nation-state politics. Most important, postloyalism as a method is *both* critical *and* self-critical: it seeks to exorcise, or more strategically, live with, the ghosts that haunt our own enchantment with, repugnance for, and conjuration of "China."

II.

I have argued that postcolonialism and postloyalism constitute the dialectic of Sinophone discourse. In this section, I pursue the question of how to position the dialectic with regard to the broader mapping of (Chinese) national literature and world literature. In 1971, C. T. Hsia (1921–2013) coined the term "obsession with China" to describe the ambivalent attitude of modern Chinese literati toward the challenges of Chinese modernity. Hsia holds that modern Chinese literati are so obsessed by national crises that they turn their repugnance for the status quo into a masochistic mentality. These literati see any given social or political malaise as a sickness unique to China, and thus grapple with Chinese modernity only negatively, by denouncing it.[13] While the "obsession with China" gave rise to a high-strung anxiety about China's fate and a sense of moral and political urgency, as Hsia criticizes, it also generated a national parochialism to the exclusion of foreign stimuli —despite (or because of) the visible impact of the West on surface. To remedy this syndrome, Hsia calls for a cosmopolitanism characterized by interaction with Western literature.

Hsia published *A History of Modern Chinese Fiction* in 1961, which remains to date the most influential book of modern Chinese literary history in the English-speaking world. Although it has been criticized, particularly among leftist circles, for endorsing Cold War ideology, Western liberal humanism, and New Criticism, one cannot overlook its polemical power. On the front of national literature, one finds that almost half a century after Hsia's critique, "obsession with China" still casts a shadow over Chinese discourse, but the phenomenon has developed in unexpected ways. Whereas writers and readers on the mainland have turned their "obsession" into something more complex, from fanaticism to cynicism, from passion to nonchalance, their radical counterparts in Taiwan have come to love hating everything about China, such that, in an ironic way, they reinstate the classic symptoms of "obsession" with China.

On the front of world literature, hindsight may find Hsia "politically incorrect" because he derives his vision of modern Chinese literature from the "great tradition" of early modern European and American classics. He cares little about the representational politics of race and region, let alone the "clash of civilizations." But one must acknowledge the fact that in the heyday of nationalism, Hsia was most keen on the mutual implication between national literature and world literature. His re-vision of Chinese literature in a cosmopolitan perspective, however debatable, appears all the more urgent in our time.

In *What Is a World?* (2016), Pheng Cheah offers a critical reappraisal of world literature by rethinking postcolonial literature. He examines the cosmopolitan vocation of recent theories of world literature by scholars from David Damrosch to Pascale Casanova, pointing out their failure at inquiring about the meaning of "world." Despite their attempt to break away with the conventional, Eurocentric model, Cheah contends, these scholars derive their concept of world literature from the global imaginary which is predicated on the circulation of cultural capitals and the constellation of national literatures. Above all, they base their imagination of the world merely in geopolitical terms, thus confining their research to the domain of spatiality.[14]

Cheah articulates a normative theory of literature's world-making power as a temporal process. Drawing his theory from an array of philosophers form Heidegger to Derrida and Ardent, he suggests that world literature demonstrates its polemical vision not by presenting the world as such but by opening up the horizons of "worlding" in the flux of time. For Cheah, literature can serve "as an active power in the making of the worlds, that is, both a site of processes of worlding and as an agent that participates and intervenes in the processes."[15]

In response to both Hsia's critique of "obsession with China" and Cheah's critique of world literature, I propose that Sinophone postloyalism provides a critical interface between the Chinese nation and the world. On the one hand, I contend that beyond China, "China" serves as the equivocal but ubiquitous signifier that delimits the contact zones of Sinophone imaginaries. On the other, in light of the circulatory power of world literature, I contend that once the "obsession with China" takes on a Sinophone dimension, a revisionist cartography of Chinese language literature surfaces. Accordingly, beyond Sinophone "obsession with China," we consider Sinophone "intervention with China."

It is at this juncture that Cheah's emphasis on worlding as a "process of time" becomes especially illuminating. Cheah finds his sources of inspiration in postcolonial fiction from areas as far as the Caribbean, Southeast Asia, and Africa. He takes pains to stress that these works are noticeable because they introduce alternative temporalities, and yet he takes issue with these alternative temporalities in view of the fact that they tend to be "undermined by global and capitalist calculations and the heterotemporalities they stage can only be sustained by conjuring with the incalculable and inhuman gift of time as the original opening of the world."[16]

In the context of Sinophone and Chinese literatures, Cheah's (and by way extension, Shih's) postcolonial intervention can be enriched by postloyalism. I stress that postloyalist imagination, as the nexus for Sinophone "heterotemporalities," opens not merely to the future but also to the past. Through the postloyalist prism, one comes to realize that Sinophone inscription takes issue with questions ranging from linguistic (national) sovereignty to enunciative subjectivity, from dynastic allegiance to diasporic disavowal, thereby directing us to the alternative modernities—and alternative histories.

It will be recalled that in light of postloyalism, China can mean the "lost" or "abandoned" heritage, and an "incomplete" or "remaining" legacy; above all, it can also mean "bequeathed" or "imposed," indicating that which has been passed on to a recipient. Through the postloyalist vocation, Chinese national literature gives way to the worlding process of Sinophone literature.

To illustrate my arguement, I introduce four examples drawn from four postcolonial and postloyalist traditions in Taiwan, Hong Kong, (the Sinophone community of) Malaysia, and Mainland China. Lo Yi-chin 駱以軍 (b. 1967) is arguably one of the most important writers of contemporary Taiwan. In *Yuanfang* 遠方 (Faraway, 2003), Lo writes the story of a Taiwanese son rushing to the mainland to look after his father, who has fallen into coma as a result of his recent homecoming trip. The remote context is the great National Divide in 1949 that resulted in the exodus more than one million mainlanders to Taiwan. They were not allowed to take a homecoming trip till martial law was lifted in 1987. In the biographical novel, Lo and his "long lost brothers," from his father's previous pre-1949 marriage, tend to the needs of their father, only to experience the sensation of both intimacy and estrangement. In the end, he transports the large, dying body of his father back to Taiwan, a symbolic gesture of farewell to the homeland.

While *Faraway* may demonstrate what the PRC scholar Li Xiangping describes a "new loyalist complex" [17] shared by writers from the émigré family background, I argue that Lo's imaginary is more complex. Lo's magnum opus *Xixia lüguan* 西夏旅館 (Western Xia Hotel; 2008) parades endless bizarre encounters that occur within the insular space of Western Xia Hotel, from a necrophilic romance to a phantasmal manhunt, from burlesque intrigues to senseless carnivals. Behind the absurdity-turned-quotidian, Lo describes the diasporic experience of a generation of Chinese exiled to Taiwan; the hotel with no exit thus becomes a topos haunted by nostalgia and hysteria. More intriguingly, Lo refers his hotel name to the Western Xia Dynasty (1038–1227) of the eleventh century, a dynasty once thriving on a hybrid civilization of Han and non-Han origins. The Western Xia was ruined by the Mongols and as a result thrown into oblivion, its short-lived cultural splendor becoming an enigma.

Lo's novel thus invokes an unlikely parallel between a postmodern haunted hotel and a premodern barbarian regime. One leitmotif of the novel is the mingling and unmingling between the Han and the *Hu* (barbarian) cultures throughout the history. For our concern, such a fact speaks to the Sinophone geopolitics of exclusion through assimilation or vice versa. The game of "Chinese" versus "barbarian" was as precarious in the Western Xia era as it is now in contemporary Taiwan. The result is a bizarre national allegory of Taiwan trapped in multiple temporalities—or multiple states of exceptions. At a time when radical Taiwan nativists are seeking a state free from Chinese experience, Lo contemplates not only the position of second-generation mainlanders as adherents—postloyalitsts—to a lost cause but also the fate of Taiwan at large.

Thanks to, and in spite of, the colonial conditions over the past century, the literary configuration of Hong Kong is closely related to its amorphous status as a *city* short of national identity. As the "deadline" of 1997 loomed over the fin-de-siècle moment, Hong Kong writers were compelled to contemplate their colonial and national identities, and to reimage the political past and future of their city. Dung Kai-cheung 董啓章 (b. 1967) is one such a case. Since the mid-1990s, Dung has created a series of works about the mysterious V (for Victoria) City. Instead of a nationalist longing, his narrator observes the rise and the fall of the metropolis from the perspective of a post-apocalyptic future. He recollects its grandeur in the vein of ancient Chinese cities such as Chang'an 長安 (Xi'an), Bianliang 汴梁 (Kaifeng), and Hangzhou 杭州, pondering the illusory and ephemeral nature of *all* cities in world history. Fiction becomes the final locus where the city can sustain its mesmerizing power.

In novels such as *Menghualu* 夢華錄 (Dream of Splendor) and *Fanshenglu* 繁勝錄 (Account of Prosperity), Dung relates in the future perfect sense the splendor and prosperity of V City that will have been ruined by a certain point of time. The titles of the two novels are of special historical significance. *Dream of Splendor* brings to mind Meng Yuanlao's 孟元老 (?–?) *Dongjing menghualu* 東京夢華錄 (East capital: dream of splendor), arguably the most famous loyalist account of everyday life in classical Chinese literature. Meng was made a refugee from Bianliang, when the thriving capital of the Northern Song fell to the hands of Jurchen barbarians in 1126. In a quasi-encyclopedic manner, his book catalogues the old capital's commercial life, seasonal products, and festivals, as well as foods, customs, and traditions, all of which had evaporated like a dream. Likewise, *Account of Prosperity* is derived from *Xihulaoren fanshenglu* 西湖老人繁勝錄 (Account of prosperity by a senior gentleman on the west lake), a book by an anonymous writer recollecting the bygone life of Hangzhou, where the Song royal house built its southern capital after the fall of Bianliang. By copying the style and structure of the two Song accounts, Dung's novels about life in Hong Kong generate the sensation of a ghostly déjà vu, while the sense of pastness of Hong Kong is projected in the time after 2046, fifty years after her return to China.[18]

By nationalist logic, the people of Hong Kong should have welcomed the restoration of the Chinese regime to the island, following one hundred and fifty-six years of colonial rule. Dung's fiction reverses such an assumption. On the eve of the return, according to Dung, Hong Kong is experiencing not so much a wish fulfilment but rather a deeper sense of loss. Instead of the jubilant, postcolonial fervor, Dung entertains a postloyalist nostalgia—most ambiguously, for the lost time of British colonial rule. By "anticipating" Hong Kong to become a ruined city like Kaifeng and Hangzhong, he enacts a historical melancholia, one that speaks to the "eternal return" of a fallen city.

We have yet to pay more attention to Sinophone literature in Southeast Asia. More than thirty million people of Chinese descent live in the area, demonstrating a variety and vitality of Sinophone cultures that can hardly be homogenized by the conventional paradigm of "overseas Chinese heritage." Particularly in Malaysia, Sinophone language and writing have long served as a token of Chinese ethnic solidarity. However, ever since the 1940s, Malay(si)an Chinese-language authors have had to negotiate between a Chinese identification—fostered by language and the inevitably powerful influence of the Chinese literary tradition—and a sense of belonging to their local environment of Malay(si)a.

Our case in point is Ng Kim Chew 黃錦樹 (1967–). Ng grew up witnessing the ever-tightening control of the Malaysian government over the Chinese community. He went to study in Taiwan in 1986 and ended up settling down on the island. Nevertheless, Ng has engaged in a literary career as if he had never left Malaysia. He remains to date a most vehement critic of Chinese Malaysian ethnic culture. On the one hand, he wants to heighten Chinese Malaysians' vigilance regarding their diasporic position vis-à-vis governmental hegemony; on the other, he lashes out at their longing for transplanting anything Chinese to a new land, likening their effort to a necrophilic ritual. Oscillating between the "wandering Chinese" complex and its disavowal, Ng demonstrates the Sinophone "obsession with China" of the most perplexing kind.

Ng has sought to turn such an "obsession with China" into an interventional move in recent years, as best evinced by *Nanyang Renmin*

Gongheguo 南洋人民共和國 (The people's republic of the South China Sea; 2011–2013). The Republic of the South China Sea is said to be a socialist state that "could have been" founded by Chinese communists on the Malay Peninsula in the 1950s. It is a phantom polity that vanished no sooner than it was conceived by leftist activists. In a way, Ng takes up where the generation of Chinese Malayan communist writers such as Jing Zhimang left off in the 1960s, when the nation-building project of the Malayan People's Republic fell through. Nevertheless, as history has proven to be other than Jin's and his fellow communists' socialist dream, all Ng can do is to describe either the "pre-history" of the republic, when the leftists underwent all trials to realize their nation-building dream, or the "post-history," when the leftists were either coopted by the Malaysian government or simply died off as time passed.

Ng's fictional project brings home the *aporia* of the postloyalist discourse we have discussed so far. It speaks to both the wildest dream and the deepest melancholy of overseas Chinese in regard to their expatriate circumstances. More than sixty years after the establishment of the Malayan Federation (1957), Ng's characters are seen as wandering ghosts on their "homeland," the Malay Peninsula, which they refuse to call home. They are citizens of the phantom People's Republic of the South Pacific or the aborted Malayan People's Republic— either merely an imagined diasporic mimicry of the People's Republic of China. Nevertheless, at a time when the PRC regime is trying to shed its image as the instigator of leftist insurgencies in Southeast Asia, these characters are destined to be denied by their "spiritual" mother country too. They are postloyalists of the most abject kind because, besides a vague "Chinese dream," they find no political legacy to pledge allegiance to. As Ng's stories become more and more fantastic, his characters' sense of loss and gratuitousness becomes more and more poignant.

Finally, we come to the Sinophone dynamics *within* mainland China, and the case-in-point is Ge Fei's 格非 (b. 1964) trilogy *Wutuobang sanbuqu* 烏托邦三部曲 (Trilogy of utopia: part 1 *Renmian taohua* 人面

桃花 (A peach blossom romance; 2005); part 2, *Shanhe rumeng* 山河入夢 (Into the dreamscape of China; 2007); *Chunjin jiangnan* 春盡江南 (Spring ends in the south of the Yangtze River; 2011). Ge Fei won his fame in the 1980s with a series of experimentalist fiction which subverts Maoist discourse at linguistic, thematic, and conceptual levels, and he has been hailed as a leading avant-garde writer of the New Era. After a long hiatus in the aftermath of the Tian'anmen Incident, Ge Fei resurfaced in the new millennium. He impressed us with a series of novels that combines both his critical reflections on the legacy of modern Chinese revolutionism and his nostalgic invocation of classical Chinse utopian dreams, tantamount of which is the legend of *Taohua yuan* or Peach Blossom Spring.

The Trilogy of Utopia casts an overarching view of the ups and downs of twentieth-century China—from the Republican Revolution to the Communist Revolution; from urban planning to rural reconstruction; from "free love" to "literary creativity." All these projects or provocations have inspired generations Chinese to pursue the vision of national as well as personal liberation, only to turn into one nightmare after another. Ge Fei nevertheless packages his narrative with romantic allusions and lyrical references, thus bringing about a series of uncanny stylistic and thematic parallels. While he frames the first novel, about the aborted revolutionary and romantic attempts in early modern China, with the Tang poet Cui Hu's 崔護 famous poem of illusory love "Renmian taohua" 人面桃花 (A face as beautiful as the peach blossom), he refers the second novel, about the disastrous consequence of a public commune on an allegorical island Peach Blossom Island, to none other than Tao Qian's 陶潛 account of Peach Blossom Spring. In the third novel, Ge Fei ushers us into the decadent world of postsocialist China, where all Moaist promises turned into their own parodies. With a title suggesting the demise (*jin* 盡) of *Jiangnan* 江南, the classical poetic topos of abundance and elegance, he sets the elegiac tone for the finale of his trilogy.

At the center of the third novel is a modernist poet who has lost his capacity to compose anything new but killing time by reading Ouyang

Xiu's 歐陽修 *Xin wudaishi* 新五代史 or *New Five Dynasties History*,
a historical account of one of the most chaotic periods of medieval
China. When the dreamland proves to be a facade for the wasteland,
utopia betrays its dystopian nature. To the critics who may blame Ge
Fei for "depoliticizing" Chinese revolutionism, he may suggest that the
depoliticized *status quo* results more from the entropy of the originary,
lyrical momentum of revolution: Hasn't Marx suggested that revolution
cannot take its *poetry* from the past but only from the future?[19] Can the
nation-state rejuvenate the dream of Peach Blossom Spring?

Combining eschatological prophecy, political satire, and nostalgic
lyricism, Ge Fei's trilogy casts a bleak vision of modern Chinese history,
and as such it pits itself against the sublime, euphoric writings mastered
by political campaigners and wishful intellectuals. What concerns us more
is how a Sinophonic view can help tease out the discordant sounding of
Ge Fei, who otherwise would have been regarded as a mainstream Han
Chinese writer. Whereas a postcolonial approach may prove strenuous or
even irrelevant, a postloyalist approach may offer something debatable.
I argue that the way in which Ge Fei envisions the history of modern
Chinese revolution has gone beyond the boundary of national history;
instead, he thinks of it in light of the turbulence within the "world" of
premodern China as a Sinitic landscape, one constituted by Han and
non-Han dynasties and empires, aborted adventures and failed dreams.
Thus he is able to let his story shuttle back and forth amid multiple
temporal schemes. At its most disturbing, his revolutionary protagonists
come across either like "loyalists" obsessed with bygone utopian dreams,
or like "postloyalists" indulging in nihilist escapade. Either way, they
dramatize the history that has lost its authenticity. Coming to mind is
the trilogy's leitmotif of Peach Blossom Spring, one inhabited by the
decedents of those who sheltered themselves from the grand, monolithic
course of history, be it spectacular or barbarous: they "didn't know the
Han, let alone the Wei and the Jin."[20]

This essay represents an attempt to broaden the scope and methodology for studying modern Chinese language literature. It does not seek to overwrite the extant imaginary of "China," but rather seeks to tease out its complexity. Is it not a paradox that critics can subscribe to a "politics of marginality" and pontificate about a "clash of empires" and "global contextualization," all the while rigidly marginalizing forms of Chinese/ Sinophone modernity and historicity that do not emerge within some preconceived mainstream? If one of the most important lessons one can learn from modern Chinese literature and history is the tortuous nature of Chinese writers' attempt to grapple with a polymorphous reality, then this knowledge can be appreciated in full only through a criticism and literary history equally exempt from formulaic dogma and geopolitical blindness. Through examining two critical models of postcolonialism and postloyalism, I argue that one must genuinely believe that Chinese and Sinophone writers have been, and still are, capable of complex and creative thought, constructing and deconstructing the nation and the world in the literary domain and beyond. From "obsession with China" to Sinophone "intervention with China," any critical endeavor in the name of Chinese literature must be unafraid to look squarely at this historical reality—a reality of contested Sinophone modernities.

NOTES

1. Shu-mei Shih, *Visuality and Identity: Sinophone Articulations across the Pacific* (University of California Press, 2007).
2. Shu-mei Shih, "The Concept of the Sinophone," *PMLA* 126, 3(2011): 709–718; "Global Literature and the Technologies of Recognition," *PMLA* 119,1 (2004): 16–30; "Theory, Asia and the Sinophone," *Postcolonial Studies* 13.4 (2010): 465–484.
3. Shih, "The Concept of Sinophone," 709–718. See also Victor Mair, "What Is a Chinese 'Dialect/Topolect'? Reflections on Some Key Sino-English Linguistic Terms," *Sino-Plantonic Papers*, 29 (1991):2–52.
4. Tu Wei-Ming, *The Living Tree: The Changing Meaning of Being Chinese Today* (Stanford: Stanford University Press, 1994).
5. Rey Chow, *Writing Diaspora: Tactics of Intervention in Contemporary Cultural Studies* (Bloomington: Indiana University Press, 1993).
6. Ien Ang, *On Not Speaking Chinese: Living between Asia and the West* (London: Routledge, 2001).
7. Kim-chew Ng, "Minor Sinophone Literature: Diasporic Modernity's Incomplete Journey," in *Global Chinese Literature*, eds., Jing Tsu and David Der-wei Wang, (Leiden: Brill, 2010), 15–28.
8. Shih, The *Sinophone Reader*, 11.
9. Jing Tsu, *Sound and Script in Chinese Diaspora* (Cambridge, MA: Harvard University Press, 2010), 23.
10. Xie Zhengguang 謝正光, *Qingchu shiwen yu shiren jiaoyou kao* 清初詩文與士人交遊考 (A study of poetry and literati circles in the Early Qing; Nanjing: Nanjing University, 2001), 6. For the definition of a Ming-Qing loyalist, see Lynn Struve, "Ambivalence and Action: Some Frustrated Scholars of the K'ang-hsi Period," in *From Ming to Ch'ing: Conquest, Region, and Continuity in Seventeenth-century China* (New Haven: Yale University Press, 1979), 327.
11. See my discussion in *Houyimin xiezuo* 後遺民寫作 (Postloyalist writing; Taipei: Ryefield, 2007).
12. Jacques Derrida, *Specters of Marx: The State of the Debt, the Work of Mourning, and the New International*, trans. Peggy Kamuf (New York: Routledge, 1994), 4.

13. C. T. Hsia, "Obsession with China: The Moral Burden of Modern Chinese Literature," appendix 1 of *A History of Modern Chinese Fiction* (New Haven: Yale University, 1971), 533–554.

14. Pheng Cheah, *What Is A World: On Postcolonial Literature as World Literature* (Durham: Duke University Press, 2016), Introduction.

15. Cheah, 16.

16. Ibid.

17. Li Xiangping 黎湘萍, *Wenxue Taiwan: Taiwan zhishizhe de wenxue xushi yu lilun xiangxiang* 文學台灣：台灣知識者的文學敍事與理論想像 (Literary Taiwan: Taiwan intellectuals'literary discourse and theoretical imagination; Beijing: Renmin wenxue chubanshe, 2003), 292–293.

18. See my discussion in "Qiannian huaxu zhimeng: Dung Kai-chueng, Meng Yuanlao, Menghuati xushi" 千年華胥之夢：董啓章，孟元老，華胥體敍事 (A thousand-year-old dream of the splendid kingdom of Huaxu: Dung Kai-cheung, Meng Yuanlao and the Huaxu narrative style), in Chen Pingyuan 陳平原，David Wang 王德威，Guan Aihe 關愛和，eds, *Kaifeng: Dushi jiyi yu wenhua xiangxiang* 開封：都市記憶與文化想像 (Kaifeng: urban memory and cultural imaginary; Beijing: Peking University Press, 2013).

19. Karl Marx, *The Eighteenth Brumaire of Louis Bonaparte* (New York: International Publishers, 1994), 18.

20. 「乃不知有漢，無論魏晉。」Tao Qian 陶潛# "Taohuayuan ji" 桃花源記 (Peach blossom spring), *Tao Yuanming quanji* 陶淵明全集 (Complete works of Tao Yuanming), vol. 6 (Shanghai: Zhongyang shudian, 1935), 76.

CHAPTER 4

A TALE WITHOUT
SHAPE OR SHADOW

THE WEDDING, THE WAR, AND THE COURT CASE
OF THE MOUSE AND THE CAT IN
TRADITIONAL CHINESE POPULAR LITERATURE

Wilt L. Idema

The great modern author Lu Xun 魯迅 (1881–1936) was no cat lover. In his "Dogs, Cats, and Mice" (*Gou mao shu* 狗貓鼠), the opening piece of his childhood memories collectively published in 1928 as *Dawn Blossoms Plucked at Dusk* (*Chaohua xishi* 朝花夕拾), he traces his aversion to cats back to the moment as a youth in Shaoxing when he realized that the house cat had killed his pet mouse. He also fondly remembered the print of "The Wedding of the Mouse" (*Laoshu chengqin* 老鼠成親) that was pasted on the wall next to his bed. "Every single mouse in it, from the bridegroom and bride down to the best man, bridesmaids, guests, and attendants, had the high cheekbones and slender legs of scholars, although they wore red jackets and green trousers."[1] Later on in the same piece, he referred to the local custom of the observance of the wedding of the mouse that in Shaoxing was celebrated on the eve of the Lantern Festival, when children were put to bed early so as not to disturb the ceremony, noting "[o]n the eve of the Lantern Festival I was always reluctant to go to sleep as I waited for that procession to emerge from under my bed. But all I saw were the same few mice wearing no clothes and parading the floor as usual, not attending any wedding apparently."[2]

In his sympathy for mice and aversion to cats, Lu Xun was very much a modern author.[3] The novelist Lao She 老舍 (1899–1966) made cats the rulers of a dystopian realm in his *Cat City* (*Maocheng ji* 貓城記) of 1933. Earlier, the poet Zhu Xiang 朱湘 (1904–1933) had depicted the cat as a pompous old fart and a coward in his "Lessons of the Cat" (*Maogao* 貓誥) of 1925. And as early as 1907, Bao Youfu 包由斧 had depicted the cat as China's archenemy Russia in his *A New History of the Rats* (*Xinshu shi* 新鼠史). Premodern authors, however, saw it as the cat's natural task to catch mice and rats; they might lament the tendency of their cats to catch butterflies and songbirds but would complain at length about any real or perceived lack of enthusiasm of their cats in their duty of exterminating rodents. Even though the rat (or mouse), occupying the first position among the twelve birth-year animals, might be venerated for its amazing fertility, and even in some regions be credited with saving mankind from starvation by stealing grain seeds from heaven, rodents were throughout Chinese recorded history primarily seen as obnoxious thieves and destructive hooligans, vermin that deserved to be exorcised and annihilated at all costs. Cats, whether the barely domesticated native wild cats or the domestic cats that reached China from the West from the Han dynasty onward, were therefore first and foremost appreciated for their value in catching mice and rats. Special texts circulated on how to select good mousers, while other texts instructed new cat owners on how to make their newly acquired animal feel at home so it would not run off. Starting from the Song dynasty (960–1278), cats, especially ornamental breeds such as the lion cats, were also greatly appreciated as pets, and during the Qing dynasty no fewer than three authors independently of each other compiled encyclopedias of cat lore.

Mice and cats may live in close proximity to humans, often sharing their homes. Not surprisingly perhaps therefore, the animosity of rodents and felines has given rise from early on to a wide variety of stories all over Eurasia and Northern Africa that have been recorded in pictures and text. From the fifteenth century BCE onward, one finds visual materials on the war of the cat and mice (or rats) in ancient Egypt, and as the domestic cat fanned out over the Middle East and Europe that story accompanied it to be adapted again and again in paintings, ballads, and mock epics. In ancient South Asia, the most popular tale on the cat and mice would appear to have been the tale of the cat that caught its prey by assuming the manner of a pious cleric. As the introduction of the domestic cat into China is closely linked to the introduction of Buddhism, this story also found its way to China in a Buddhist guise. But by far the most popular story on the animosity between the mouse and the cat in late imperial China was the tale of the underworld court case of the mouse against the cat. This tale not only amused but also instructed, and its message must have been that crooks and bullies may present themselves as decent, law-abiding citizens but that eventually their crimes will be unmasked and justice will be served. In the most elaborate written version of the underworld court case of the mouse against the cat as *A Tale without Shape or Shadow* (*Wuying zhuan* 無影傳), this tale would also include as prequels accounts of how the cat disturbed the wedding of the mouse and of how the mice were defeated by the cats when they rose in revolt. Nowadays such texts that feature speaking animals may be appreciated as fairy tales in China, but until the advent of the twentieth century such fantastic texts could only survive in popular literature as elite poetics demanded truth from its authors. In popular literature these tales of the wedding, the war, and the court case of the mouse and cat locally are popular to this very day.

The Wedding of the Mouse

Partly because the wedding of the mouse (or rat) had been described by Lu Xun,[4] the custom has been studied extensively by Chinese scholars. It would appear that the custom, called in some places *laoshu jianü* 老鼠嫁女 (the mouse marries off his daughter) and in others *laoshu quqin* 老鼠娶親 (the mouse brings home a bride), was and still is observed widely all over China.[5] Children were put to bed early so as not to disturb the wedding, and in some places a little bit of food was placed outside mouse holes as a contribution to the festivities. The date, however, can vary from the final days of the last month of the lunar year to the earliest days of the second month. Stories about the custom tend to be quite simple in many places: if one disturbs the wedding, the mice will be a pest throughout the year. It is thus far better to allow the mice to leave the house *en masse*, whether to send off the bride or to fetch her.[6] The earliest references to the observance of the wedding of the mouse only date from the Qing dynasty, but it is a safe guess that this custom goes back to ancient exorcist rituals. Several early sources contain a detailed description of a rat exorcism that was to be conducted in the first month of the year. "During that month at dawn before the sun came out, the head of the household was to 'behead' or cut open a rat, suspend it in the middle of the house, and chant an exorcistic prayer."[7] In more civilized times, however, one left the dismemberment of the mice and rats to the cat. Lu Xun neglects to mention that the print in his room also will have included a large cat that is about to eat its fill.

The absence of a more developed story in many places is reflected in the design of the New Year's prints on the wedding of the mice. Their design is usually limited to that of a cat observing a wedding procession of mice. The musicians and carriers in the procession may be dressed in human garb, and the bride and groom may appear in human shape or as mice.[8] In one print, titled *Cat Mountain* (Limaoshan 貍貓山), in which they appear in human shape, they also appear as rats in clouds above their heads as they have been frightened out of their wits and back into their original shape by the appearance of not one but five cats. The print includes the following poem:

> The mouse demons are strong by nature
> And make their home in granary rooms.
> Having selected the bride-fetching day,
> The groom brings home the bride today.
> He only thinks he has to travel forward,
> When suddenly he sees the kings of cats:
> Each of them with its maw wide open—
> It scares the mice into a frantic flight![9]

In one more elaborate print, titled *The Bottomless Cave* (*Wudidong* 無底洞), which has been studied repeatedly by Mainland scholars, the designer of the print, for lack of a better story, has linked the theme of the wedding of the mouse with the theme of the amorous pursuit of the monk Xuanzang 玄奘 on his pilgrimage to the Western Paradise by the White Mouse Demon as told in chapters 80–83 of the *Journey to the West* (*Xiyou ji* 西遊記). This means the amorous mouse first has to satisfy the cat by feeding him with plenty of fish before she can set out in a grand procession to marry the monk (who, according to the long accompanying poem, will be saved in the nick of time by the intervention of bodhisattva Guanyin 觀音 in the shape of a vegetarian cat).[10]

A number of places know more elaborate stories in connection with the wedding of the mouse. The story that has attracted most scholarly attention is the story of the selection of the groom. When their mouse daughter has reached a suitable age for marriage, her mouse parents want to choose the most powerful person in the world as her husband, but when they approach the sun, it declines the marriage proposal because it is less powerful than the cloud that can obscure it; the cloud declines in favor of the wind; the wind declines in favor of a wall; and the wall declines in favor of a mouse, because it can undermine any wall by digging its holes. This story is encountered not only in China but also in Korea and Japan, and it is obviously derived from South Asia. The

Indian fable collection *Pantacantra* (second century–fifth century) for instance contains an elaborate version of this tale. In it, an ascetic saves a baby mouse from the claws of a raptor and turns it into a girl. When she reaches the age of twelve, he starts to search for a husband for her and ends up selecting a mouse as the groom for his ward by the same aforementioned process of elimination, whereupon the girl happily turns back into a mouse.[11] In versions of this story that are found in Sichuan and Hainan, the holy man is occasionally still encountered, now in the guise of an immortal, which would suggest that the tale entered China by different routes from the south.[12] Whereas most Chinese versions (as well as the versions encountered in Korea and Japan) omit the holy man, some Chinese versions, probably inspired by the New Year's prints featuring a cat, add the cat to the list of grooms: If the mouse is the most powerful being on earth and still fears the cat, the cat must be the perfect groom for the ambitious mouse parents. The cat will happily accept the proposal and eventually lovingly store the mouse bride in its stomach. Readers of the Grimm brothers know of course that nothing good can come of a shared household of cat and mouse.

The tale of the selection of the groom originally circulated in the oral circuit as folktale and folksong; nowadays it is one of the well-known Chinese fairy tales. It is, however, rare to encounter adaptations of this tale in the many genres of late-imperial popular literature (*suwenxue* 俗文學). One of the rare examples is a drum ballad (*guci* 鼓詞) that was recorded in the 1950s. In this text, titled *The Rat Marries a Cat* (*Haozi qu mao* 耗子娶貓), the rat parents of a grown-up son rejects the matchmaker's sensible proposals of marriage to a weasel, a hamster, and a rabbit, and insists on a female kitten as bride for their son. The widowed mother of the kitten is initially deeply offended by the proposal because she thinks the rats are taking advantage of her in her straitened circumstances, but the little dog that acts as matchmaker persuades her there may be some profit in the match for her. On the day set for the wedding, the cat and her daughter patiently wait for the arrival of the bride-fetching party:

The old cat upstairs was just dozing off
When she heard outside that loud noise.
There was no need for anyone to tell her:
She knew the mice came to seek their death!
    She opened her mouth and called Little Dottie,
Saying, "Dear Little Dottie, listen to mommy.
Get up, little darling, now please get up:
A fat pig is delivered right at our door."
    When the little cat had heard this sentence,
She stretched her nails and tested her waist.
Mother and daughter burst from the room
Like a pair of tigers from southern mountains.
    They jumped on this procession of rodents.
Bean hamster at first sight fled the battle ground.
The new father-in-law jumped from his able horse,
The bride-fetching guests jumped from the saddle.
    Now do you think that this new daughter-in-law was bashful?
She ran forward and swallowed them all with hide and hair!
Now wouldn't you think this new bride was a terror?
She ingested the groom while he was still alive!
    This is the piece of the mouse that married a cat,
Next comes the tale of the mouse lodging an accusation.[13]

But the final couplet gives away a secret: this drum ballad was not conceived as an independent story, but as a prequel to the tale of the court case of the mouse against the cat, and that was a tale, as we will find, that was repeatedly adapted in the popular literature of the final century of the Qing dynasty and beyond.

THE COURT CASE OF THE MOUSE AGAINST THE CAT

The story on the antagonistic relation between the mouse and the cat that was repeatedly adapted in various genres of popular literature of late-imperial times was the tale of the court case of the mouse against the cat. This story is most commonly known as "The Mouse Lodges an Accusation" (*Laoshu gaozhuang* 老鼠告狀) but also circulates under a variety of other more or less similar names. Whereas the wedding of the rat was a popular theme on New Year's prints (because the image was expected to scare mice and rats away from the house), the tale of the court case was only very rarely depicted. I actually know only one New Year's print on this topic, which provides a summary account of the tale in eight scenes.[14] The popularity of the theme of the court case of the mouse against the cat in the nineteenth century is suggested by the fact that two different versions were translated into English verse: one, from the Beijing area, by George Carter Stent as "The Rat and the Cat in Hades",[15] and one, from Yichang, by Archibald Little as *The Rat's Plaint*.[16] While we also have a version from the Guangdong area in which the animals face off before the famous Judge Bao 包公,[17] usually the action takes place in the underworld court of King Yama. King Yama has heard complaints of animals at least since the ninth and tenth centuries, but initially these animals all complained about the treatment they had received at the hands of their human owners, hunters and cooks.[18] The case of the mouse against the cat may have been the most popular case of animal against animal, but one can also find cases of other animals fighting each other in court, even of animals as small as the bedbug, the flea, and the louse. The highly formalized procedure of a court case, with its set roles for the various participants, is one of those social occasions that apparently has held a great appeal to authors of beast epics East and West. In the West, one can quote the *Ysengrimus* and the *Reinaerdt de Vos*; while in China, one can point to the *Rhapsody of the Swallow* (*Yanzi fu* 燕子賦), in which a swallow fights a sparrow in the court of the phoenix, the king of the birds.[19] Such parodic works have in the Chinese case also to be read against the background of an extensive legal literature and of the stories about the incorruptible judges of the past, such as Judge Bao, that in their different adaptations as ballads, plays, short stories, or novels often would include detailed descriptions of court sessions (which in traditional China were conducted in public). In the absence of a recognized legal profession, many daily-use encyclopedias

provided models for all kinds of legal documents, starting from formal
accusations of murder.

One of the earliest literary versions of the court case of the mouse
against the cat that has been preserved consists of a case file, all in prose.
It includes the statement of the mouse, accusing the cat of unmotivated
murder of the mouse; the counter statement of the cat, in which it lists the
damages caused by rodents and expounds on its own duty to exterminate
the race; and the final statement of King Yama, in which the mouse is
condemned to hell, the cat is sent back to earth to continue his work of
killing vermin, and the dog that had served as witness for the mouse is
given a beating. The text is concluded by a quatrain:

> The mouse is the most criminal creature in the world of men:
> How can it be allowed to breed without end in house and wall?
> It may be as cunning as can be and have a thousand dirty tricks—
> In the end it will fall into the sea, attacked by nail and claw.[20]

More common, however, are the adaptations in verse (or in verse
interspersed with prose) in the many genres of "prosimetric literature" (*shuochang wenxue* 說唱文學). The earliest known version of this
kind is the *Scroll of the Accusation of the Mouse against the Cat* (*Laoshu gao
limao juan* 老鼠告狸貓卷) that is found in a precious scroll manuscript
of 1803.[21] This text, which quite recently has been published by Shang
Lixin and Che Xilun, limits itself to a description of the court case. King
Yama is at first moved to pity by the statement of the mouse, which
presents itself as the innocent victim of unprovoked cruelty, and sternly
berates the cat once it has been summoned to his court, but eventually
also has to accept the arguments of the cat when it describes the material
and social damage caused by rodents. At a loss how to decide the case
he sends both mouse and cat back to earth:

> The rat lodged a most cunning accusation;
> The cat then countered by telling the truth.
> But King Yama, at a loss how to investigate,

Ordered both of them to live in harmony.[22]

In later versions King Yama does not show himself so befuddled and judges clearly in favor of the cat.

Until now I have been able to collect well over twenty different versions of the tale of the court case of the cat and the mouse. Some of them are woodblock editions of the nineteenth century. These texts are very rare nowadays, but a few of them are quite easily accessible these days as some major Japanese collections of traditional Chinese popular literature have been digitized in recent years.[23] While there also exist some lithographic editions from the first half of the twentieth century, a large number of texts is made up of works that circulated either in manuscript or orally in the final decades of the twentieth century and were collected in the context of the nationwide campaigns of the 1980s and beyond to document the heritage of oral and popular literature. Some of these texts can be found in the massive tomes that were printed at the national level, some are found in local collections, and some were put on the web by local aficionados. Contemporary performances in several genres can be viewed on YouTube and Baidu.

While a few of these versions are very short, most of these versions exhibit a tendency to expand the simple story of the confrontation in court. Summarizing, one may say that the authors and performers of these versions employ three strategies to expand their text. The first is simply to expand the length of the statements of both the mouse and the cat (or to allow them to respond to each other's statements). The second strategy is to add more episodes to the court case itself. And the third strategy is the addition of a prequel that will tell how the mouse ended up in the underworld court so that it could appeal to King Yama. When expanding its accusation of the cat, the mouse may for instance paint its own lifestyle as modest and harmless in order to stress the cruelty of the cat, which also may be developed at length. In order to counter the argument that it is a common thief, the same mouse may claim a long-established privilege to take its share of any harvest, and to explain its improbable privilege it may tell various stories of how it saved mankind from famine (by stealing seed grain from heaven), or how it once saved Emperor Taizong 唐太宗 of the Tang, either from a food shortage during his Korean campaign, or when his enemies had hatched a plan to kill him with a huge bomb hidden in a massive candle. The cat can of course expand its statement by providing more examples of the gluttony and destructiveness of the rodents (and the social consequences as students are scolded by their teachers for destroying books and girls are punished for messing up their silk). It may also narrate the story how it was brought to China from the Western Regions by Xuanzang to protect the sūtras against their destruction by rats,[24] or by Judge Bao from the Western Paradise to end the rampage in the Eastern Capital of the Five Rats.[25]

When the narrative of the court case of the mouse against the cat is expanded by the addition of new episodes the favorite moment is when an enraged King Yama, persuaded by the appeal of the mouse, orders the cat to be summoned. In some adaptations the cat arrives in court the moment it is summoned, but in other cases ghostly runners or Horseface and Oxhead are dispatched to arrest him. In some versions, Horseface and Oxhead are at a loss how to find the one cat that is accused among the millions of cats in the world. To solve their problem, they may appeal to the local god of the soil. Once they have found the cat, these ghostly runners may try to make some money on the side by extorting the cat, especially if the cat asks for a delay of a few days so it may engage the services of a litigation master to draw up its counter statement. On its way to the court of King Yama, the cat, like any visitor of the underworld, may be treated to a tour of hell to witness the tortures the sinners have to suffer there. One version ends with the addition of a scene of the revival of the cat upon its return from the underworld, to the great joy of its female owner who had believed it dead.[26] But we also have a version in which the mouse on arrival in the underworld finds that he has no money on him to pay the clerk for drafting his statement, so has to return and steal a gold pin in order to be able to appear to the court for justice.[27]

While many authors and performers apparently feel that the enmity between the mouse and the cat is commonly known and needs no elaboration, others expand their tale with a prequel in which the mouse is killed by the cat and arrives in the underworld. These prequels can be quite diverse in contents and length. One adaptation starts with a discussion between a rat and a mouse in which they both vaunt their unlimited power to create mischief, until they are surprised by a cat—while the rat makes its escape, the mouse is swallowed by the cat.[28] If the mice deplore their poor living conditions, they also may indulge in fond memories of the past when their ancestors like the White Mouse Demon and the Five Rats held great power. In the *Precious Scroll of the Mouse* (*Laoshu baojuan* 老鼠寶卷) from Western Gansu the mice not only nostalgically remember these days of transgressive glory, but also try to take revenge for their father which earlier had been killed—only to become the victims of the cat on this mission.[29] A Minnanese ballad of ca. 1920 starts with extended descriptions of the meetings of the mice and their negotiations with cats in order to achieve some kind of truce, apparently satirizing the many peace conferences of warlord-era China.[30] Most of these prequels are focused on the rodents and narrate the events as experienced by them; as such these are clearly intended to make the readers or the audience temporarily forget the common behavior of these rodents so they, like King Yama, can be filled with sympathy for these small creatures as the victims of the unwarranted violence of the cat(s). This applies especially to those adaptations that start with an account of the wedding of the mouse and start out in the happy atmosphere of the wedding preparations only to culminate in the cat's brutal murder of bride and groom.

In view of the apparently unprovoked violence of the cat(s), one will also feel an initial sympathy for the mice and rats when they want to free themselves from feline oppression by raising their troops and engaging their archenemy in battle. So there are adaptations in which the tale of the court case is preceded by a narrative of the war between the mice and the cats.

THE REVOLT OF THE MICE

In world literature the theme of the war between the mice and the cats can be traced back to ancient Egypt. From the fifteenth century BCE and later one encounters pictures of mice and cats at war (as massed armies and in individual combat), cats serving mice, and mice seeking peace with cats. These pictures have been interpreted as the illustration of an involved story of a war of the mice against the cats, the initial victory of the mice over the cats (and their enslavement of the cats?), and a final revolt of the cats resulting in their victory over mice and rats. Unfortunately, so far no text has been discovered that corresponds to such a story, and the interpretation of these ancient Egyptian materials is largely based on stories of the war between the mice and the cats that were popular all over the Middle East over the last one thousand years.[31] From earlier times we have a number of Aesopian fables that take a war between the mice and the weasels (or cats) for granted, and one papyrus has preserved fragments of a Hellenistic Greek mock epic on the war between the mice and the weasels (or cats) in the style of the *Batrachomuomachia* and probably of an earlier date.[32] From the twelfth century or later we have versions in Byzantine Greek,[33] Arabic,[34] Persian, and Turkish.[35] Especially the Persian narrative poem on the war between the cat and the mice, often ascribed to the fourteenth century satirist Obeyd Zakani has enjoyed a great popularity wherever Persian/Farsi was and is used, and it has repeatedly been translated into English starting from the beginning of the twentieth century.[36] According to the second-century Latin poet Phaedrus the war between the mice and the weasels (or cats) was painted on the walls of every inn, and in medieval Europe one encounters both frescoes and manuscript illustrations of the war between the mice and the cats.[37] From the sixteenth century onward we have prints of the war between rodents and felines,[38] as well as by mock epics in Latin (by Andrea Dazzi, 1473–1548), Italian (anonymous), and Polish (by Ignacy Krasicki, 1735–1801).

One cannot exclude the possibility that some of the Middle Eastern works on the war of the mice against the cats might have made their way to China, but it is difficult to trace such influence. The introduction of the domestic cat in China would appear to be closely linked to the introduction and spread of Buddhism (one legend, as we already saw, credits the introduction of the cat in China to no one less than Xuanzang).[39] With Buddhism, Indian tales about the cat made their way to China. While cat and mouse have a cameo appearance in the *Mahabharata*, the most popular cat and mouse tale in South Asia would appear to be the tale of the cat that captures its prey by feigning to have adopted an ascetic lifestyle, an adaptation of which is already included in the *Pancatantra*.[40] That story was also taken up in Indian visual art, for instance in the famous rock relief of the Descent of the Ganges, which shows a cat standing on one leg surrounded by mice.[41] A Buddhist version was recorded in China already in the seventh century, but it became especially popular in Tibet.[42] The motif also was known in medieval Persia: In Zakani's poem, the cat is accepted as their ruler by the mice when it pretends to be a pious Muslim.

In the Chinese world, the theme of the war between the cat and the mice made its appearance only at a relatively late date.[43] The only treatment of this work as an independent text that I am aware of is *The Revolt of the Mice* (*Shujing zuofan* 鼠精作反). I only know this drum ballad from a song book that must have been printed sometime in the 1920s.[44] Interestingly enough, this text introduces itself as a prequel to the tale of the court case of the mouse and the rat:

> The end of spring: the Third Month's weather
>   is so bright and sunny;
> The Cold Food Festival[45] is here and sacrificial money
>   turns to smoke.
> As royal sons and noblemen roam at Golden Horse Gate,
> Celestial fairies and jade maidens fly high on their swings.
>   But I am bored as I sit in this simple lane, since time began,
> And having nothing else to do I read some of these song-books.

I read the story of that rat that fights the cat in court:
How come it always is the second part and never the beginning?
   Because I have the leisure time, I want to move my brush:
The tiger's modeled on a cat—it's only a fantastic fiction.
I write about the night's first watch: the moon shines in the east
And in its hole a little mouse is crying without end.

In desperation over its situation this mouse, House-Dweller, decides to call all rodents to arms. In the second watch the cat becomes aware of the army that has been assembled against it and sharps it nails. In the third watch the mouse addresses a rousing speech to its troops:

In the third watch the moon is as bright as can be:
The commander-in-chief of the rats gives his orders.
   When speaking its words, it addresses its officers,
"You my generals, now listen to my instructions!
Today, marching forth, we will engage in battle,
On first arrival, I assure you, we will be victorious.
   That old cat, it is bound to lose this engagement:
As of today we will never suffer from destitution.
If today in this battle we do not achieve victory,
We, old and young, count as a blown-out candle!"
   The rats set out their battle lines most perfectly,
But when on the other side the cat meowed only once,
The mice at first sight lost all their determination
And madly squealing they ran from this disaster!

In the fourth watch the shattered mice are literally devoured by the cats that continue to eat till they burst.

In the fifth watch the sky turned clear and bright
That House-Dweller had died quite a bitter death!
Its soul didn't disperse and lodged an accusation:
The cat had to appear to state its side of the case.
   It visited all courts of hell in the world of darkness:
Virtue is rewarded, evil punished without any fail.
This book today is called "the chapter of the mice",

It is a bunch of nonsense that may cure the blind.

Many drum ballads are based on earlier "youth books" (or bannermen's tales; *zidishu* 子弟書), and the opening eight lines of *The Revolt of the Mice* very much reminds me of a typical opening poem of a youth book, but so far I have not been able to identify a nineteenth-century version of this tale.[46] In the twentieth century, however, *The Revolt of the Mice* would appear to have exerted some influence. In a folksong from Shandong on the court case of the mouse against the cat, which also uses the framework of the five watches of the night, the mouse makes up its mind to raise its troops in the first watch, and by the end of the second watch the impressive army he had mobilized has been utterly defeated by the cat.[47]

In the first half of the nineteenth century, however, we already encounter the war between the mice and the cat as an episode in *A Tale without Shape or Shadow* (*Wuying zhuan* 無影傳), to which we will have to turn now.[48]

A Tale without Shape or Shadow

A Tale without Shape or Shadow, written in an alternation of prose and verse, is the most detailed account of the antagonistic relation between the mouse and the cat, covering not only the court case in great detail, but also the disrupted wedding and the war. The text was popular in Northern China, especially Shanxi, and circulated in manuscript. Shang Lixin and Che Xilun list three copies of this text in their study of precious scrolls of Northern China under the heading of the *Precious Scroll of the Mouse*,[49] but there is no reason to classify this work as a precious scroll: while most of the action takes place in the underworld, the work has no religious content, it does neither include an opening poem inviting buddhas and bodhisattvas to come to earth in order to attend the reading of this text, nor a final poem in which these divinities are sent off. The earliest manuscripts listed by Shang Lixin date from the Tongzhi and Guangxu periods (1870, 1883).[50] In recent years some manuscript copies have also been offered for sale on the web, one of which dates from the Daoguang period (1841). To these mostly incomplete and inaccessible manuscripts should be added two journal publications. In 1989 the January issue of the journal *Minjian wenxue* 民間文學 published a version titled "The Mouse Accuses the Cat" (*Laoshu gao limao* 老鼠告狸猫), collected by Hao Wanhui 郝万慧.[51] This text does not identify itself as a version of *A Tale without Shape or Shadow*, but can be identified as such as it follows the broad outline of the story of *A Tale without Shape and Shadow* and at times reflects its text, but the version as published would appear to be based on an oral performance version.[52] The second publication is titled "A Tale without Shape or Shadow" (*Wuying zhuan*) and is found in the January issue of the *Shanxi minjian wenxue* 山西民間文學 of 1992. This is a version of the text as reproduced by a certain Zhong Shengyang 钟声 扬 on the basis of his memory of his father's manuscript copy of *A Tale without Shape or Shadow*, as we learn from his note at the end of the text:

> I love popular literature. The story of the rat marrying a bride (*A Tale without a Shadow*) is popular all over northern China. In my youth I often heard my father tell this story, and I almost knew it all by heart. In those days we at home had my father's hand-written copy. Later I carried that with me, but in the early days of the Cultural Revolution I inadvertently lost it, so now I have recorded it on the basis of my memory, so it may serve as a small literary memory of my late father to remember him by.[53]

My comments on *A Tale without Shape or Shadow* are based on the recently acquired manuscript copy in the Rare Books Collection of the Harvard-Yenching Library. It consists of thirteen folded sheets, and is written in an experienced and quite legible hand. Phonetic substitutions are rare (while these are quite common in some other manuscripts of *A Tale without Shape or Shadow* to judge from the sample scans that are posted on the Kongfuzi jiushu website). The cover page mentions the name of the copyist,[54] but the manuscript includes no precise date. Most likely the manuscript dates from the early decades of the twentieth century. At one point in time someone apparently made a repeated attempt to destroy this manuscript by tearing it in two, but fortunately the torn pages were kept together by their binding and luckily the full text is preserved. In translation the full text runs to twenty-two single-spaced pages A4.

A Tale without Shape or Shadow starts with a scene in which the mice parents discuss the upcoming marriage of their son. Because the road to the home of the bride-to-be is fraught with dangers, it is decided to hire an armed party to protect the bride-fetching procession and to proceed furtively at night. When the bride-fetching party is about to set out, the father mouse for added security provides Sharphead, the leader of the party, with a detailed route map. All to no avail: as the bride-fetching party carefully makes its way to the home of the bride, it is noticed by one of the cats, which immediately warns the brothers. Under the leadership of the eldest of them, the cats ambush the mice and devour all of them, except Sharphead, who manages to hide itself. Meanwhile, back at the home of the groom, the father of the groom busies itself with the master of ceremonies (the yellow weasel) about the preparations of the wedding banquet. As the bride-fetching party fails to return, the servants start to grumble. It is only on the next day that Sharphead returns to bring tidings of the murder of the groom and the death of its companions. On this news the wedding guests all disperse.

After a while the father of the groom pulls himself together and decides to take revenge. Following discussions with the hare, he mobilizes all his troops, and has a formal declaration of war delivered to the cats. The line-up of the multitudinous troops of the rodents is described with epic grandeur:

> Old Mouse went home and called out to his wife,
> "The way this is going today really pleases me well.
> I will set up my battle line on the Southern Slope,
> With the aid of Weed Hare and Hopping Rabbit."
>   All the youngsters of the tribe called to each other
> That they wanted to wage a battle against the cats.
> Fat Mouse volunteered to serve in the front line,

Slim Mouse insisted on serving as the vanguard.
  Sharphead transported grain without any slacking,
Weed Hare set up his camp and waited in ambush.
Hopping Rabbit inspected the ranks and patrolled,
Granarymover protected the grain and the fodder.
  These massed mouse soldiers were filled with rage;
Each and every mouse soldier showed his might.
The seven-*li* command banner hung in the army;
The eight great flags preceded the encampment.
  Nine layers of swords and spears arranged blades;
The ten seating towers dominated the battalions.
Once Old Mouse had transmitted all his orders,
He took his seat in the center, holding his flag.
  He set out a single-stroke long-snake battle line
Like the Dashing King when attacking Beijing.[55]
The troops, old and young, took up their posts;
Upon three canon shots, they then made camp.

But for all their number the rodents are quickly defeated by the cats
when the two armies meet in battle. The assembled cats decimate their
opponents, and the father of the groom too is killed. When his wife is
informed of his death, she collapses for grief, and when she revives she
praises her husband as a good provider in a lengthy lament, rejects the
possibility of remarriage as she is already too old, and commits suicide
to join her husband in the underworld.

Once the mother mouse has caught up with her husband, it informs her
it will accuse the cat in the underworld court of King Yama in an ultimate
attempt to achieve revenge. It has a statement of accusation drafted
by the responsible clerk, in which the cats are accused of unmotivated
murder.[56] When the cat has been summoned to the underworld it has
no cash on him to pay the clerk to draft his counter statement, but a
Student Hu 胡生 volunteers to draft his statement for free. When the cat
wants to decline this offer, Student Hu insists on doing so, and reveals
himself to be no one else but the Hu Di 胡迪 who, in a fifteenth-century
tale, had accused the highest worldly and otherworldly authorities of

miscarriage of justice in the case of Qin Gui 秦檜 (1090–1155) and Yue
Fei 岳飛 (1103–1142).[57] But when the cat submits its statement, the clerk
on duty that day is the Lunar Lodge Rat, who, intending to protect his
relative the mouse, refuses to accept his documents because the cat is
unable to pay the customary fee. Fortunately the cat finds a protector in
the Lunar Lodge Tiger. King Yama is eventually convinced by the plea
of the cat, so he rejects the accusation of the mouse and finds in favor
of the cat. The cat is ordered to still make its rounds to catch rodents,
and the old mouse thinks to himself:

> "Only in death I realize now that I have been wrong:
> I never should have made this accusation of the cat."

[King Yama] also commented,

> If you had fetched no bride, you had not suffered any harm,
> You made the wrong decision, so you have no one to blame.
> Lodging this accusation in the underworld you earned to die:
> A mouse that accuses a cat for murder makes no sense at all.

As the aforementioned summary shows, *A Tale without Shape or Shadow*
is a highly original treatment of the themes of the wedding, the war, and
the court case of the mouse and the cat. The anonymous author (and
subsequent copyists of the text) has come up with highly original accounts
of the wedding and the war, greatly enlarging the cast of characters.
In addition, the description of the court case contains highly original
touches. Not only do both the mouse and the cat have their relatives in
court who try to help them in the lunar lodges of the rat and the tiger, but
we also only in this text encounter Student Hu, who insists on helping
out the cat by writing its counter statement. The appearance of Student
Hu in this text is rather surprising because otherwise the text has made
an effort to limit the cast to animals and deities. The animals have names
and functions that correspond to their animal characteristics, and in a
world of constant rebirth the animals are as common in the underworld
as humans. The setting too is a world of animals: while the mice live in

their holes, the cats enjoy the warmth of the *kang* 炕, the heated brick platform that is such a typical feature of traditional northern Chinese architecture. On their way to the home of the intended bride, the bride fetching party passes by places such as Shithouse Pass, Throughton, Gate Lintel Mountain, Tableton, Mt. Granary, Fatmutton Fort, Wokstand Cliff, etc. Student Hu, however, is not any anonymous human being but a very specific, ostensibly historical character. As a well-known champion of justice, he declares that the injustice suffered by the cat is equal to the injustice suffered by Yue Fei! Perhaps we should read this only as irony, but then it may call for a political reading of some kind of *A Tale without Shape or Shadow*. Perhaps the comparison of the army of the mice to the troops of the Dashing King Li Zicheng on his way to Beijing is less accidental that it might seem as first sight. But if the rats stand for the rebels that wrecked the Ming dynasty, one wonders whether the cat might stand for the Manchus who were brought in by Wu Sangui to defeat them, and had been forced to stay afterwards to maintain law and order. But then the reference to the Dashing King also may only be a local memory of his army that swept through Shanxi. Many texts on the war between rodents and felines from outside China too have been interpreted as political allegories at some time, but the object of satire has almost always turned out on closer inspection to be quite elusive and difficult to ascertain.[58]

Even so, the most original aspect of the court case in the Harvard-Yenching Library manuscript of *A Tale without Shape or Shadow* may well be its treatment of the cat. In its long statement before King Yama the cat enumerates of course all the crimes of the rodents, but also includes a highly original account of the Five Rats upsetting the Eastern Capital, not as seen (as is usual) through the eyes of Judge Bao but as seen through the eyes of the cat. In the first words of its oral statement the cat immediately introduces itself as pious monk from the Western Regions:

> Wildcat stepped forward and then hurried to kowtow,
> Then cried out, "Your Lordship, please kindly listen!

I the cat while alive didn't have any inherited fields;
I am not a locally established citizen of these parts.
   My home is the Thunderclap Monastery in the West,
Where I nourished my nature by reciting the sūtras.
I have never paid any attention to wine or to sex
And never concerned myself with money or honor."

The cat follows this up by expanding on the havoc created by the Five Rats inside and outside Kaifeng, and then evokes its own blessed and peaceful existence in the Western Paradise where it devoted its life to religious exercises. When Heavenly Master Zhang (Zhang Tianshi 張天師) and Judge Bao came to the Western Paradise to borrow a cat from the Buddha, they were allowed to take it with them down to earth, but only the condition that they would return it as soon as it had accomplished its mission of exterminating the Five Rats. But because the cat had slackened for one moment, it had allowed one rat to escape and so had been ordered to wait outside the rat's hole until it would have finished the job. Because the escaped rat turned out to be pregnant, the rodents could again proliferate, resulting in the permanent banishment of the cat to earth. Actually our cat is even more to be pitied because Heavenly Master Zhang and Judge Bao first had received another cat from the Buddha, which they had allowed to escape because they doubted its power, after which it had become the ancestor of all tigers. Eagerly longing for its blissful existence in heaven, our cat now finds itself, as a victim of its skills, condemned for all eternity to catch mice and rats, and it ends its catalogue of the crimes of the rodents with the following description of its tragic fate:

They steal the grain and beans that's stored in granaries,
And so abuse authorities, a crime that is not minor.
Their many crimes are way too many to be counted—
And then they blocked the chance that I go home.
   They wrecked my magic power that I can't complete,
And broke my Great Completion that I can't achieve.
I had conceived this deep-seated hatred for their kind:
How could I allow them to bring home a bride again?

I gaze upon the Western Paradise that I will never see,
I long for that old road back home that I can't travel.
These things can all be documented and be proven,
That false and wrongful accusation is one blatant lie.

But after the cat has stressed its foreign origin, the mouse uses that argument against the cat in its reaction to the cat's counterstatement:

The cat is not a local citizen who owns some land,
But is a person who arrived from Western Regions.
He is here in the Eastern Capital a foreign resident,
Because we let him as a stranger live amongst us.
    I never had an issue with him over any kind of business,
So I don't know what is the cause of his deep hatred.
But when I see him, I make sure to cede the road—
In contrast it is he who wants to seek my traces.
    But even though we tolerate his hatred and his grudge,
He is too cruel in the way in which he will abuse us.
Whenever any of my rodent sons or brothers will go out,
I urge them many, many times to flee his presence.
    Because if once by chance you fail to flee from him,
He'll swallow you all equally, both young and old alike.
The road to fire and water[59] so is constantly obstructed,
As we at home all close the door, afraid to go outside.

This is the only adaptation of the court case that I have seen in which such stress is placed on the foreign origin as the cat, and in which its foreign origin is used against the cat in a court of law. This reminds one of course of the two accounts of court case of the swallow against the sparrow, both titled *Rhapsody of the Swallow*, that were discovered among the Dunhuang manuscripts.[60] In those texts the bullying sparrow that has occupied the nest of the swallow during its winter absence tries to strengthen its own position in court by stressing the status of the swallow as an immigrant and therefore apparently less entitled to the protection of the law. Like the Phoenix in the *Rhapsody of the Swallow*, King Yama is not taken in by this arguments and judges against the mouse, in this case especially because of its unlimited proliferation:

> Now tell that when Lord Yama had heard Old Mouse tell his story, he slapped the table in his rage, and said, "When after in the Song Dynasty the Five Rats had created havoc and you had been the only one to survive, you should have fled faraway to hide yourself. You should not have stayed in the Eastern Capital and made it your home. You should have adhered to the common law in order to compensate for your former sins. How could you dare bring home a bride and sire sons in order to harm the common people? No one is more detestable!"

In the 1883 manuscript of *A Tale without Shape or Shadow*, which is incomplete, we unfortunately never reach the cat's entry into the underworld. The text printed in the January 1992 issue of *Shanxi minjian wenxue* still mentions Student Hu as the person who drafts the counter statement of the cat, but does not disclose his identity, and in its description of the battle of the mice against the cats it does not compare the mice to the army of Li Zicheng. The mouse does stress the foreign origin of the cat, but does so in his own opening statement, not in reaction to the lengthy statement of the cat, in which the cat stresses its status as "an invited guest". In the version printed in 1989 in *Minjian wenxue* the focus during the confrontation in court shifts to the mouse. No Student Hu is mentioned in this version. While the scene of the battle between the rodents and felines is very much developed (the mice have the support of a fierce marten, but the cats are saved from defeat in the nick of time by the intervention of a chained-up guard dog that breaks free), the description does not include any historical reference. In the court scene King Yama is clearly on the side of the mouse, so the cat thinks it wiser to keep silent, but the mouse ruins its own case by chewing a hole in the cloth that covers the table of the judge. Once King Yama notices that the mouse can't even stop itself from damaging his belongings, he immediately turns around and judges against the mouse and in favor of the cat. If the author of the version of *A Tale without Shape or Shadow* as found in the Harvard-Yenching Library copy did indeed attempt to insert a political message in the text, such message was lacking in other versions, or ignored in the process of transmission.

CONCLUSION

The enmity between the mouse and the cat was noticed and used in all settled agricultural societies. The enmity between the mouse and the cat also became a popular theme in the visual and literary arts, first in the Near East, and eventually all over Eurasia, including the British Isles and Japan. But while the theme of the war between rodents and felines may have followed the migrations of the domestic cat out of Egypt, the literary treatments would appear to show little sign of mutual influence. Despite the popularity of some of these works, such as the Persian poem ascribed to Obeyd Zakani, none of them would appear to have had any impact beyond its own linguistic borders. Whereas in South Asia the tale of the cat that feigned to be an ascetic in order to catch its prey would appear to have become the most popular tale on the enmity of the cat and the mouse, in late-imperial China (where the tale of the war between cats and rodents also was known) by far the most popular tale on the enmity of the mouse and the cat focused on their underworld court case before King Yama.

The most elaborate adaptation of the tale of the court case is found in the anonymous *A Tale without Shape or Shadow*, which combines its account of the court case with accounts of the disturbed wedding of the mouse and the war between rodents and felines. If we were better informed about the date of composition of *A Tale without a Shape or Shadow* one might perhaps entertain the thought that it was the source for the three stories as they circulate independently. Under the present conditions I very much doubt whether that is the case. In the universe of traditional popular literature texts rarely carry dates, and if they carry dates, these tend to be the dates of copying, not of composition. Many accounts of the court case limit themselves to an account of the court case and try to develop their tale by adding episodes to the court case.

When adaptations of the court case include a prequel, it may be the story of the disturbed wedding, only rarely is an account of the war, and can also be a quite different story. Personally I would prefer to see *A Tale without Shape or Shadow* as an integrated version of three stories that originally circulated independently of each other.

Despite its originality and obvious literary quality *A Tale without Shape or Shadow* was of course doomed to a highly marginal existence in traditional China. Whereas in other cultures animal tales and beast epics could achieve a major position in their literary histories, there was little chance of that in China. In the eyes of the literati, who were wedded to a conception of literature that demanded truth of fact and emotion, it could only be "a tale without shape or shadow", that is to say, an unfounded tale without any value, as it advertised its own blatant fictionality by featuring a cast of speaking animals.[61] In Chinese animal fables by elite authors of the imperial period animals may be imbued with moral feelings and failings and exemplify virtues and vices, but they rarely if ever speak and engage in a dialogue. And if the tale of the wedding of the mouse and the story of the court case of the mouse against the cat have achieved any status at all in modern times, it is in the world of contemporary Chinese children's literature (including children's drama) once it abandoned *The Twenty-Four Exemplars of Filial Piety* (Ershisi xiao 二十四孝) in favor of fables and fairy tales, both foreign and domestic.[62]

NOTES

1. Lu Hsun, *Dawn Blossoms Plucked at Dusk*, trans. by Yang Hsien-yi and Gladys Yang (Peking: Foreign Languages Press, 1976), 12. The term *laoshu* (and its synonym *haozi* 耗子) refers both to mice and rats (and a host of other noxious rodents). I will use both "mouse/mice" and "rat(s)" in my translation, depending on context.
2. Ibid.
3. For a general discussion of Lu Xun's treatment of animals see Clint Capehart, "The Animal Kingdom in the Legacy of Modern Chinese Literature: Lu Xun's Writings on Animals and Bio-Politics in the Republican Era," *Frontiers of Literary Studies in China* 10/3 (2016): 430–460.
4. For a detailed discussion of Lu Xun's (and his brother Zhou Zuoren's 周作人 [1885–1966]) comments on the wedding of the mouse, see Ma Changyi 马昌仪, *Shu yao tian kai* 鼠咬天开 (Beijing: Shehui kexue wenxian chubanshe, 1998), 301–318.
5. The term *laoshu chengqin* as used by Lu Xun would appear to be much less common.
6. Ma Changyi, "Zhongguo shuhun gushi leixing yanjiu" 中国鼠婚故事类型研究, *Minsu yanjiu* 43 (no. 3, 1997), 60–71; Ma Changyi, "Wudi shuhun suxin yu yishu" 吴地鼠婚俗信与艺术, *Minjian wenxue luntan* 4 (1997), 8–15; Ma Changyi, *Shu yao tian kai*, 1998. The wedding of the mouse has inspired many forms of folk art, such as paper cuts. In some villages, local inhabitants dressed as mice nowadays stage elaborate wedding processions on the festival day.
7. Roel Sterckx, *The Animal and the Daemon in Early China* (Albany: State University of New York Press, 2002), 65.
8. Zhang Daoyi 张道一, *Laoshu jianü: shu minsu ji qi xiangguan yishu* 老鼠嫁女鼠民俗及其相关艺术 (Jinan: Shandong meishu chubanshe, 2009), 80–91, reproduces a selection of New Year's prints dedicated to the wedding of the mouse. John Lust, *Chinese Popular Prints* (Leiden: E.J. Brill, 1996), 227–228 provides a superficial characterization of this type of prints.
9. Maria Rudova, *Chinese Popular Prints* (Leningrad: Aurora Art Publishers, 1989), Pl. 102.
10. Gao Jiyan 高紀言, ed. *Suzhou Taohuawu muban nianhua* 蘇州桃花塢木版年畫/ *Taohuawu Woodblock New Year Prints, Suzhou* (Nanjing: Jiangsu

guji chubanshe/Hong Kong: Colorprint Publishing House, 1991), 72, Pl. 44; Zhang Daoyi, *Laoshu jianü: shu minsu ji qi xiangguan yishu* 老鼠嫁女鼠民俗及其相关艺术 (Jinan: Shandong meishu chubanshe, 2009), 92–94.

11. In folktale studies stories of this type are classified as AT 2031. For a translation of the *Pantacantra* version see Visnu Sarma, *The Pantacantra*, trans. by Chandra Rajan (London: Penguin books, 1993), 325–331. For the popularity of this story in China, see Ding Naitong 丁乃通, *Zhongguo minjian gushi leixing suoyin* 中国民间故事类型索引 (Wuhan: Huazhong shifan daxue chubanshe, 2008), 356–357; Jin Ronghua 金榮華, *Minjian gushi leixing suoyin* 民間故事類型索引, 3 vols. (Taipei: Zhongguo kouchuan wenxue xuehui, 2007), vol. 2, 649–651; Gu Xijia 顾希佳, *Zhongguo gudai minjian gushi leixing* 中国古代民间故事类型 (Hangzhou: Zhejiang daxue chubanshe, 2014), 263. For studies of the spread of this story-type in East Asia see Ji Xianlin 季羡林, "'Maoming' yuyan de yanbian" 猫名寓言的演变, in Ji Xianlin, *Bijiao wenxue yu minjian wenxue* 比較文學與民間文學 (Beijing: Beijing daxue chubanshe, 1991), 72–77; Nomura Junichi 野村纯一, "'Laoshu jianü' de dongjian beishang—Ri-Zhong minjian gushi bijiao yanjiu" 老鼠嫁女的东渐北上—日中民间故事比较研究, in Jia Huixuan 贾蕙萱 and Shen Ren'an 沈仁安, eds. *Zhong-Ri minsu de yitong he jiaoliu* 中日民俗的异同和交流 (Beijing: Beijing daxue chubanshe, 1993), 33–48; Zhong Jingwen, "Zhong-Ri minjian gushi bijiao fanlun" 中日民间故事比较泛论, in Jia Huixuan 贾蕙萱 and Shen Ren'an 沈仁安, eds. *Zhong-Ri minsu de yitong he jiaoliu* 中日民俗的异同和交流 (Beijing: Beijing daxue chubanshe, 1993), 5–32. Whereas the *Pancatantra* enjoyed a great popularity in Southeast Asia and was adapted into Persian by the seventh century (and from there spread throughout the Near East and eventually reached Western Europe), the collection was never translated into Chinese in premodern times. As a result, only a few individual tales found their way to China. See also Liu Shouhua 刘守华, "Yindu *Wujuanshu* he Zhongguo minjian gushi" 印度五卷书和中国民间故事, *Waiguo wenxue yanjiu* no. 2 (1983), 63–69.

12. Dong Xiaoping 董晓萍, "Laoshuxing gushi de kuawenhua yanjiu—jianlun Zhong Jingwen yu Ji Xianlin xiansheng guanyu tongxing gushi de yanjiu fangfa" 老鼠型故事的跨文化研究—兼论钟敬文与季羡林先生关于同型故事的研究方法, *Guangxi shifan daxue xuebao* 48 no. 6 (Dec. 2012), 1–10; Jiang Yuxiang 江玉祥, "'Laoshu jianü': cong Yindu dao Zhongguo—yan xinan sichouzhilu jinxingde wenhua jiaoliu shili

zhi yi" 老鼠嫁女从印度到中国—沿丝绸之路进行的文化交流实例之一, *Sichuan wenwu* 6 (2006), 61–64; Li Pengyan 李鹏燕 and Zun Shikai 遵世凯, "Qianlun 'Laoshu jianü' gushi zai Zhongguo de liubian" 浅论老鼠嫁女故事在中国的流变, *Jiaozuo shifan gaodeng zhuanke xuexiao xuebao* 30 no. 2 (Jun. 2014), 28–30; Zhu Jingwei 朱婧薇, "Zhongguo shuhun gushi qingjie leixing de xingtai jiegou fenxi" 中国鼠婚故事情节类型的形态结构分析, *Yalujiang* no. 3 (2016), 69–70.

13. Chen Xin 陈新, *Zhongguo chuantong guci jinghui* 中国传统鼓词精汇. 2 vols. (Beijing: Huayi chubanshe, 2004), 1120–1122. See also Li Yu 李豫, Li Xuemei 李雪梅, Sun Yingfang 孙英芳, and Li Wei 李巍, comp. *Zhongguo guci zongmu* 中国鼓词总目 (Taiyuan: Shanxi guji chubanshe, 2006), 126, which suggests that the text was recorded in Shenyang in the 1950s.

14. A rare New Year's print devoted to the court case of the cat against the mouse, produced by in 1920 by the Qingchuncheng huadian 慶順成畫店 in Wuqiang, depicts the court case in eight scenes: 1) the mice destroy books and food; 2) the mouse is killed by the cat; 3) the soul of the mouse request someone to write its accusation statement; 4) the mouse presents its accusation to King Yama; 5) King Yama dispatches runners to summon the soul of the cat; 6) the cat details the crimes of the mouse that is thereupon thrown into hell; 7) the cat returns to the world of light; 8) and pursues its duty of killing mice and rats even more vigorously. See Zhang Daoyi, *Laoshu jianü*, 63–65 for a reproduction and transcription of the texts inscribed on the picture, based on the reproduction in Zhang Chunfeng 張春峰, ed. *Hebei Wuqiang nianhua* 河北武強年畫 (Shijiazhuang: Hebei renmin chubanshe, 1996).

15. George Carter Stent, *Entombed Alive and Other Song, Ballads, Etc., From the Chinese* (London: William H. Allen and Co., 1878), 115–135. Stent's rendition is based on *Haozi gao mao* 耗子告貓 (*Xinkan Laoshu hanyuan Yanwang shen mao duan* 新刊老鼠含冤閻王審貓段/*Xinkan Haozi gao limao quanduan lianhualao ci* 新刊耗子告狸貓全段蓮花落詞). Beijing: Baowentang, 19th century.

16. Archibald Little, *The Rat's Plaint* (Tokyo: Hasegawa, 1891).

17. *Xinben Laoshu gaozhuang* 新本老鼠告狀, 19th century, woodblock edition. Tokyo University Library. "Laoshu tong mao gaozhuang" 老鼠同貓告狀, from Maoming city; performed by Li Shichang 黎世昌; recorded by Yang Qiangwen 杨强文 (*Zhongguo geyao jicheng Guangdong juan* 中国歌谣集成广东卷. Beijing: Zhongguo zhongxin, 2007), 667–678.

18. Stephen F. Teiser, *The Scripture on the Ten Kings and the Making of Purgatory in Medieval Chinese Buddhism* (Honolulu: University of Hawai'i Press, 1994), 175, pl. 8b.

19. Wilt L. Idema, "Animals in Court," *Études chinoises* 34 no. 2 (2015), 251–258.

20. *Xinbian Maoshu gaozhuang* 新編貓鼠相告 (Shiwentang 世文堂, 19th century). This text is reproduced in Wu Shouli 吳守禮, ed. *Qing Daoguang Xianfeng Minnan gezaice xuanzhu* 清道光咸豐閩南歌仔冊選注 (Taipei: Wu Zhaowan, 2006), 90–94, who provides a typeset edition on pp. 123–126. For a full English translation see Wilt L. Idema, "Animals in Court," 265–270.

21. Shang Lixin 尚丽新 and Che Xilun 车锡伦, *Beifang minjian baojuan yanjiu* 北方民间宝卷研究 (Beijing: Shangwu yinshuguan, 2015), 542. But on p. 72 of the same publication the manuscript is dated to 1788. Shang and Che classify the text as a "small scroll" (xiaozhuan 小傳), a short and often humorous intermezzo.

22. "Laoshu gao limao juan" 老鼠告狸貓卷, attached to an 1803 copy of *Ciyun baojuan* 慈雲寶卷. Modern edition in Shang Lixin and Che Xilun, *Beifang minjian baojuan yanjiu*, 542–543.

23. The following title can be added to those already mentioned: *Gaomao Haozi shenyuan* 告貓耗子伸冤 (Beijing: Ronghuantang 榮煥堂, 1882; reproduced in *Suwenxue congkan* 俗文學叢刊 vol. 98, 89–108). For translated extracts from this version see Wilt L. Idema, "Animals in Court," 272–277.

24. Isobe Akira 磯部彰, "Daitō Sanzō seiten kyokyō densetsu no keisei—Tō, Godai in okeru Genshō sanzō no shinkakuka wo megutte" 大唐三臧西天取經傳說の形成―唐五代における玄奘三臧の神格化をめぐって, in *Sōdai no shakai to bunka* 宋代の社會と文化, Tokyo: Kyuko shoin, 1983, 197–236.

25. The tale of the Five Rats creating havoc in the Eastern Capital first circulated in prosimetric format as a ballad-story (cihua 詞話), but starting from the late sixteenth century it was repeatedly rewritten as a novel, a chapter in a novel, a short story, and verse narratives. See André Lévy, "Le motif d'Amphitryon en Chine: "Les cinq rats jouent de mauvais tours à la capitale orientale," in his *Études sur le conte et le roman chinois* (Paris: École Française d'Extrême Orient, 1971), 115–146; Pan Jianguo 潘建國, "Hainei guben Mingkan *Xinke quanxiang wushu nao Dongjing* xiaoshuo kao" 海內孤本明刊新刻全像五鼠鬧東京小說考, *Wenxue yichan* no. 5 (2008), 90–102; Pan Jianguo, "Ming shuochang cihua *Xinkan Songchao*

gushi wushu danao Dongjing ji kao—zailun "Wushu nao Dongjing" zhi gushi liubian ji qi xueshu yiyi" 明说唱词话新刊宋朝故事五鼠大闹东京记考—再论五鼠闹东京之故事流变及其学术意义, *Wenxue yichan* 2 (2015), 116–127; Yamamoto Noriko 山本範子, "*Goso dō Tōkei* seiritsu kō" 五鼠鬧東京成立考, *Hyōfū* 飆風 37 (2003), 88–106. For translations see for instance Anonymous, "The Song of the Five Rats Wreaking Havoc in the Song Palace," trans. by. Wilt L. Idema, *Taiwan Literature: English Translation Series* 31–32 (2013b), 117–140; George Hayden, trans., "The Jade-Faced Cat," in Y.W. Ma and Joseph S.M. Lau, eds., *Traditional Chinese Stories: Themes and Variations* (New York: Columbia University Press, 1978), 456–462.

26. This is the version translated by Stent.

27. Idema, "Animals in Court," 284–286.

28. Ibid. 278–279, "Laoshu gaozhuang" 老鼠告狀, in Wei Ren 韦人, Wei Minghua 韦明铧, comp., *Yangzhou qingqu* 扬州清曲, Shanghai: Shanghai wenyi chubanshe, 1985, 110–113.

29. *Laoshu baojuan* 老鼠寶卷. In Fang Buhe 方不和, ed. *Hexi baojuan zhenben jiaozhu yanjiu* 河西宝卷真本校注研究 (Lanzhou: Lanzhou daxue chubanshe, 1992), 301–313. According to an editorial note the text had been collected by Xu Zhude 徐祝德 in the area of Shandan county, and copied out by Ren Yumei 任玉梅 and Yan Fujiang 阎富江. A similar text is included in He Denghuan 何登焕, comp., *Yongchang baojuan* 永昌宝卷, 2 vols. (Yongchang: Yonchang xian Wenhuaju, n.d.), 783–789; Wang Xuebin 王学斌, comp., *Hexi baojuan jicui* 河西宝卷集粹, 2 Vols. (Beijing: Zhongguo renmin daxue chubanshe, 2010), vol. 2, 900–912; Xu Yongcheng 徐永成, comp., *Jin Zhangye minjian baojuan* 金张掖民间宝卷, 3 vols. (Lanzhou: Gansu wenhua chubanshe, 2007), Vol. 1, 238–244; Zhang Xu 张旭, comp., *Shandan baojuan* 山丹宝卷, 2 vols. (Lanzhou: Gansu wenhua chubanshe, 2007), vol. 2, 21–26. A complete English translation is included in Wilt L. Idema, *The Immortal Maiden Equal to Heaven and Other Precious Scrolls from Western Gansu* (Amherst NY: Cambria Press, 2015), 355–396. See also Idema, "Animals in Court," 281–284.

30. *Zuixin Maoshu xianggao quange* 最新貓鼠相告全哥 (Xiamen: Huiwentang, ca. 1920).

31. Emma Brunner-Traut, "Der Katzmäusekrieg in Alten und Neuen Orient," *Zeitschrift der Deutchen Morgenländichen Gesellschaft* 104 (1954): 347–351; Emma Brunner Traut, *Egyptian Artists' Sketches: Figured Ostraka from the Gayer-Anderson Collection in the Fitzwilliam Museum*

Cambridge. PIHANS XLV (Leiden: Nederlands Instituut voor het Nabije
Oosten, 1979); Emma Brunner Traut, *Altägyptische Tiergeschichte und
Fabel: Gestalt und Strahlkraft* (Darmstadt: Wissenschaftliche Buchge-
sellschaft, 1980).

32. Herman S. Schibli, "Fragments of a Weasel and Mouse War," *Zeitschrift
für Papyrologie und Epigraphik* 53 (1983): 1–25; Herman S. Schibli,
"Addendum to 'Fragments of a Weasel and Mouse War'," *Zeitschrift für
Papyrologie und Epigraphik* 54 (1984): 14; Martin Litchfield West, *Home-
ric Hymns, Homeric Apocrypha, Lives of Homer* (Cambridge MA: Harvard
University Press, 2015), 258–261.

33. Herbert Hunger, *Der byzantynische Katz-Mäuse Krieg: Theodoros Pro-
dromos, Katomyomachia, Einleitung, Text und Übersetzung* (Graz: Verlag
Hermann Böhlaus, 1968).

34. Victor Lebedev, "Cats, Mice, Thieves, and Heroes in Ara-
bian Nights Genizah Tales," *Genizah Fragments* 24 (Oct. 1992),
2, www.lib.cam.ac.uk/Taylor-Schlechter/GP/Geniza_Fragments_24.pdf;
Enno Littmann, "Katze und Maus. Ein arabisches Streitgedicht. Zum
ersten Male aufgezeichnet un übersetzt," in *Aus der Welt des Buches:
Festgabe zum 70. Geburtstag von Georg Leyh* (75. Beiheft zum Zentral-
blatt für Bibliothekwesen). Leipzig: Otto Harrasowitz, 1950, 241–259;
Joseph Sadan, "Arabic *Tom 'n Jerry* Compositions: a Popular Composition on a War between Cats and Mice and a *Maqāma* on Negotiations and
Concluding Peace between a Cat and a Mouse," in Albert Arazi, Joseph
Sadan, and David J. Waserstein, eds. *Compilation and Creation in* Adab
and Luġa: *Studies in Memory of Naphtali Kinberg (1948–1997)*. Israel Oriental Studies XIX (Tel Aviv: Eisenbrauns, 1999).

35. Georg Jacob, *Türkische Volksliteratur: Ein erweiterter Vortrag* (Berlin:
Mayer und Müller, 1901), 8.

36. Dick Davis, *Faces of Love: Hafez and the Poets of Shiraz* (Washington:
Mage Publishers, 2012), 217–223; *The Mice and the Cat, Ascribed to
'Ubayd Zākānī: Facsimile of the Original Manuscript from the National
Library of Tunis.* Preface by Ali Muhaddis; trans. into English and
Swedish by Bo Utas (Uppsala: Department of Linguistics and Philol-
ogy, Uppsala University, 2011); Obeyd Zakani, *Cat and Mouse*, trans.
and introd. Paul Smith (Campbell's Creek: New Humanity Books/ Book
Heaven, 2012).

37. Ursula Schubert, "Zwei Tierszenen am Ende der ersten Kendicott-Bibel
La Coruña, 1476, in Oxford," *Journal of Jewish Art* 12–13 (1986–1987):
83–88.

38. Sheila O'Connell, *The Popular Print in England 1550-1850* (London: British Museum Press, 1999), 49–50, 122–124.
39. T.H. Barrett, *The Religious Affiliations of the Chinese Cat: An Essay towards an Anthropozoological Approach to Comparative Religion*. The Louis Jordan Occasional Papers in Comparative Religion No. 2 (London: The School of Oriental and African Studies, 1998); T.H. Barrett, "The Monastic Cat in Cross-Cultural Perspective: Cat Poems of the Zen Masters," in James A. Benn, Lori Meeks, and James Robson, Eds., *Buddhist Monasticism in Asia: Places of Practice* (London: Routledge, 2010), 107–124.
40. In the *Pantacantra* the animals that request a judgement are the partridge and the hare (Visnu Sarva, *The Pancatantra*, 290–296). See also Laurits Bødker, *Indian Animal Tales: A Preliminary Survey* (Helsinki: Suomalainen Tiedeakatemia, 1957, 25, no. 135). In folklore studies, stories of this type are classified at AT 113B. Ding Naitong, *Zhongguo minjian gushi leixing suoyin*, 13–14; Jin Ronghua, *Minjian gushi leixing suoyin*, Vol. 1, 40–41; Gu Xijia, *Zhongguo gudai minjian gushi leixing*, 17.
41. At about the same time the story was also depicted on the Mendut Temple on Java. See Marijke Klokke, "Dierenfabels van India naar Java, Tweede eeuw voor tot vijftiende eeuw na Christus," in Wilt Idema, Mineke Schipper, and P.H. Schrijvers, eds. *Mijn naam is haas: Dierenverhalen in verschillende culturen* (Baarn: Ambo, 1993), 199–200.
42. Liu Shouhua 刘守华, *Fojing gushi yu Zhongguo minjian gushi yanbian* 佛经故事与中国民间故事演变 (Shanghai: Shanghai guji chubanshe, 2012), 175–178; 201–207. The feigning cat is also included in a late-Qing New Year's print titled "The Mouse Marries off its Daughter in Western Style" (Xiyang laoshu jianü 西洋老鼠嫁女). The main body of this print is, as usual, taken up by the wedding procession of the mouse. In the lower left-hand corner, one sees Xuanzang and his companions making their way toward the Bottomless Cave in the upper right hand corner. In the upper left-hand corner, a large cat is reading the sutras while a long row of mice parades past the cat in front of it—the last one in the queue, we know, will be eaten. Zhang Daoyi, *Laoshu jianü*, 94.
43. In Japan too, the theme of the war of the mice against the cats only shows up in the visual and literary arts of the nineteenth century. The National Diet Library holds a copy of a little black-and-white illustrated booklet titled *Neko-nezumi gassen* of the early nineteenth century. Utagawa Yoshitsuya treated the theme in a single print of 1843, while Utagawa Yoshitoshi (1839–1892) treated the theme in a series of six prints of

1859. The theme was revived during the Sino-Japanese war of 1894–1895, when the victorious Japanese were depicted as cats and the defeated Chinese as rats.

44. *Shujing zuofan* 鼠精作反, in *Maolü guai xifu, Shujing zuofan(Gaomao qianduan)* 毛驢拐媳婦 鼠精作反告貓前段, Beijing: Republican period, 1–3, shanben-ioc.u-tokyo.ac.jp/file/D85330000/PDF/0250032.pdf.

45. The Cold Food Festival was an ancient festival that was celebrated on the 105th day following the winter solstice. Later it became identified with the Clear and Bright festival of early April.

46. I also know of only one New Year's print on the subject of the war between the mice and the cats. Pu Songnian 蒲松年, *Zhongguo nianhua shi* 中国年画史 (Shenyang: Liaoning meishu chubanshe, 1986), 108 provides a (very poor) reproduction of a print titled *The Great Battle at Cat Mountain* (Dazhan Mao'ershan 大戰貓兒山) from Shaanxi. Pu Songnian, *Zhongguo nianhua yishu shi* 中国年画艺术史 (Changsha: Hunan Meishu chubanshe, 2008), 131 transcribes the poem on the print, which may be translated as "The mice had after many years become a demon plague:/How could the king of cats upon his mountain live with this?/ When he in rage set out the battle lines to capture them alive,/ The mice lost their commanders and they also lost their troops."

47. "Laoshu gaozhuang" 老鼠告狀, in *Linqu minjian wenxue jicheng (ziliao ben diyi juan)* 临朐民间文学集成资料本第一卷 (Linqu: Linqu xian minjian wenxue jicheng bangongshi, 1989), 383–388. According to an editorial note, this song was performed by "Ma Yiqin 马一琴, female, illiterate, aged 68, from Sanyuan village in Chengguan town" and had been recorded and edited by Ma Tongxiu 马佟秀. For a very similar text see "Laoshu gaozhuang" 老鼠告狀, in Zhang Daoyi, *Laoshu jianü*, 58–62, quoting *Minjian wenxue* 民间文学 (1982) no. 8. That version was provided by an old peasant in Yitang Township in Linyi County, Shandong Province. For a short extract in translation from the first text, see Idema, "Animals in Court," 279–280.

48. The text does not comment on the title, but I take it that *wuying* (without a shadow) here is short for *wuxing wuying* 無形無影 (without shape or shadow), which means "without rhyme or reason, totally unfounded". According to Mi Cheng 米成, ed. *Fanshi fangyan suyu huibian* 繁峙方言俗语汇编 (Taiyuan: Shanxi renmin chubanshe, 2013), 560 the expression *wuying zhuan* (locally pronounced *wuying zuan*) may refer either to "unlimited bragging, unfounded lies, and unrealistic rubbish" or to "a

kind of prosimetric storytelling which specializes in narrating nonsensical things to make people laugh."

49. Shang Lixin and Che Xilun, *Beifang minjian baojuan yanjiu*, 543.

50. Professor Shang has kindly provided me with scans of the 1883 manuscript, which unfortunately ends in the middle of the text of the accusation statement of the mouse.

51. *Minjian wenxue* 1 (1989): 3–7.

52. It should be pointed out that Shang Lixin lists the title of the 1870 manuscript of *A Tale without Shape or Shadow* as *Laoshu gao limao quanbu* 老鼠告狸貓全部, and describes it as "apparently based on a rewriting of the Yuan-dynasty tale *Wuying zhuan*." (Shang Lixin and Chen Xilun, *Beifang minjian baojuan yanjiu* 543) which makes one wonder whether the text as edited by Hao Wanhui may reflect this version of the *Wuying zhuan* . Unfortunately, Hao Wenhui does not explain where and how (s)he collected this text.

53. Zhong Shengyang 钟声扬, "Wuying zhuan (Laoshu gao limao)" 无影传 老鼠告狸猫, *Shanxi minjian wenxue* 61 (1992, no. 1): 26–30. On the web, this version also has the subtitle "The Rat Marries a Wife" (Haozi qu xifu 耗子娶媳妇); see http://blog.sina.com.cn/s/blog_a36441e80102 v563.html.

54. The inscription reads *guixian yuan ji* 貴銑袁記, which most likely should be read as "copied by Yuan Guixian".

55. The Dashing King (chuangwang 闖王) is Li Zicheng 李自成who in 1644 toppled the Ming dynasty when he entered Beijing with his troops. He would soon be defeated by the invading Manchus who founded the Qing dynasty once Wu Sangui 吳三桂 (1612–1678) had opened the Shanhaiguan Pass.

56. *A Tale without Shape or Shadow* includes the full prose text of both the accusation by the mouse and the counter statement by the cat.

57. Zhao Bi 趙弼, *Xiaopin ji* 效顰集 (Shanghai: Gudian wenxue chubanshe, 1957), 51–57.

58. Weinuogeladuowa 维诺格拉多娃, "Songzang yu quqin: Zhong E muban nianhua zhong maoshu de xingxiang yu yinyu 送葬与娶亲：中俄木板年画中老鼠的形象与隐喻," *Nianhua yanjiu* 年画研究 2013: 99–107.

59. Shops where one fetched water or a burning coal in case the fire at one own place had gone out.

60. Idema, "Animals in Court," 251–258.

61. On the Internet one can still encounter the statement that Lewis Carroll's *Alice in Wonderland* in 1931 was outlawed in China because it featured

talking animals. *Alice in Wonderland* was never prohibited in China, but a traditional official did complain in that year about the prevalence of talking animals in the new primary school books, and that piece of news eventually resulted in this persistent "urban legend." See Mark Burnstein and Zhongxin Feng, "Another Ben Trovato," *Knight Letter* 94 (2015): 10–11. The authors of this informative note create their own urban legend when they claim that the official concerned "accused the primary school textbooks of his day of not conforming to Communist standards." The Guomindang official concerned actually expressed his fear that the lack of proper terms of address would "advocate communism" as is clear from the Chinese text of the original press coverage of his speech as reproduced by Burnstein and Feng.

62. Xu Guangyu 徐广宇, "Minjian dongwu gushi zhetan" 民间动物故事摭谈, *Zhongguo Xiaowai jiaoyu* 26 (Sept. 2016), 104–105.

Chapter 5

Maligned Exchanges

The Uyghur-Tang Trade in the Light of Climate Data

Nicola Di Cosmo

Introduction

The Uyghur Khaganate (745–840), founded on the ashes of the second Türk Khaganate (682–744), is *sui generis* in the history of Inner Asian empires in ways that still remain unexplained. With their conversion to Manicheism, the Uyghurs were the first steppe people who accepted a non-native religion, setting a precedent for other conversions, by their own Uyghur descendants, and by Khitans, Tanguts, and Mongols, all of whom adopted Buddhism as their main faith. It was notably the first steppe empire that not only collaborated with the Tang dynasty (618–907) but also actively defended it against internal and external foes, first and foremost among them the expanding Tibetan empire.

The alliance between China and the Uyghurs, as is well known, included a commercial agreement known as the horses-for-silk trade, which resulted, over the decades, in the transfer of massive amounts of Chinese silk to the Uyghurs, and from there to the Silk Road markets, in exchange for hundreds of thousands of horses needed by the Tang military.[1] At the apex of Uyghur society, the native Turkic aristocracy partnered with Central Asian (Sogdian) prominent families in a commensality that combined the former's political and military power with the latter's commercial reach and financial clout. The development of what may appear as a fully integrated military-commercial complex was complemented by another innovation in the history of the Inner Asian empire, that is, the establishment of a large capital city—the largest ever built in Mongolia in premodern times—and other urban centers surrounded by agricultural fields. Uyghur urbanism under the aegis of imperial rule enabled the rapid transition to the establishment of sedentary "oasis-kingdoms" on the Silk Road by Uyghur refugees, who were forced to move from Mongolia after the dissolution of the empire in 840. [2]

So many "firsts" produce a rich trove of questions that suggest that something special happened in the near hundred years of Uyghur rule. One such question, bearing directly on the issue of the horse-silk trade, concerns the widespread notion, repeatedly suggested, that the Uyghurs were an economic parasite that the Tang tolerated only because their enervated military would otherwise become easy prey to the fierce attacks of foreign forces. In particular, the Uyghurs were faulted for presenting to the court emaciated and worthless horses, the greater number of which would sooner die than see any battlefield. In exchange, the northern barbarians exacted a hefty price in precious silks, coveting it above all else and being insatiably greedy for it.

What was the truth behind these allegations? In particular, why were the horses that reached China in such a wretched state? Attempting to answer such questions, this essay aims to reexamine the Tang-Uyghur relationship in light of climatic studies, on the basis of which a new hypothesis can be presented to reconstruct the conditions under which the horses-for-silk exchange was carried out, and the foundations of the Tang objections to the trade.

A Brief Survey of the Economic and Political Reality of the Horse-Silk Trade

Several issues have been raised in relation to the historical assessment of the trade, and in particular to its fairness and relative importance to both Uyghurs and Tang. Masaru Saitō has pointed out the Tang loss of horse-breeding regions in Hexi and Longyou (along the Gansu corridor).[3] These areas had been conquered by the Tibetans by 765, and their loss had made China more dependent upon the northern nomads to supply horses.[4] The historical documentation does indeed support the notion that the Uyghurs brought to court thousands of horses to be sold for silk at the nominal price of forty rolls, or bolts, per horse, with a bolt being normally four *zhang* in length (12 meters by 54 cm).[5] The supposedly extortionate cost of the horses has been questioned by Sechin Jagchid and Christopher Beckwith, who provide slightly different calculations as to the actual number of silk rolls exchanged per horse but fundamentally agree that the Tang needed to import horses for military purposes to preserve the viability of their military defense.[6] Moreover, the Tang court on occasion could not pay the price in full, thus accumulating debts. [7]

Another issue that makes it difficult to estimate the Tang disbursement is the conversion from cash to silk, which made it possible to lower the actual value by paying with low-quality, less expensive silk, while retaining the same exchange rate by continuing to provide the nominal forty (and at times less than that) rolls of silk per horse. The low quality of silk was cause for Uyghur protestations no less than the poor health of the horses for Tang complaints. Finally, when the Uyghurs were no longer able to provide horses, following the collapse of their state, their price rose as an effect of reduced supply.[8] Incidentally, the horse trade may have been interrupted already around 829, which is the date of the last reported Uyghur trading mission to China.[9]

The historical literature on this topic is in agreement on the fact that the cost extracted by the Uyghurs per horse was not excessive, given the Tang's dependency on them. The real problem was that the Chinese were paying for what they claimed to be useless. The Chinese argument was articulated by officials and statesmen, and in the works of eminent literary figures. In the following section we shall review the historical documentation, and the poems written by Bai Juyi and Yuan Zhen on the Uyghur trade, both of which were searing denunciations of its ills and trials. Bai Juyi's poem is especially relevant for its environmental observation.

Tang Perceptions of the Uyghur Horse Trade

The trope of the greedy, covetous barbarian was frequently associated with the Uyghurs, as in the memorial of the then President of the Board of Rites Li Jiang, dated 808 CE: "The northern barbarians are insatiably greedy, and only care for profit. Recently bringing horses [into China] used to be the norm, [but] for two consecutive years they have not arrived [here]; do they [suddenly] detest the profits from silken fabrics?"[10] This statement echoed earlier protestations, recorded in various sources, according to which as early as 758 the Uyghurs began to trade horses for silk, as a reward for the military assistance provided to the Tang. The Uyghur's envoys arrived frequently bringing horses and asking for silk in exchange: "the foreigners (fan) were insatiable in getting silk, we got horses that could not be used."[11] In a separate report, dated 768, it is stated more specifically that the horses could not be used because they were too weak.[12]

The literati's case against the rapacious Uyghurs was made most prominently by the poet Bai Juyi (772–846) in the poem "Yinshan Route," which is worth quoting in full as an example of a view undoubtedly widely shared in China not just in regard to the trade relationship with the Uyghurs, but especially in terms of the trade's economic and social consequences within China.[13]

The poem's opening lines show a picture of natural devastation left by numberless horses that arrive at the destination in pitiful physical shape:

紇邏敦肥水泉好。
每至戎人送馬時
道旁千裡無纖草。
草儘泉枯馬病羸,
飛龍但印骨與皮。

Steppe shrubs are thick and rich, springs are plentiful.[14]
Yet every time *Rong* men come to present horses
By the sides of the road for a thousand *li*
 there is not the wispiest of grass
With the grass spent and springs dried up,
 the horses become sick and emaciated
The flying dragon [seal] is merely a stamp on bones and skin.

The archaizing and surely not endearing term *Rong*, redolent of classical tropes from the ancient Spring and Autumn annals (*Chunqiu*) to imperial historiography as the epitome of China's northern barbarians, connoted, from the dawn of Chinese civilization, a cultural, political, and moral distance. By associating the Uyghurs with China's historical antagonists (fearsome nomadic warriors) rather than describing what they actually were (military allies and commercial partners), that moral distance was resuscitated and validated by historical precedent. The contrast between the fabled qualities of these horses, branded as "flying dragons," and the pitiful skin-and-bone creatures that reached the court and military stables could not have been starker.

In the next lines, the price paid in silk, given here at fifty rolls per head —which in other Tang sources is given at forty—was probably correct in the early ninth century and is meant to shock the reader as exorbitant for creatures whose mortality and injury rates could reach up to 60 or 70%.

五十匹縑易一匹,
縑去馬來無了日。
養無所用去非宜,
每歲死傷十六七。

Fifty rolls of silk to pay for one horse,
The silk goes and the horses come without missing a day.
Raising them is useless and sending them (back) inappropriate,
Every year the dead and injured [horses] are six or seven out of ten.

The subsequent four lines are meant to express the misery of the Chinese female workers, who were forced to weave day and night and even cut corners to satisfy the demand. Hence, the quality of the exported silk—thinner (not double-thread as it should have been) and in rolls shorter than the standard length (three *zhang* instead of four)—was compromised, causing the Uyghurs to protest.

縑絲不足女工苦，
疏織短截充匹數。
藕絲蛛網三丈餘，
回鶻訴稱無用處。

Silk not being sufficient, the female workers suffered,
Sparsely weaving, they cut it short
　　to make up for the number of bolts.
Silk like lotus root and cobwebs
　　[merely] over three *zhang* of length,
The Uyghurs protested that they had no use [for it]

Therefore, adjustments were needed, favored by the diplomatic intervention of emperor Tang Dezong's daughter, the Chinese Princess Xian'an, who had long before been sent in marriage to the Uyghur *qaghan* and had been the wife of three *qaghans* in succession.[15] The difference in value was compensated by gold disbursements, while better silk was requisitioned from the southern provinces, in accordance with normal standards:

鹹安公主號可敦，
遠為可汗頻奏論。
元和二年下新敕，
內出金帛酬馬直。

仍詔江淮馬價縑，
從此不令疏短織。

Princess Xian'an, whom they called *qatun*,
From faraway on behalf of the *qaghan* frequently memorialized.
In the second year of Yuanhe [807] a new decree was issued
The Court would pay gold and silk for the horses' price
And also ordered that silk for horse-price from Jiang and Huai
From then on [silk] was not allowed
　　[to be woven] thin and cut short

Hence, the Uyghur generals were able to get their fill of wealth, opening, to the surprise of the Chinese, their "greedy hearts". But peace was cold comfort because the higher value of the payment only begot more horses, but whether their quality also improved is intentionally omitted:

合羅將軍呼萬歲#
捧授金銀與縑彩。
誰知黠虜#貪心，
明年馬多來一倍。
縑漸好，
馬漸多。
陰山虜，
奈爾何。

The Heluo[16] Generals cried out "Ten Thousand Lives"
Extending their hands received gold, silver, and variegated silks
Who would have known that those cunning barbarians
　　could open their greedy hearts?
Next year the horses will have a one-fold increase
As the silk gradually improves
The horses gradually increase.
The Yinshan barbarians:
What can one do [with them]?

The predicament expressed in the poem, which condemned China to a doomed exchange of treasure for large numbers of useless horses, was of great concern to Bai Juyi, who was distressed at the economic pressures of the trade. The suffering of the indentured weavers echoes the chagrin of the Tang court.

A less obvious point is the contrast between the lush vegetation, described as rich *hela* grass and plentiful water, and the depleted landscape after the passage of the herds. The inference is to very large herds; so numerous were the horses that their passage left the land along the trail barren of grass and water, and as a result the horses arrived at the capital so malnourished that two-thirds of them did not survive.[17]

According to Jagchid, the poor health of the horses was due to "transportation conditions" under the Tang administration.[18] In this he seems to refer to the situation denounced by Yuan Zhen (779–831) in the poem "Yin Mountain Route," exactly the same title as Bai Juyi's, which he composed in 809. The poem is complementary to that of his close friend Bai, in the sense that it does not contradict it, but places the blame of the imbalance more squarely on the moral and structural shortcomings of the various Tang agents. Yuan Zhen denounces the graft of officials, great families, and merchants who profited from business deals. Such cliques and clans were responsible for extravagant consumption of silk.

This poem has been studied in depth in a recent essay by Tan Mei Ah, to whose translation I will refer.[19] What concerns us here is above all the issue of the mortality of the horses. According to the introductory lines of the poem, every year horses were brought to China via the Yin Mountain route, and since horses died on the Yin Mountain, silk was squandered for nothing.[20] This statement is not quite as informative as Bai Juyi's more detailed account. The dead horses may refer to those that died upon arrival, or after they were purchased. It is also possible that horses were accounted for on the northern frontier because they probably crossed through the Tiande or Zhenwu military districts (Tiandejun, Zhenwujun) located respectively to the north and to the northeast sectors of the territory within the great bend of the Yellow River.[21] Those horses that died in Tang territory, before arriving at their destination (Chang'an or

Taiyuan), were still included in the purchase.[22] Frontier military garrisons, which would have been natural gateways into China, were sufficiently close to the Yin Mountains to be regarded as part of the general route. Therefore, the sense of the poem may be reconstructed as saying that many horses died on the trek from the Yin Mountain to their destination in Tang territory, but those that died within China, after a reckoning had been made at the crossing stations, were still going to be included in the purchase price. Sharing the risks would have been a fair arrangement so that the Uyghur side would not have had to absorb the entire volume of the losses incurred en route.

The central question, however, regardless of the amount of silk paid for the horses and how many horses were paid for, is why the level of mortality was so high. This fact was central to the Chinese protestations and fomented the Tang belief in the fundamental unfairness of the trade. However, no explanation has been offered for the obviously very trying conditions on the trail. While a presumed cunningness of the Uyghurs can be dismissed offhand, since it is not realistic that they would expose themselves to high financial losses just to trick the Chinese, the issue of malnutrition and mortality deserves a closer look. To investigate this question, we need to turn to an environmental study of the territory that the horses had to cross before reaching their destination.

MID-TANG CLIMATIC DOWNTURN

In a letter to the Uyghur Khan composed by Bai Juyi on behalf of the emperor, we find an intriguing passage "due to floods and droughts in recent years, regrettably there have not been enough provisions for the army and the state."[23] The poor weather conditions were blamed for having depressed productivity in China. Indeed, several reports in the sources testify to the worsening of China's climatic conditions in the late-eighth and early ninth centuries. Both floods and droughts as well as a steep cooling of the temperature caused disasters across northern China.

Recently, proxy data from natural archives enable us to look more closely at the conditions on the region south of the Yin Mountains and more specifically within the bend of the Yellow River (*hetao*) such as the Ordos general region and, in the southern portion of it, the Mu Us Desert.[24] Numerous scientific studies attest to the turn of climate in the mid-Tang, around 800 CE or slightly earlier, towards a colder and more arid climate, which led to a first period of serious desertification of the Ordos region, with a second taking place in the Ming dynasty (1368–1644). A recent study based on sediment analysis in the Mu Us Desert within the bend of the Yellow River, with the support of archaeological documentation, shows that several cities were abandoned in the later Tang, attesting to the deteriorating climatic conditions and increase of desert areas. The data show that desertification began around 800, with sand dunes developing around existing cities by 820.[25] The study, which focuses on the area between the Yinshan mountain chain, running east to west to the north of the Yellow River, and Taiyuan, located to the east of the Yellow River, provides evidence of a depleted environment along the "Yin Mountain Route".

A climatological study on the temperature of the Tang dynasty, based on historical records, also shows that early ninth-century northern China, especially the area of Chang'an, was one of the coldest periods on record until the Ming dynasty, during which we have a sharp cooling coinciding with the Little Ice Age.[26] Based on parameters such as exceptional snowfalls, unseasonal frosts, and freezing of rivers and coastal waters, the study's findings show in particular that both severity and recurrence of cold events increased sharply in the early ninth century. Additional evidence is based on historical sources that document the aridization of the Mu Us Desert and its depopulation in the late Tang, after an early Tang phase of demographic and economic growth.[27]

While historians and archaeologists also have argued for anthropogenic desertification as the result of environmental overexploitation, the most recent data provide evidence for climatic change as the chief cause for the aridization of the Ordos region.[28] The reconstruction of climate in northern China, based on speleothems from the Shihua cave, shows that "desertification occurring after the 790s in northern China followed by decreasing biological productivity after 820s in Central China led to the decline of the Tang dynasty, and their former domains fell under the control of warlords."[29] While mechanistic understandings of the interaction between human and natural systems are not historically acceptable—and therefore theories that climatic change might be responsible for the downfall of the Tang dynasty would be exceedingly dubious—the climate data showing that increased aridity occurred in northern China from around 790 cannot be ignored as a possible cause of economic losses, depopulation, or, as in the case at hand, more trying conditions in the transportation of horses.

Additional evidence is provided by a paleoclimatic record with nearly annual time resolution from a sediment core from Lake Huguang Maar in southern China.[30] This records correlates with records from the Hulu (Jiangsu Province) and Dongge (Guizhou Province) caves to show that, in the late eighth century, periods of low summer monsoon strength caused a substantial decrease in the amount of precipitation in northern China.[31] Therefore, one possibility is that drought conditions in north-central China (and beyond) were caused by a variation in the strength of the summer monsoon and the rain they carried to the north.

Moreover, tree-ring-based moisture reconstructions show that Mongolia was hit by a severe and protracted drought from 783 to 850.[32] While it would be incorrect, for the same reasons just mentioned, to attempt to correlate directly the drought with the collapse of the Uyghur empire, it is possible to infer from the climatic data that the megadrought altered the productivity of Mongolia, and presumably affected the well-being of the animals. Moreover, recent studies show that the greatest losses of livestock in Mongolia due to natural disasters occur when a sudden cooling of the fall and winter temperatures is preceded by a summer drought, because the animals are unable to store enough fat to

survive the heavy snowfalls and frosts.[33] We do not have temperature
data from Mongolia, but an analysis of temperatures from northern
China indicate that the period of the drought also coincided with lower
temperatures.[34] These sources do not reflect temperature conditions in
Mongolia, but nonetheless we do have evidence of winter disasters in
the Mongolian region. Indeed, the downfall of the Uyghur empire was
precipitated, together with an ongoing political crisis, by a very harsh
winter that caused high losses of livestock and famine and disease among
the populace.[35] Incidentally, it is noteworthy that the Kyrgyz, who finally
routed the Uyghurs and occupied their capital in 840, did not settle in
Mongolia, preferring to return to their homeland in the Yenisei region
in southern Siberia.[36] It is possible that the political vacuum created in
central Mongolia after centuries of Turkic political rule was caused by
unfavorable climatic conditions and the long-term effects of the drought.

A significant issue in relation to the movement of herds is, of course,
seasonality. Here we must note a considerable variability in the timing of
the trade missions. Based on the data collected by Colin Mackerras, the
early missions tended to arrive in the fall, as we would expect for horses
that would leave Mongolia at the peak of their shape, that is, at the end
of the summer.[37] However, later missions (from 816 to 829) tended to
arrive in the early months of the year, which must have been far less
convenient. Without additional information, it would be pointless to
speculate about the shift, except that it may depend on a change of route
or on a greater distance from pastures in Mongolia.[38]

Finally, one may ask why the comments reported in the sources about
the poor health of the horses apply also to a period in time that precedes
the onset of the climatic turn. Should we not expect, if climatic conditions
are key to the well-being of the horses, that the period before the drought,
from 760 to approximately 790, would have been favorable to the trade,
and the horses should not have been negatively affected? A possible
answer is not climatic but historiographical—namely, that the standard
histories, written in the tenth (*Jiu Tangshu*) and eleventh (*Xin Tangshu*)

centuries, were redacted to paint the whole trade with the same brush, according to the greedy Uyghur trope that, by the end of the Tang, had become widely known. Thus, they may not accurately reflect differences in the condition of the horses between the periods before and during the drought. However, according to paleoclimatic data from the Shihua cave, northern China started to experience drought conditions already in the second half of the eighth century, and while these were not as severe as after 790, they might have affected the passage of horses.[39] If so, what the early records may be telling us is that from the beginning the journey across arid lands was arduous and the horses arrived weak, while the actual mortality rate was probably not as high as in the latter period, when the drought reached peak severity. Additional data specific to the area of southern Mongolia and the Yinshan mountains would be required to help clarify the degree of aridity from 760 to 790.

CONCLUSION

Environmental issues are present in Bai Juyi's moral and political considerations: malnourished horses died as soon as they were exchanged for silk because even a region with abundant natural resources could not suffice to feed and sate the number of mounts sent by the Uyghurs. Yuan Zhen also reports on the mortality of horses but does not dwell on its causes. Tang historical sources are more explicit, albeit not univocal, in the condemnation of an unfair trade and the harm that it did to China: the Uyghurs appear as greedy and cunning, and their moral failings were ultimately responsible for the moribund horses that they delivered, since they seemed to be indifferent to their fate. Both literary and historical sources also register the Uyghurs' remonstrations for the poor quality of the silk, and Chinese sources occasionally show a keen attention to climatic conditions in the steppes and their economic and political impact on the nomads. A memorable quote of the seventh century (629), in reference to the Türks—then the Tang's northern enemies—has it that "the Türks rise and fall solely according to their sheep and horses".[40]

To answer one specific question at the heart of Sino-Uyghur relations—namely, how it was possible that the horses the Tang badly needed, and the Uyghur were eager to exchange for precious silk, died in large numbers on the Yin Mountain trail, we have put forward an environmental hypothesis, based on combined natural data and historical sources.

First of all, these natural proxies illuminate the climatic conditions of the region the horses were to pass through, showing clearly the progressive aridization of northern China, which lasted from the last decade of the eighth century to the middle of the ninth century. During this time the area within the great bend of the Yellow River experienced an expansion of desertification, and routes that connected Chang'an to the northern frontier suffered from greater aridity and vegetation changes. Such phenomena were largely hydroclimatic, that is, due to a decrease in precipitation. However, floods were also registered, indicating an uneven distribution of rainfall.

The progressive aridification of northern China coincided, according to historical sources, with a general cooling of the temperature that caused unseasonal frosts, heavy winter snowfalls, and generally lower-than-average temperatures. As a result, the productivity of the land decreased and water became scarcer, thus lowering the ratio between the carrying capacity of the land and the animals that could be supported. These problems in themselves may have been sufficient to increase the mortality of the horses, but another factor further aggravated the situation. From 783 onwards Mongolia also experienced a drought that, in terms of severity and duration, had not been registered for centuries. Assuming that grassland productivity decreased during the drought, the horses might have been underfed when they started their trek to China. The long journey across an arid territory that afforded meager pasturage, aggravated by early frosts and low temperatures, thus account for above-average mortality rates.

It is surprising that the Uyghurs continued to trade horses under such trying conditions, undoubtedly knowing that many animals would be lost. A possible answer to this question is that the Uyghur elites required the international currency of the age, silk, to feed their own depleted economy and were willing to take substantial risks in order to acquire it. Eventually, in 830, the horse-for-silk trade came to end, with a final record mentioned in the sources regarding 10,000 horses brought to China by the Uyghurs.[41] In addition to the protracted and severe drought, a contributing cause to the deteriorating climate, might have been the cold conditions induced by the Katla volcanic eruption of 822–823, which may have been responsible for very low temperatures between 821 and 826.[42] One might wonder whether volcanic forcing might have affected grassland productivity in the 820s as well and be responsible (together with the drought) for the end of horse exports.

It is significant in the history of Inner Asian empires that the Uyghurs preferred to continue to export horses rather than using them to build up their military power and force China to pay a tribute in silk, as was the case, for instance, with the Xiongnu empire. Not that the Uyghurs ceased completely to be warriors, since military expeditions continued in other parts of their realm, but their foreign policy towards China was never based on conquest or the threat of it. The Uyghurs' mercantilist, rather than militarist, orientation, could be attributed to a number of causes, such as the growing influence of commercial interests represented by the highly influential Sogdian merchants, or a partial turn of the Uyghur aristocracy away from military pursuits under the influence of Manichaeism and partial sedentarization. After 821, the renewed marriage alliances with the Tang court, the peace treaty with Tibet, and the large volume of trade, indicate a deliberate choice away from military ventures.[43]

Such overarching political questions cannot be given a climatic answer, but the more limited question regarding the high mortality and poor health of the horses certainly can. The climatic downturn of the second half of the Tang dynasty, between c. 790 and 850, strained the economies of both China and the Uyghurs, and it may have played a role as a possible factor in the long-term weakening and eventual downfall of the Uyghur empire. In the final analysis, the study of climatic conditions, and their effects on the horse-silk trade, allows us to establish more clearly the economic, cultural, and political contexts of Sino-Uyghur relations.

NOTES

1. On Uyghur-Tang relations see Colin Mackerras, *The Uyghur Empire, According to The T'ang Dynastic Histories: A Study in Sino-Uyghur Relations 744–840.* Columbia: University of South Carolina Press, 1973).
2. For an overview of the Uyghur empire see Roman K. Kovalev, "Uyghur Khaganate." *The Encyclopedia of Empire.* Wiley Online Library, 2016. DOI: 10.1002/9781118455074.wbeoe093;
3. Saitō, Masaru, "Tō-Kaikotsu kenba kōeki saikō." *Shigaku zasshi*108.10 (1999): 1749–1774. This point is also made by Tan Mei Ah, "Exonerating the Horse Trade for the Shortage of Silk: Yuan Zhen's 'Yin Mountain Route,'" *Journal of Chinese Studies* 57 (July 2013): 49–96.
4. Horlemann, Bianca, "A Re-Evaluation of the Tibetan Conquest of Eighth-Century Shazhou/Dunhuang," in *Tibet, Past and Present: Tibetan Studies, I*, edited by Hank Blezer. (Leiden: Brill, 2002): 49–66.
5. Sheng, Angela. "Determining the Value of Textiles in the Tang Dynasty in Memory of Professor Denis Twitchett (1925–2006)." *Journal of the Royal Asiatic Society (Third Series)* 23.02 (2013): 183.
6. Beckwith, Christopher I., "The Impact of the Horse and Silk Trade on the Economies of T'ang China and the Uyghur Empire: On the Importance of International Commerce in the Early Middle Ages," *Journal of the Economic and Social History of the Orient/Journal de l'histoire economique et sociale de l'Orient,* 34.3 (1991):183–198; Jagchid, Segchid, "The Uyghur Horses. of the T'ang Dynasty," in *Gedanke und Wirkung, Festschrift zum 90. Geburtstag von Nikolaus Poppe,* edited by W. Heissig, K. Sagaster (Wiesbaden: Harrassowitz, 1989):175–188.
7. Beckwith, "Impact of the Horse and Silk Trade," 188–189.
8. Ibid., 192.
9. Mackerras, Colin. "Sino-Uyghur Diplomatic and Trade Contacts (744 to 840)." *Central Asiatic Journal* 13.3 (1969): 215–240.
10. *Xin Tangshu,* 6126–6127. See also Jagchid, 182.
11. *Jiu Tangshu,* 5207. See also Jagchid, 178.
12. *Xin Tangshu,* 6120.
13. Some translations of this poem can be found in Jagchid, 181; I express my gratitude to Professor Stephen West for advice on the rendering of some passages. Otherwise, the translation is mine.

14. I follow here the reconstruction of the word *hela*, obviously of foreign origin, as camelthorn, or sheepthorn, from a Persian loanword, proposed by Sanping Chen. This rendering seems to fit the picture of a lush steppe environment. See Chen Sanping, "Bai Juyi and Manna," *Central Asiatic Journal* 58.1-2 (2015): 17–25.

15. Pan Yihong, "Marriage Alliances and Chinese Princesses in International Politics from Han through T'ang." *Asia Major* (1997): 120.

16. In my view the term *heluo* refers to the Heluo River, which in rare instances is referred to as the original homeland of the Uyghurs and therefore is used here metonymically to indicate the Uyghur generals. On the Heluo river as the original land of the Uyghurs, see *Zizhi Tongjian* 7968.

17. On this point see Tan, "Exonerating the Horse Trade," 69. She perceptively notes that the horses were not necessarily undernourished when they started their journey, but they became so after crossing the deserts; this may explain why they ate more when they reached the Yin mountains.

18. Jagchid, *op. cit.*, 180.

19. Tan, "Exonerating the Horse Trade."

20. Ibid., 53.

21. See Tan Qixiang, *Zhongguo lishi ditu ji*, vol. 5, map 40–41, 3–6 and 3–9.

22. According to Tan Mei Ah (p. 68), the horses were brought to Taiyuan, where the transaction would take place. This is possible given that they needed pasture land, although one imagines some of them would be taken also to other locations, and possibly take also different routes, such as the route through the Fengzhou and the Xiazhou regions, which was a critical military route to the northern frontier. See Ai Chong, "Tangdai Xiazhou cheng tong wang Fengzhou quyu de daolu kaoju," *Zhonguo bianjiang shidi yanjiu* 24.3 (2014):107–113.

23. Tan, "Exonerating the Horse Trade," 66.

24. The Mu Us Desert and the Ordos Desert are often used as synonymously.

25. Huang, Yinzhou, et al. "Historical Desertification of the Mu Us Desert, Northern China: A Multidisciplinary Study." *Geomorphology* 110.3 (2009): 115.

26. Man Zhimin, "Guanyu Tangdai qihou leng ruan wenti de daohua Disiji yanjiu," *Quatermary Sciences* (1998) 1: 20–30.

27. Du Zhongchao et al., "Changcheng yanxian Maowusu shadi xingcheng, kuozhan ji qi huangmohua xiaoying," *Shui tu baode yanjiu*, 13.3 (2006): 227.

28. A representative of human impact in the historical desertification of the Ordos as a "man-made desert" (*renzao shamo*) is Wang Weilin, "Maowusu shamohua niandai wendi zhi kaogxue guancha," *Kaogu yu wenwu* 5 (2002): 80–84. While natural causes are regarded as a contributing factor, the opening to human immigration is considered by Wang the major and primary cause of environmental depletion. On the basis of preliminary archaeological investigations, Hou Renzhi, while cautious in his conclusion, also endorses the human impact theory; see his "Cong Hongliu he shang de gucheng feixiu kan Maowusu shamo de bianqian," *Wennwu* 1 (1973): 35–41.

29. Wang, Xunming, et al. "Climate, Desertification, and the Rise and Collapse of China's Historical Dynasties." *Human Ecology* 38.1 (2010): 164.

30. Yancheva, Gergana, et al. "Influence of the intertropical convergence zone on the East Asian monsoon." *Nature* 445.7123 (2007): 74–77.

31. Wang, Y. J. et al. "A High-Resolution Absolute-Dated Late Pleistocene Monsoon Record from Hulu Cave, China." *Science* 294 (2001): 2345–2348; Dykoski, C. A. et al. "A High-Resolution, Absolute-Dated Holocene and Deglacial Asian Monsoon Record from Dongge Cave, China." *Earth Planet. Sci. Lett.* 233 (2005): 71–86.

32. See Di Cosmo et al., "Environmental Stress and Steppe Nomads: Rethinking the History of the Uyghur Empire (744–840) with Paleoclimate Data," *Journal of Interdisciplinary History* (forthcoming, 2018).

33. Begzsuren, S., et al. "Livestock Responses to Droughts and Severe Winter Weather in the Gobi Three Beauty National Park, Mongolia." *Journal of Arid environments* 59.4 (2004): 785–796. Rao, Mukund Palat, et al. "Dzuds, Droughts, and Livestock Mortality in Mongolia." *Environmental Research Letters* 10.7 (2015): 074012.

34. Man Zhimin, "Guanyu Tangdai qihou leng ruan wenti," 26.

35. Michael Drompp, "The Uyghur-Chinese Conflict of 840–848," in *Warfare in Inner Asian History (500-1500)* (Leiden: Brill, 2002), edited by N. Di Cosmo, 75 [73–103]. See also Mackerras, *The Uyghur Empire*, 122–125.

36. Michael. R. Drompp, "Breaking the Orkhon tradition: Kirghiz Adherence to the Yenisei region after AD 840." *Journal of the American Oriental Society* 119.3 (1999): 390–403.

37. Colin Mackerras, "Sino-Uyghur Diplomatic and Trade Contacts", 239.

38. If the breeding grounds had been moved to a different area of Mongolia, and the route had become longer, this may explain the later arrival time. However, it is impossible to provide an explanation for the difference in travel time.

39. Wang Xunming et al., "Rise and Collapse of China's Historical Dynasties." While the authors date the turn towards desertification in northern China after 790, the graph on page 163 shows an earlier downward trend onset for northern China.
40. *Jiu Tangshu* 62, 2381.
41. Beckwith, "Impact of the Horse and Silk Trade," 188.
42. Büntgen et al. "Multi-Proxy Dating of Iceland's Major Pre-Settlement Katla Eruption to 822–823 CE." Geology (2017). DOI: 10.1130/G39269.1
43. On the marriage alliance between the Taihe Princess and the Uyghur Kaghan Chongde see Pan Yihong, "Marriage Alliances and Chinese Princesses in International Politics from Han through T'ang." *Asia Major* (1997): 121. On the peace treaty with Tibet see Janoush Szerb, "A Note on the Tibetan-Uigur Treaty of 822/823 AD," in *Contributions on Tibetan Language, History and Culture, Vol. 1,* edited by E. Steinkellner and H. Tauscher (Delhi: M. Banarsidass, 1995): 357–374. On the increased number of horses brought to China in the 820's, see Mackerras, "Sino-Uyghur Diplomatic and Trade Contacts," 239.

CHAPTER 6

IMAGERY OF ARCHERY AND ACCOUTREMENTS IN EPICS FROM SOUTHWEST CHINA

Mark Bender

INTRODUCTION

Since the 1950s, groups of Chinese folklorists and other researchers have documented long narratives in poetic from among many ethnic minority groups in southwest China. A number of edited versions of these narratives were published in the late 1950s and early 1960s, and many were republished in the late 1970s and the 1980s after the Cultural Revolution (1966–1976). All told, dozens of long narrative poems have since been collected and processed into various written and published formats, and more recently into electronic ones. Although often ignored or dismissed by Western researchers because of concerns over collecting and editing practices, these texts have come to form a major component of published ethnic minority folk literature that have both scholarly and general audiences. Recent projects concerning such long poems employ improved collecting and editing strategies, exemplified by the rigorous and innovative efforts of scholars in the Institute of Ethnic Literature in the Chinese Academy of Social Sciences in Beijing.

These long narratives are often termed "epics" (*shishi* 史诗) by Chinese scholars and are frequently classified into two major categories related to content, geographic distribution, and ethnic affiliation.[1] Epics that concern heroes who fight human enemies and monsters are regarded as heroic epics, or *yingxiong shishi* 英雄史诗. Transmitted among groups dwelling in the northern and western regions of China are the Tibetan and Mongol versions of the story of the demigod King Gesar, the Mongol epic *Janggar*, and the Kirghiz epic *Manas*. Heroes are typically described as riding a super horse—sometimes with wings—and having various accoutrements such as helmets, armor, swords, bow and arrows, and possibly other weapons. Narrative poems and folktales from smaller northeastern groups such as the Daur 达斡尔, Olunchun 鄂伦春, and Hezhe 赫哲 feature hunter heroes (called *mergen*, as is sometimes the case with Mongol heroes) who typically ride horses and have dogs or eagles in tow, along with their bow and arrows and swords or hunting knives.[2]

In the south and southwest many epics tell of the creation of the sky, earth, and the plant and animal inhabitants, including humans. These *chuangshi shishi* 创世史诗, or origin epics, share many similar motifs. They are, in essence, cosmogonic myths in the format of long narrative poems or epics. In some cases they are delivered orally in an antiphonal performance involving two or more singers. They are often associated with funerals, wedding feasts, house raisings, community festivals, and other such communal events. Within the larger plots of the creation stories are subplots—which are sometimes told as discrete tales—concerning human characters, or gods with human characteristics. Several of the epics that have received scholarly attention are products of the large and

diverse ethnic groups officially designated as Yizu 彝族 and Miaozu 苗
族.[3] These characters are sometimes martial heroes, like the Yi culture-
hero Zhyxge Axlu discussed later, or the Miao/Hmong hero King of Yalu
(*Yalu Wang* 亚鲁王).[4] Non-martial characters, which can be considered
"heroic" in other ways, appear in some of the narrative poems. Epics
scholar Lauri Honko suggested such characters may serve as "exemplary
characters" or as role models.[5] In some cases, female characters are
prominent in the southern creation narratives. These include *Mais Bangx*
or Butterfly Mother, a figure in Miao/Hmong epics from southeastern
Guizhou 贵州 province, who lays the eggs from which protohumans and
many other creatures hatch; the creator goddess *Miloto (Miluotuo* 密洛
陀) of the Yao 瑶 of Guangxi 广西, who is extremely active in the creation
of humans and other life forms; the shape-shifting Zyzy Hninra in the
Nuosu ritual chant "Origin of Ghosts" (*Nyicy Bbopa*); and the figures
Gamo Anyo and Ashima who are central in bridal capture narratives of
various Yi subgroups in Sichuan and Yunnan, respectively.[6] Two well-
known Yi creation epics from Chuxiong 楚雄 Prefecture in northern
Yunnan are *Meige* 梅葛 and *Chamu* 查姆 are both rich in imagery of
traditional material culture, much of which parallels recent items and
practices. Weapons, especially various sorts of archery equipment and
hunting tools (including snares, nets, and clubs) also appear in all of
the previously mentioned verse narratives, as well epics of other ethnic
groups and many other folksongs and stories.

My purpose in this chapter is to draw attention to the almost pervasive
presence of imagery of material culture in Chinese ethnic minority
oral literature and how it meaningfully relates to verifiable contexts of
vernacular culture in a fading or not-too-distant past. I will focus on
objects of warfare and hunting, which are prominent in many epic texts,
often in concert with the actions of a hero or other exemplary character.

TRADITIONAL REFERENTIALITY AND MARTIAL/VENATIC IMAGERY

Ethnic groups in southwest China have been affected by waves of social and technological changes since the mid-nineteenth century and increasingly since 1949. Items related to warfare and hunting that are mentioned in living or moribund oral traditions and oral-connected written texts from ethnic minority cultures in the southwest are no longer common in everyday life due to the introduction of technologies such as muzzleloaders and modern cartridge firearms which made bows and spears obsolete by the 1930s or earlier, in addition to more recent restrictions on any sort of firearms. Yet the situation of working with imagery of material culture in these southwestern epics is unlike that of studying the same in historically or culturally disconnected texts like *Beowulf* or Homer's epics. The chronological proximity of the southwestern epics is often close enough to the actual period of use that many items can be readily identified and contextualized within remembered social situations by living informants or actual items can be observed firsthand in recently assembled collections in museums or occasionally in private hands. That said, some observations on these two classic Western epic traditions will contribute to our discussion of items of warfare and hunting in the oral and oral-connected literature of southwest China.[7]

Speaking of the imagery of warfare and warriors in the ancient English epic of *Beowulf,* Clark has noted in his discussion of the symbolic meanings of arms and armor:

> ...the multitudinous references and allusions to arms and armor pervading *Beowulf* constitute an imaginative whole, a symbol for the heroic life. Arms and armor, the tools of war and violence, are highly appropriate indices of the poem's re-creation of the heroic world and delineation of heroic ideal. The symbolic value arms and armor attain in *Beowulf* depends upon the contextual meanings the poem allows them and the associations these meanings carry.[8]

Andrew Lang, in a prescient discussion of shields and greaves in Homer in his classic *Homer and His Age*, comments discerningly on the appearance or absence of weapons in the narrative and their relation to the knowledge of the poets and their chronological relation to the text and archeological evidence.[9] Lang notes, among other things, that just because a Homeric poet does not mention an item in the text does not mean he is ignorant of it—rather, in John Miles Foley's idea of "traditional referentiality," such knowledge need not be wholly represented—a representative item or what might be called a constellation of "meaningful items" can act in the principle of metonymy to conjure a fuller dimension of the story context.[10] That said, to what extent the singers are consciously critiquing the historical accuracy of their texts is a question that can only be answered by fieldwork with knowledgeable informants.[11] A related issue is the aspect of the process of oral composition as it relates to the chronological currency of imagery in individual versions of oral and oral-connected texts. Does an individual text reflect items of material culture that were current at the time that the retelling got recorded, or is the text a vessel for images that may have existed in an earlier time and were obsolete at the time of collection? Ruth Benedict talked in her study of Zuni oral tradition of the phenomenon of items in a story that do not "tally with culture," which she suggested can sometimes be associated with what she called "cultural lag"—and what Barre Toelken might call the conservative dimension of the folklore process.[12]

Among the southwestern oral traditions in which imagery of martial and venatic items appear are origin stories, creation myth-epics, ritual and folk songs, bridal capture tales, migration and colonization narratives, legendary accounts of wars, personal narratives/hunting tales, folk dramas, festival, crafting narratives, etc. Specific imagery includes a variety of longbows and crossbows, spears, swords, knives, leather armor, horses and tack, dogs, traps, nets, and occasional references to firearms (cannons or smaller muzzle-loading weapons) and other similar weapons. Indeed, many of these items, such as crossbows, snares, and various traps were used in rural areas all over southern China and had counterparts in Northeast China, Korea, Japan, Southeast Asia, and elsewhere.[13] Such items of weaponry of war and the hunt are often gender specific and present in situations in which males commit heroic acts that range from shooting down suns, taming lightning, and killing or downsizing monsters, to rescuing female kin from raiders, killing fierce wild beasts (especially tigers) and transformational (shape-shifting) animals. In other instances, such items appear in tests of folk knowledge or contests of skill, often involving both male and female characters.

Archeological Evidence and Epic Correlates

Evidence from archeology and observable modern-era hunter-gatherer groups strongly suggests that such hunters typically utilize an array of "weapon systems such as bow and arrow, spears, clubs, nets, and snares."[14] This general assemblage of weapons corresponds quite well with items that are detailed in the oral and oral-connected literature from southwest China. Although virtually all of the ethnic groups in southwest China have been sedentary agriculturalists or seminomadic herders for the last few centuries, hunting has until quite recently supplemented the protein supply in many areas. Certain battle weapons can be utilized in some forms of hunting. Hunting has often been considered a practice for war among the peoples of East Asia, including the ruling elites.

A weapon type widely depicted in oral literature from China's ethnic minorities (as well as texts of the Han 汉 majority) is the bow and arrow, appearing in the form of longbows of various sorts and cross-bows. According to recent research, longbows and arrows seem to have originated between 30,000 and 60,000 years ago in the Upper Paleolithic and Middle Stone Age, with the earliest evidence found in Sibudu Cave, South Africa.[15] According to Stephen Selby, several types of bows were used in various places and eras of Chinese history.[16] Composite bows made of layers of horn and wood seemed more popular in the north and steppe areas, while wooden self-bows (made of one material) may have been more popular in the south due to the effects of humidity on the natural glues and materials used to make composite bows, causing them to delaminate.

Crossbows, mentioned in some recently collected narratives and songs from the southwest, may have originated in ancient China. Examples of bronze crossbow triggers and handheld stocks date to the 6th century BCE in Qufu 屈服, Shandong 山东 Province and the origin is likely much earlier.[17] Many examples of bronze crossbow triggers have been found in archeological excavations across the country. These include the tomb of the Marquis of Yi of Zeng (Zeng Hou Yi 曾侯乙) dating from about 433 BC in Hubei 湖北, southern China, and at the tomb site of China's first emperor, Qin Shi Huangdi 秦始皇帝, which dates to around 221–206 BC.[18] Dong Sun culture sites in northern Vietnam, on the fringes of the Chinese cultural orbit, date to as early as 100 BC.[19] Motifs of mythic archers and other instances of heroes and more common folk using weapons and tools of war and the hunt appear in various narrative situations within oral literature from the Yi 彝, Qiang 羌, Miao 苗, Yao 瑶, Zhuang 壮, Wa 佤, and many other ethnic groups of China's multicultural southwest.

Perhaps the most widespread motif in the mythology of the ancient Han people involving bows and arrows is that of a hero who shoots down extra suns that are overheating the earth and making it uninhabitable for life. Such accounts date to the early Han dynasty (206 BC–220 AD) with certainly much earlier antecedents in works like the *Shanhaijing* 山海经 (Classic of Mountains and Seas) and *Huainanzi* 淮南子 and relate how a heroic archer shoots down ten suns.[20] In Han traditions, a common name for this archer is Hou Yi 后羿. However, a hero who engages in similar actions appears in many non-Han mythologies, especially in southwest China. One example is the heroic figure Zhyxge Axlu who shoots down suns and moons that are overheating the earth in the epic called the *Book of Origins* (*Hnewo tepyy* in Nuosu language) associated with the Nuosu people of the Liangshan Mountains of southern Sichuan province. Representations in modern paintings, frescoes, and sculptures—which may be employing artistic license—usually depict him wielding a recurve bow similar in general outward appearance to Han, Mongol, and Manchu laminated recurve bows, which are different from the straight longbows collected among the Nuosu in the twentieth century, some of which are in museum collections.[21] Another version of the sun-shooting motif, as well as accompanying imagery of bows and arrows, is found in a cycle of Miao/Hmong epics from southeast Guizhou, discussed in detail later in this chapter. The relations between these ethnic minority myths and the remnants of Han mythology in texts and frescoes is still unclear, though the parallels are obvious. It can be assumed that the various myths and their versions are related to what epic scholar Lauri Honko has called a "pool of tradition" dating to early times on the landmass now called China.[22] The following sections will detail various situations in which imagery of bows, arrows, and accoutrements appear in these two epic traditions, which in some instances have parallels in recent vernacular culture.[23]

EXAMPLE ONE: BOOK OF ORIGINS

As the Nuosu epic of the creation of the earth and sky unfolds, the story introduces Zhyxge Axlu, the great culture-hero, who is a chimera combining human and dragon-eagle blood.[24] According to many versions, one day Zhyxge Axlu's mother Pupmop Hnixyyr was weaving under the eaves of her home when several dragon-eagles flew above her. Drops of their blood fell from the sky and she was impregnated. The resulting child acted strangely, so she abandoned it in the wild, where it was raised by dragons. Later, as the precocious Zhyxge Axlu grew up, he progressively began making and using bows and arrows of increasing power and efficiency. As the narrative notes, in his first year he made a child's bow of bamboo and grass stalks:

> One year after
> Zhyxge Axlu's birth,
> while out with those tending pigs,

he made a bow from a strip of bamboo,
using grass stalks as arrows.

By the time he was two he was using a bow made out of a bamboo stalk —a weapon with a much heavier draw weight than the bamboo strip of his first bow, and could presumably be used to protect the sheep he was herding. By his third year he was using a wooden bow, engaging in battles with rivals, and steadily engaging in proficiency. By his fourth and fifth years he was ascending in his role as culture-hero, investigating what I have called elsewhere his "eco-genealogy" by searching for his roots in the sky and earth. His accoutrements include not only four sets of magical bow and arrows, but magical armor and dogs and horses, all in sets of four.

A defining act of the mature hero is his setting the boundaries of the Yi areas (presumably in Sichuan, though possibly in the ancient Yi homeland associated with the border of Yunnan and Guizhou). The boundaries are established by the act of shooting arrows in each direction, with the spot each arrow falls marked by a stone. This proficiency with the bow in boundary-marking presages the act of shooting down the extra suns and moons created earlier in the epic. As time passes, the earth begins to parch and life-forms die off. In order to remedy the situation, Zhyxge Axlu attempts to stand atop a series of plants and trees in order to gain a shooting platform to down the celestial objects. In each case he stands atop a bush or tree which fails to hold him, and the plant consequently gains a feature (such as a bent stem) that distinguishes it down to today. Finally, the hero climbs atop a fir tree on mythical Turlur Mountain and is able to hit his marks. The fir tree consequently benefits humans in many other ways, including shingles for homes and shade for cattle. After demonstrating his skill with the bow to help humans, Zhyxge Axlu next uses another sort of weapon for the benefit of humans. In this case it is his fists, which he uses to smash snakes, frogs, and insects—which seem once to have been the size of dinosaurs—into the sizes they are today, and press them into their respective ecological niches.

Much later in the *Book of Origins*, after a great flood again destroys the world, a descendant of the survivor of the flood, named Shyplip Wote, is traveling about looking for his father. Before this time, Yi children supposedly did not know their fathers, so this is a part of the myth which Marxist-influenced Chinese researchers associate with the rise of patrilineal culture. On the way he encounters the daughter of a great local ruler, a *tusi* 土司 (Chinese term for local ruler appointed by Chinese state) or *nyzmo* (an Yi term approximating "*tusi*"), who poses several questions to him in order to gain her hand. With the help of his younger sister, Nyingemop Alat (who "knows everything"), Shyplip Wote correctly answers all of the questions, the latter of which has to do with small rectangular plates of stiff, lacquered leather that are laced together to form lamellar armor carapaces. The answers to the questions reveal detailed technological details about the construction of the armor:

> The upper part of the war armor—
> the war vest with the front and back—
> is missing a piece made from antler skin.
> The mid-part of the war armor—
> made of 6,600 leather plates—
> but lacking one,
> is made of the thick skin on a wild boar's neck.
> The rear part of the armor—
> that has two plates—
> is the skin of a water buffalo's knee.

In other words, each of the pieces in the armor references a very specific animal part suited to a specific purpose. The antler skin is from the very long pedicles (antler bases) on certain species of musk deer native to the Eastern Himalayan region to which the Yi would have access. The skin from the boar's neck and shoulder is in fact a very dense carapace of skin and integument well known among boar hunters worldwide today, who must take care in directing their shots to avoid it. Likewise, the skin on the knee of a water buffalo is very thick.[25] Thus, these images are excellent indices of the high level of place-specific knowledge of material culture associated with the epic tradition.

Despite receiving the correct answers, the *tusi*'s daughter decides not to marry Shyplip Wote, and he is later introduced to another potential mate. In this process, the motif of archery in relation to virtue is mentioned regarding his impolite treatment of his future in-laws, noting that when shooting arrows he did not properly attend to the needs of his friends. This strategy allows him to break off the unwanted engagement with this undesired bride. Later, however, he is introduced to a woman he is willing to marry, and again archery is used as an index of his treatment of his future relatives. This time he shoots arrows alongside his future relatives and inserts an arrow in his topknot when dressing up to accept the marriage.[26]

Although the entire accoutrements of the traditional Nuosu Yi warrior (*re ke*) are not mentioned (or at least not in as great a detail as some Mongol, Tibetan, or Han narratives), the images that are presented would likely work metonymically to stimulate images of the warriors in listeners' minds in terms of Foley's "traditional referentiality"—at least for those conversant in traditional warrior ways. What a fully dressed elite warrior would have looked like is hinted at by items on display in several museums in Sichuan today.[27] Moreover, in some communities in southern Sichuan Nuosu, males dress in traditional warrior garb (sometimes holding heirloom weapons) during parades held during the summer Torch Festival.

The images of martial culture in the oral literature support Professor Liu Yu's argument that the Nuosu, who controlled a rather large portion of the uplands of southern Sichuan and parts of Yunnan for several hundred years, had a strictly stratified society of elites, commoners, and slaves that was the basis of a "heroic age" with an ethos that included the demonstration of martial valor and ability in interclan raiding and warfare that ended with the breakup of the traditional order by the government in the 1950s. One saying reflecting the ethos of the former elites (the *nuoho* class) is, "One who deceives his own kin will be fined nine armloads of arrows; one who deceives his own family will be fined good horses."[28]

EXAMPLE TWO: HMONG ORAL EPICS

Hxak Hlieb/Miaozu shishi 苗族史诗/*Hmong Oral Epics*, is a trilingual volume based on narrative poems collected from Miao/Hmong groups in southeast Guizhou province beginning in the 1950s. The published text is comprised of a series of transcriptions based on oral performances of a number of singers. The collectors and editors were careful to retain the original wording and content of the passages, including rich imagery of material culture, which is supported by lengthy notes. The original sections of the epic, which no one singer knew in entirety, were woven together by the editors to form a sort of master text which was published in 2012. The printed volume exists as a monument to the oral epic tradition, which is in serious decline, and also serves as a potential resource for contemporary and (optimistically) future singers.[29]

The scene involving shooting down the extra suns and moons is the culmination of a long description of how the ancient mythic grandfathers searched the rivers and landscapes for gold and silver, which are described as children of mother earth. Once obtained, the metals are transported by boats to a construction site, then smelted and cast into orbs which are ultimately hung in the sky. After a while, however, the earth begins to overheat. The lines tell us that, "the soil looked like a bubbling cauldron of vegetable soup" (295).[30] An archer named Hsangb Sax becomes furious at the grandfathers and threatens to kill them. They counter, saying they had so enjoyed their work that they made too many orbs, then decided to make them come out at turns. But because the orbs were hard of hearing they all came out at once. Thus, Hsangb Sax decides that the extra suns and moons had to be killed, and he was the one to do it. On the way to carry out his deed, he encounters two young men who give him an ancient barbed arrow they had found in a field, its shaft marked with burn marks.[31] The lines in the following passages relate that[32]:

   ...
The two said to Hsangb Sax:
"While clearing the fields on the cliff tops,
we found a great arrow;
on the shaft are eleven burn marks,
on the head are eleven steel barbs.
Take it and shoot down the suns and moons!"

Hsangb Sax takes the arrow, but soon encounters another young man who claims that the arrow is inadequate—only good for shooting down smaller birds—and that he has a much larger one at home, and a crossbow to propel it:

   ...
Hsangb Sax ran into a young fellow,
clearing fields below a well-spring:
Old Fellow, where are you going?"
"I'm going up to shoot down the suns and moons!"
"That arrow is only for shooting owls,
for killing turtledoves for breakfast,
it won't do for shooting down the suns and moons.
If you want an arrow to shoot down the suns,
Come home with me to sleep the night;
I have a crossbow to shoot the suns and moons
It takes seven men to cock it,
and seven men to carry the arrow—
one pull of the trigger and it will hit the sky."

When Hsangb Sax went to shoot the precious objects,
he stood on the prow of a boat;
but the boat rocked back and forth;
it was hard to aim from the boat.

Where did he climb to shoot?
He scrambled up the cliff tops;
but on the cliff tops he couldn't stand steadily,
it was too hard to aim from the cliffs.

> He quickly climbed up a horse-mulberry tree;
> the horse-mulberry tree really obeyed him.
> In a flash it grew nine times its size
> until it was half as high as the sky.
>
> Hsangb Sax hurriedly mounted an arrow on the bow.
> he aimed an arrow at the head of each sun,
> and shot an arrow at each sun's heart;
> and shot an arrow at each moon's heart.
> The suns and moons all fell to the ground

In the aforementioned lines, Hsangb Sax, like Zhyxge Axlu in the *Book of Origins*, must find a suitable perch from which to shoot. In this case it is a horse-mulberry tree, which in today's world is a lowly shrub. What is of interest in terms of weaponry is the description of the working of the crossbow and the details of aiming, which suggest parallels with crossbows once used throughout China for warfare and those in recent use in for hunting in the southwest and Southeast Asia. In particular, the lines mention cocking the bow—a main feature in the mechanics of a crossbow—and pulling the trigger. The bow is aimed, with some difficulty, while on the rocking boat, likely in a stance similar to that of using a firearm, the tool that eventually displaced the bow and arrow in battle and hunting by the early twentieth century.[33]

In other instances in the epic, it seems that longbows, rather than crossbows are used. For example, after taking eleven years to successfully shoot down the excess suns and moons, Hsangb Sax returns home and asks his wife about their sons. In a scene that also has parallels in Han myths of Hou Yi, Hsangb Sax learns that one of his sons had gone out to hunt that day. He soon discovers the mistake he made on the way home. The lines go:

> On his way home Hsangb Sax had seen a young boy:
> "What are you up to, lad?"
> "I'm here to shoot geese."
> "Let's see you shoot."

"Grandfather, where do you wish me to shoot?
Do you want me to shoot out that owl's eye,
or shoot that goose's leg?
Whatever you say, I'll shoot it."
"Alright, shoot out the owl's eye!"

The boy drew and released his bow,
hitting an owl's eye dead center.
Hsangb Sax then drew an arrow:
"Only I can rule this place,
what are you still doing here?!"
...

Years later, after securing his place as the alpha-male of the area, Hsangb
Sax, his wife, and remaining son die and become three stars in the sky
—what Westerners call the belt of Orion, the hunter. Contradicting this,
the epic later on claims that they became various sort of insects found
in the rice paddies.

There are a number of other references to archery and hunting in the
Hmong Oral Epics. Hunting dogs play a key role in the passage entitled
"Hunting to Sacrifice to the Ancestors," which appears in a section
titled "Hxak Bangx Lief" ("Song of Butterfly Mother"). The song was
performed during lengthy rites to honor the ancient ancestors Butterfly
Mother (Mais Bangx), who laid eggs from which many life forms hatched,
including the progenitor of humans, Jangx Vangb, who survived the
Great Flood and married his own sister.[34]

In regard to the appearance of items of material culture that have
parallels in recent culture, there are repeated uses of a pattern that
directly compares practices and objects from contemporary times with
those in the mythic past. For instance, the rites detailed in "Hunting
to Sacrifice to the Ancestors" involve placing a wild animal skin upon
one of the drums used in the ritual. The passage details the hunt for the
drum skin, which is the skin of a wild goat, or similar animal. The epic
notes that dog and goat had once been sisters working together husking

rice in a treadle mortar, but got in a spat when the goat stole the dog's horns.[35] The epic recounts that when it was time to get the skin for the drumhead, Jangx Vangb went searching for an appropriate hunting dog. In the pattern, the epic relates that in present times hunters customarily go to the market to purchase a dog—but in the ancient mythic times Jangx had to purchase one from another mythic man named Liangx Tongb for 17 ounces of silver. As things came to pass, Jangx obtained a fierce dog with a hair whorl on its left side—which means it is good at chasing game up mountains, not the easy way, downhill, as a whorl on the right would indicate.[36]

After obtaining the dog the hunt ensues and finally the wild beast is chased up a mountain and cornered. At this point the lines question what sort of hunting weapon will be used to dispatch the prey[37]:

> As the wild beast was chased up the mountain,
> with what did Liongx Tongb point?
> With what did Jangx Vangb kill it?
> Liongx Tongb pointed with his finger;
> Jangx Vangb brought a horse knife to the kill.
> If an arrow had been used, it might have broken a leg;
> if sliced with a knife, it might have damaged the skin.
> They still wanted the skin to cover the drum,

A horse knife is a large utility knife; very large knives were used to sacrifice water buffaloes in the ancestor sacrifice rites. It is unclear what sort of arrow might have been used, though possibly a crossbow dart (a quarrel). In the end, Jangx Vangb used his fist to strike the animal dead. What seems important is that the skin should not be damaged when the animal is killed and skinned, with nothing more than the needed cuts. The passage in the Miao epic also describes how the prey, a goat, is caught in a fish nest (used to guard young fish fry) and is carried off by another tool—a wooden carrying pole, made of gallnut and birch, specific local species of wood. The final lines of the section state that, "Once caught, the buck goat had to be shared," suggesting the sharing

ethos of the real-life hunt.[38] This episode echoes an earlier one in which
an otter (the teeth and pelt of which are highly prized) was accidentally
caught in a fish net cast to find gold and silver. The captured animal was
clubbed to death rather than killed with weapons.[39]

The last section of the Miao epics recounts a perilous migration
westward of early Miao groups from their overcrowded homeland in the
east westwards through river valleys into eastern Guizhou. Along the
way, the migrants face many difficulties. At one point amidst hills that
have been scorched bare by wildfires and eroded by rushing waters—
which may be a reference to the downside of slash-and-burn agriculture—
they encounter a huge parasol tree protected by the Thunder God and
decide to make boats from it. However, in the tree is the nest of a giant
eagle, who wishes to protect its young and thus threatens the migrants
with the promise that it will "eat your mother" if they proceed. The
elders decide that this creature with "a beak as thick as fire tongs/ and
claws as long as harrow spikes" must be killed. But a few questions had
to be asked and answered:

> They needed to kill the mountain eagle.
> What wood was used for the bow?
> What vine was used for the bowstring?
> What wood was used for the arrow shaft?
> *Nongx hniangb* wood was used for the bow;
> *nongx eb* vine was used for the bowstring;
> *nongx hniub* bamboo was used for the arrow shaft,
> to make the bow and arrow to kill the old eagle.

However, the eagle is still alive. It is decided that it must be tried for its
crimes, the trial and sentencing presided over by an oriole, who wanted
only the eagle's chin as a reward. Thereafter the eagle was chopped to
pieces and boiled in a wormwood stalk—though listeners are told that if it
were today, a cooking pot made by the "skilled Han people" would have
been used. Once cooked, the eagle's parts were divided between two men
who spoke strangely afterwards.[40] The passage specifically mentions

the components of the longbow and arrows. Each of the components is very strong and durable, though I am as yet unclear if any of them was used in bow and arrow making in the past. The *nongx hliangb* wood is used to make carrying poles (which are bow shaped, but much heftier than normal bows); the *nongx eb* vine is a species of cane that lives in moist areas; and the *nongx hniub* bamboo is a solid heart species that would seem to lend itself to shaft making. It is interesting that a bow is employed to dispatch this creature of the sky, possibly echoing Hsangb Sax's shooting down of the extra suns and moons early in the epic cycle and the shooting of his dove-and-goose-hunting son. The reference to the Han people supplying cooking pots is only one of many references to cross-cultural trade and technological influences among numerous ethnic groups that appear in many narrative poems from the southwest. Among the objects that appear are items of metal such as pots, jewelry, and swords, and fabrics of cotton, silk, and hemp.

As material objects, the bows mentioned in the Nuosu epics are longbows, as supported by actual objects documented in recent use. In the *Hmong Oral Epics*, however, the bow used by Hsangb Sax to shoot down the suns and moons is clearly a crossbow, though the longbow is used in other sections of the epic, as well as one instance that references a pellet bow (a bow, often longbow in configuration that launches small round pellets instead of arrows). This difference in bows suggests different martial and venatic traditions, though crossbows do appear in some Yi narrative poems such as *Meige*, from Yunnan and have been documented among many ethnic groups in the southwest and contiguous border areas. Another factor to consider is that ancestors of both contemporary Yi and Miao encountered Manchu troops during the seventeenth to nineteeth centuries and possibly Han, Tibetan, Mongol, and Southeast Asian armies at much earlier times) and such engagements may have resulted in various sorts of cultural transfers, including weapons systems.[41]

CONCLUSION

This brief survey can only raise a few points about the imagery in the epics and its relation to real life that may have carried over from earlier ages, and later strata of content that suggests an accretion of imagery from contemporary society as the process of epic creation and transmission proceeds telling by telling in emerging cultural situations. In some cases, these poems may act as vessels which contain hints of earlier material technologies, some of which may be obsolete or obsolescent, and may also include images that "tally with" more recent practices and associated objects, some of which may still be current. One factor to consider is the different rhetorical traditions of the epics, some of which are more conservative in both transmission and performance, and others which typically display an emergent dimension that may encourage incorporation of contemporary imagery.

For researchers, major challenges in approaching this body of ethnic minority epic literature includes dealing with a diverse range of individual recitals and performance formats and differing processes of collection, editing, translation (many are translated into Standard Chinese), and publication. The published versions range from printed versions based on single performances to the common format of weaving several performances together to create a master text. It is understanding this process of textualization, as Honko has called it, that provides a backstory on a given text, shedding light on how to understand, evaluate, and appreciate the provided content and context.

For instance, in the 1950s, the texts were often written down word for word, sometimes translated on the spot in situations involving two or more languages and without the use of electronic recording equipment. In recent decades, improvement in collection technology has alleviated some problems inherent in that process, but other challenges remain. One big challenge is the loss of tradition-bearers who are competent in the local traditions of epic performance, have deep knowledge of the material culture that often forms the imagery, and can communicate their knowledge to researchers who in turn must be sensitive to the meanings and practices surrounding the objects.

As noted earlier, projects undertaken by the Institute of Ethnic Literature under the leadership of epic scholars Chao Gejin 超戈金, Bamo Qubumo 巴莫曲布嫫, and others have melded Western ethnographic and folkloristic theory with methods derived from Chinese fieldwork realties, creating such innovations as epic research field stations in the border areas of the country, the utilization of teams of experts to collect and process the epics and associated materials, and the use of current recording and archiving technology.

More research needs to be done on identifying the material objects found in oral literature of ethnic minority groups in China and about the technological processes, social contexts, performative, and creative dynamics associated with them. By doing so, we will more deeply comprehend the rich fabric of traditional technology girding the imaginative processes of narratives in these diverse oral and oral-connected traditions of literature, and enable further comparisons on many levels with other bodies of traditional lore within and without the region of East Asia.

NOTES

1. The following texts treat the subject of epics of the ethnic minority peoples of China: Zhu Yichu 朱宜初 and Li Zixian 李子贤, *Shaoshu minzu minjianwenxue gailun* 少数 民族 民间 文学 概论 [Introduction to Ethnic Minority Literature] (Kunming: Yunnan renmin chubanshe, 1984); Wu Zhongyang 吴重阳 and Tao Lifan 陶立璠, *Zhongguo shaoshu minzu minjian wenxue zuopin xuanjiang* 中国少数民族民间文学作品宣讲 [Selected Talks on Chinese Ethnic Minority Literature] (Kunming: Yunnan renmin chubanshe, 1984); Ma Xueliang 马学良, Liang Tingwang梁庭望, and Zhang Gongjin 张公瑾, *Zhongguo shaoshu minzu wenxue shi* 中国少数民族文学史 [History of Chinese Ethnic Minority Literature] (Beijing: Zhongyang minzu chubanshe, 1992); Lihui Yang, Deming An, and Jessica Anderson Turner, *Handbook of Chinese Mythology* (Oxford: Oxford University Press, 2005); Wu Bing'an, "Chinese Creation Myths: A Great Discovery," in *China's Creation and Origin Myths: Cross-cultural Explorations in Oral and Written Traditions*, ed. Mineke Schipper, Ye Shuxian, and Yin Hubin. (Leiden: Brill, 2011),177–196; "The Epic Traditions," in *The Columbia Anthology of Chinese Folk and Popular Literature* ed., Victor Mair and Mark Bender (New York; Columbia: 2011), 213–278.

2. Yu Xiaofei. *Kiki-ni hinsita chugoku syosuu minzoku-no gengo to bunka* [Crisis and Extinction of a Chinese Ethnic Minority Language and Culture] (Tokyo: Akashi shoten, 2005), 18–20.

3. For details on how Yi and Miao epics have been "processed" in the move from oral or oral-connected text to print and more information on the performance contexts of the epics, see Mark Bender. "Butterflies and Dragon-Eagles: Processing Epics from Southwest China," *Oral Tradition* 27/1 (2012): 231–246. For more information on narrative texts associated with funerals in Yi communities in northern Yunnan, see Erik Mueggler. *Songs for Dead Parents: Corpse, Text, and World in Southwest China* (Chicago: University of Chicago Press, 2017).

4. Mark Bender. "King of Yalu in Mashan, Guizhou: An 'Epic' in Contemporary Contexts," *Chinoperl Papers* 33 (2014): 82–93.

5. Lauri Honko, ed. *Textualising the Siri Epic* (Helsinki: Suomalainen Tiedeakatemia Academia Scientiarum Fennica,1998), 100–106.

6. Wu Yiwen 吴一文 and Jin Dan 今旦, ed., *Hxak Hlieb/Miaozu shishi* 苗族
史诗/*Hmong Oral Epics*, trans. Mark Bender, Wu Yifang, and Levi Gibbs
(Guiyang: Guizhou minzu chubanshe, 2012); Mark Bender, "Ashima and
Gamo Anyo: Aspects of Two 'Yi' Narrative Poems," *Chinoperl Papers* 27
(2007): 209–242; Bamo Qubumo, "Traditional Nuosu Origin Narratives:
A Case Study of Ritualized Epos in Bimo Incantation Scriptures," *Oral
Tradition* 16 (2011): 453–479.

7. "Oral-connected" texts, which are written texts that are closely related to
oral tradition by ways of origin and performance, are common in many
Chinese traditions. See Mark Bender and Victor Mair, "I Sit Here and
Sing for You: The Oral Literature of China," in *The Columbia Anthology
of Chinese Folk and Popular Literature*, ed. Victor Mair and Mark Bender
(New York: Columbia University Press, 2011), 9.

8. The quote is from p. 409 in George Clark, "Beowulf's Armor," *ELH* 32
(1965): 409–441.

9. Andrew Lang. *Homer and His Age* (CreateSpace Independent Publishing
Platform, 2006 [Reprint of 1905 edition]), 105–133.

10. For discussions of "traditional referentiality" and related concepts of
"metonymic referentiality" and "word power," see John Miles Foley, *How
to Read an Oral Poem* (Urbana: University of Illinois Press, 2002), 122–
123, and John Miles Foley, *The Singer of Tales in Performance* (Bloomington: University of Indiana Press, 1995), 95–98.

11. A related set of questions about the nature of traditional referentiality
and the oral literature of China's ethnic minority southwest is how references to weapons at one time in the past conjured images in the minds
of listeners who had, we can assume, a greater understanding of the
actual objects mentioned in the lines than contemporary listeners. Contemporary audiences, however, though deprived of the context of traditional lore, may have access to the recontextualized and assembled
displays of ethnic items in museums or private collections. Some with
access to other media may draw on the imagery of weapons—which may
amount to templates of what a bow and arrow might look like—provided
by various media such as the World of Warcraft game, kungfu movies,
or even traditional Chinese operas to create their internal visualizations
of what the characters and their accoutrements look like. In other words,
what sorts of imaginary worlds do contemporary audiences construct
based on templates of bows and arrows or spears and swords in the
hands of characters from other cultures and mediums in comparison to
imagery and referential systems of deeply familiar native contexts of the

imaginative? How do images and templates from other media "interfere" with existing story worlds an auditor may possess that are based on native, traditional experience with the local narrative tradition? While such questions are beyond the scope of this chapter, the factor of audience reception is certainly an issue.

12. For a discussion on Ruth Benedict's idea, see Robert A. Georges and Michael Owen Jones, *Folkloristics: An Introduction* (Bloomington: Indian University Press,1995), 163–164. See also Barre Toelken, *The Dynamics of Folklore* (Logan: Utah State University Press, 1996), 37.

13. For accounts of hunting tools in East Asia, see Chris Coggins, *The Tiger and the Pangolin: Nature, Culture, and Conservation in China* (Honolulu: University of Hawai'i Press, 2003), 216–230; Hiroyuki Sato, "Ethnoarchaeology of Trap Hunting Among the Matagi and the Udehe, Traditional Hunting Peoples Living Around the Sea of Japan," in Shiro Sasaki, ed. (*Human-Nature Relations and the Historical Backgrounds of Hunter-Gatherer Cultures in Northeast Asian Forests, Russian Far East and Northeast Japan.* Osaka: National Museum of Ethnology, 2009), 33–34.

14. Marlize Lombard, "Quartz-tipped Arrows Older than 60 KA: Further Use-trace Evidence from Sibudu, KwaZulu-Natal, South Africa," *Journal of Archeological Science* 8 (2011): 1918–1930, http://www.sciencedirect.com/science/article/pii/S0305440311001233.

15. Lombard, "Quartz-tipped," 1918–1920.

16. Stephen Selby, *Chinese Archery* (Hong Kong: Hong Kong University Press, 2010), 88–89, 154–155.

17. Stephen Selby, 2001, "A Crossbow Mechanism with Some Unique Features from Shandong, China," http://www.atarn.org/chinese/bjng_xbow/bjng_xbow.htm.

18. See Xiuzhen Janice Li, Marcos Martinon-Torres, Nigel D. Meeks, Yin Xia, and Kun Zhao, "Inscriptions, Filing, Grinding and Polishing Marks on the Bronze Weapons from the Qin Terracotta Army in China," *Journal of Archaeological Science* 38 (2010): 492–501, http://www.sciencedirect.com/science/article/pii/S0305440310003225.

19. Charles Higham, *Early Cultures of Mainland Southeast Asia* (Chicago: Arts Media Resources, Ltd, 2002), 176.

20. See Anne Birrell, *Chinese Mythology: An Introduction* (Baltimore: John Hopkins University Press, 1993), 77–79, and Lihui Yang, Deming An, Jessica Anderson Turner, *Handbook of Chinese Mythology* (Oxford: Oxford University Press, 2005), 232–233.

21. I have examined four Nuosu longbows, including one in the David Crockett Graham collection at the Smithsonian Institution. Rather than the typical composite bows of the Mongol, Manchu, Han, the Yi bows were made of single piece of hardwood and share a basic form. Cylindrical in cross-section they ranged in length from about 1.2 to 1.5 meters. As I have been told by local informants, some bows were left as natural wood, others were painted with black lacquer to prevent insect damage and increase strength. Fine threads of cow skin or hemp were woven into bowstrings. Although not recurved like Mongol-Manchu-Han bows, the straight limbs do exhibit a slight deflex. I will provide more details in a future study.

22. See Lauri Honko, "Text as Process and Practice: The Textualization of Oral Epics," in *The Textualisation of Oral Epics*, ed. Lauri Honko (Berlin: Mouton de Gruyter, 2000), 3–56.

23. Please note that Nuosu Yi and Miao/Hmong names are given in romanizations which employ roman letters as tone markers. These tones markers appear at the end of a syllable. Thus, the name Zhyxge Axlu contains an "x" at the end of the syllables "Zhy" and "A," which indicates a mid-high tone. These markers are not pronounced, per se. Rather they indicate the tonal profile. Some scholars do not include these final tone markers in writings in English as with some oft-used names or terms. For instance, Zhyxge Axlu could be represented as Zhyge Alu. The letters marking tones in Northern Yi (Nuosu) are: t (high), x (high-mid), unmarked (mid), p (low falling). More information can be found in Ma Linying, Dennis Elton Walters, and Susan Gary Walters, ed. *Nuosu-Yi-Chinese English Glossary* (Beijing: Nationalities Publishing House, 1991). In Southeast Guizhou Miao/Hmong, the markers, with corresponding numbers (first to eighth) are b, x, d, l, t, s, k, f. see Wu, et al., *Hxak Hlieb*, 711.

24. The observations presented here are based on a version of the narrative that Prof. Luo Qingchun 罗庆春 of Southwest University of Nationalities in Chengdu and I have been researching in cooperation with Jjivot Zopqu, a local tradition-bearer who rescued the text from oblivion in the 1990s by hand-copying a scroll belonging to a *bimo*, or traditional ritualist, and incorporating it into his own repertoire of oral and oral-connected texts. For more on this text see Mark Bender, "Snow Tribes: Animals and Plants in the Nuosu Book of Origins," *Asian Ethnology* 67 (2008), 5–42, and Mark Bender, "Butterflies and Dragon-eagles: Processing Epics in Southwest China," *Oral Tradition* 27 (2012): 231–246.

25. See Bender, "Snow Tribes," 2008, 39n47.

26. It is noteworthy that the bow is bronze, and that the hero has stuck an arrow in his hair. Though I have yet to correlate bronze to actual bows, the metal would certainly be a prestige material that could be associated with sincerity or social rank. The "arrow in the hair" motif is intriguing. Among the Apatani, a Tibeto-Burman speaking group in Arunachal Pradesh in Northeast India, the *mobi* shamans insert a small arrow (or "skewer") in their topknots. Certain aspects of an Apatani creation myth also corresponds to the story of the birth of Zhyxge Axlu, especially the motif of a vital liquid (in this case, semen) falling from the sky while the mother is weaving. See Stuart Blackburn, *The Sun Rises* (Leiden: Brill, 2010),145, 227.

27. Many museum displays in southwest China feature folk hunting tools and weaponry. One of the best exhibits is held in the main library on the campus of Southwest University for Nationalities (Xinan minzu daxue 西南民族大学) in Chengdu 成都, Sichuan 四川. Other museums with collections of hunting tools and weapons are the Liangshan Yi Slave Society Museum (Liangshan Yizu nuli shehui bowuguan 凉山彝族奴隶社会博物馆), Xichang 西昌, Sichuan; a small museum in the textile arts academy in Zhaojue 昭觉, Sichuan; Lake Lugu Mosuo Folk Customs Museum (Luguhu Mosuo minsu bowuguan 泸沽湖摩梭人民俗博物馆), Lake Lugu, Sichuan; Yunnan Nationalities Museum (Yunnan minzu bowuguan 云南民族博物馆) in Kunming 昆明, Yunnan; the early 20th century Yunnan Military Academy (Yunnan lujun jiang wu tang 云南陆军讲武堂) in Kunming; Guizhou Provincial Museum (Guizhou sheng bowuguan 贵州省博物馆); and a number of other local-level museums in the southwest provinces. From my own observation, it is noteworthy that the Yi weapons (several bows, arrows, leather carapaces, and helmets) collected by the American missionary David Crockett Graham in the early 20th century and housed in the Smithsonian Institution collections are very similar to the Nuosu Yi martial and venatic items on display in the Liangshan Yi Slave Society Museum and other collections in China. Moreover, many ethnic tourist sites in southwest China allude to aspects of traditional warfare or hunting activities and as late as the early 2000s it was quite common to see homemade muzzle-loading muskets at Miao and Dong 侗 tourist sites in Guangxi and Guizhou (See Andreassi, Katia, "China's Last Gunslingers," *National Geographic*, July 18, 2013, accessed May 4, 2017, http://news.nationalgeographic.com/news/2013/ 07/pictures/130706-china-guns-guizhou-culture-minorities/); bows and

arrows (modern ones) are often part of tourist activities throughout the southwest at places like the Qingyan Ancient Town (Qingyan guzhen 青岩 古镇) fortress west of Guiyang and around the Shangrila area of NE Yunnan. I wish to thank Carrie Beauchamp and Timothy Thurston of the Smithsonian Institution, Washington DC, for escorting me into the archives to examine the David Crockett Graham collection, and Yu Ming 余鸣 of the Yunnan Nationalities Museum (Yunnan minzu bowuguan 云南民族博物馆), Kunming for information on the Nu 怒, Tibetan, and Mongol crossbows, longbow, and quiver (respectively) in their collection.

28. Liu Yu, "Searching for the Heroic Age of the Yi People of Liangshan," in *Perspectives on the Yi of Southwest China*, ed. Stevan Harrell (Berkeley: University of California Press, 2001), 112.

29. The project dates to the1950s, when Jin Dan 今旦 and other young researchers, under the guidance of the groundbreaking ethno-linguist Ma Xueliang 马学良, began collecting parts of a creation epic that is performed in both single singer and antiphonal formats, the former means of transmission being primarily a teaching tool for novitiate singers. The project was disrupted during the chaos of the late 1950s through the late 1970s, but was revived by Ma and Jin in the late 1970s, resulting in the publication of a Chinese translation of the text. In the early 2000s, Jin and his son Wu Yiwen 吴一文 and daughter Wu Yifang 吴一方 again revived the project with the goal of creating a trilingual version. Although this manner of dealing with oral texts differs from other ways of treatment, the volume is nevertheless a valuable source of materials on traditional vernacular life among certain Miao groups in Southeast Guizhou. For more details, see Wu, et al., *Hxak Hlieb*, 689–696.

30. Wu, et al., *Hxak Hlieb*, 295.

31. This is an interesting detail of "folk archaeology" that suggests the Miao were aware of peoples who had lived in their regions beforehand.

32. Wu, et al., *Hxak Hlieb*, 297–301.

33. Robert D. Jenks notes on pp. 35 and 157 in *Insurgency and Social Disorder in Guizhou: The "Miao" Rebellion, 1854–1873* (Honolulu: University of Hawaii Press, 1994) that in the mid-19th century the Miao were armed with crossbows, swords, spears, and "fowling pieces." The latter were patterned after matchlock guns introduced by retreating loyalists seeking refuge after the fall of the Ming. Long-barreled smoothbore fusils (light muskets, or fowling pieces) are still in use today in a few ethnic areas of Guizhou, though their use was officially restricted throughout southwest China around 2000. I engaged in a shooting match with

Yi (Lolopo 倮倮泼) villagers in Chuxiong, Yunnan, in 1986. The participants were armed with crossbows, homemade fusils and a few 19th
century Enfield-style muskets. The guns used percussion caps and were
loaded with black powder (which was distributed to the contestants from
a common container), and steel ball bearings as projectiles.

34. Wu, et al., *Hxak Hlieb* 557–566.
35. Ibid., 561.
36. Ibid., 563.
37. Ibid., 565–567.
38. Ibid., 567.
39. Ibid., 197–201. The lines roughly parallel a section of the Yi epic *Meige*
    from the Chuxiong area of northern Yunnan, in which a muntjac is
    killed by hunters with stones, as detailed in: Yunnan sheng minzu min-
    jian wenxue Chuxiong diaocha dui 云南省民族民间文学楚雄调查队
    [Yunnan Province Chuxiong Ethnic Minority Literature Investigation
    Team] ed., *Meige* 梅葛 (Kunming: Yunnan renmin chubanshe), 68. See
    also: Mark Bender, "Slinking Between the Realms: Musk Deer as Prey in
    Yi Oral Literature," in *Centering the Local: A Festschrift for Dr. Charles
    Kevin Stuart on the Occasion of his Sixtieth Birthday*, Gerald Roche, et al.
    ed. (Creative Commons, Attribution 2.0: *Asian Highlands Perspectives* 37,
    2015), 99–121.
40. Wu, *Hxak Hlieb*, et al., 631.
41. In another dimension, based on ethnographic research among contem-
    porary hunters and gatherers, questions arise about the use of bows
    and arrows in traditional societies alongside other less refined and often
    "findable" weaponry. In several instances, prey or enemies depicted in
    the Yi and Miao texts are pounded with fists or rocks, rather than shot
    with arrows. (See Bender, "Slinking," 2015 for specific examples.) I have
    heard several contemporary oral accounts where rocks or logs have been
    used to dispatch musk deer or other creatures. In one instance, I was
    told about a college student from upland southwest China who, with her
    brother, encountered a beast along a river and clubbed it to death. They
    sold the pelt of what turned out to be a river otter for enough money
    to aid in college expenses. While factors of narrative interest and multi-
    layering of source materials in the storytelling process may be key in
    determining what sorts of implements are used in stories, it is interest-
    ing to imagine the non-use of arrows as a sort of economy of resources.
    Arrows are difficult and time-consuming to make and quite readily break
    if the target is missed, or snapped by the weight of the animal when

it falls. Thus, clubbing is a practical and effective alternative, especially when animals are immobilized by nets or entangled in vines, as we saw in one example earlier. Studies of traditional hunting societies support this idea.

CHAPTER 7

PASSING FOR CHINESE

READING HYBRIDITY IN WANG TAO'S 王韜 "THE STORY OF MARY" (*MEILI XIAOZHUAN* 媚麗小傳)[1]

Emma J. Teng

She exchanged her [Western clothes] for Chinese dress in order
to make herself into a Chinese woman...and no one knew that
she was a Western beauty.
　　　　　　　　—Wang Tao, "The Story of Mary," ca. 1887

Passing forces reconsideration of the cultural logic that the physical
body is the site of identic intelligibility.... For both the process
and the discourse of passing challenge the essentialism that is
often the foundation of identity politics, a challenge that may
be seen as either threatening or liberating but in either instance
discloses the truth that identities are not singularly true or false
but multiple and contingent.
　　　　　　　　—Elaine K. Ginsberg, *Passing and the Fictions of Identity*, 1996

In the late 1880s, eminent Chinese literatus and pioneering journalist Wang Tao 王韜 (1828–1897) penned a fanciful story for the Shanghai illustrated periodical *Dianshizhai's Pictorial* about an Englishwoman named Mary, who married a Chinese scholar, Feng, and returned with him to China.[2] The heroine of this classical tale performs two acts of boundary crossing: first, by marrying across the color line; and second, and perhaps more remarkably, by assimilating herself to Chinese custom —so well, in fact, that she manages to "pass" for Chinese.[3] Known for his blending of journalism with entertainment fiction, Wang Tao may have been inspired by the case of Ho Kai 何啟 (1859–1914), who married Alice Walkden, an Englishwoman, and returned with her to Hong Kong at the time when Wang resided in the colony.[4] The story, however, is imaginative fantasy in the *chuanqi* 傳奇 (tales of the strange) tradition, blending romance with foreign adventure and elements of the female knight-errant, "bewitching creature," and other character types.[5] Passing or masquerade was a well-established literary trope in this genre, and through the device of passing, "The Story of Mary" playfully calls into question the certainty of identity and the construction of "Chinese" (*zhong* 中) and "Western" (*xi* 西) as essentially distinct and mutually oppositional categories. It furthermore enables Wang to upend the convention of "gender inversion" commonly found in premodern Chinese literary and ethnographic representations of the foreign, suggesting the possibilities for domestication of the Other.

Wang Tao wrote this tale against the backdrop of emerging controversy among Chinese elites concerning the intermarriage of Chinese overseas students (*liuxuesheng* 留學生) to Western women, which was touched off by a number of marriages between Chinese scholars and Western women during the 1870s and 1880s.[6] Whereas cultural conservatives argued that such transnational marriages inevitably spelled Westernization and deracination for Chinese men, however, Wang's "Story of Mary" conversely playfully provided a fictional example of a Western wife who became Sinicized. During an age of mounting anxiety concerning Western imperialism and hegemonic cultural influence, Wang Tao thus offered his audience, in Shanghai and beyond, a means of imagining the transmission of cultural flows in the opposite direction, from China to the West.[7] The mode of fiction enabled Wang Tao to do something that could not be achieved through journalistic reporting with its privileging of "fact," for in literature, as Homi Bhabha has argued, one has the power to posit the counterfactual, the "what if?"[8]

The "what if" of Wang Tao's tale, in suggesting a model of transculturation as a two-way process between China and the West, speaks to issues that are still relevant in our own age, when the pace of global migration and cultural flows far exceeds that of the nineteenth century. Emigration continues to raise anxieties regarding deracination even as host countries wring their hands over failures of integration or assimilation. The very notion of assimilation also raises anxieties, and contestations over competing visions of national identity. It further forces us to ask what kinds of unevenness govern presumptions about "immigrants" versus "expatriates," and the respective expectations for assimilation that accompany such categories. Unlike assimilation, which is generally treated as a one-way process of cultural change toward the dominant culture, the notion of transculturation emphasizes the subordinate or peripheral culture's agency and creativity, and the notion of mutual, rather than unidirectional influence. In this respect, it comes close to the concept of cultural hybridity as theorized by Bhabha, with both colonizer and colonized changed through the imperial encounter. Both transculturation and hybridity are useful concepts for a contemporary reading of Wang Tao's "Story of Mary," though it was set in the semi-colonial context of Shanghai rather than a colonial context, per se. Especially noteworthy is the fact that hybridity in Wang's tale is embodied not only by the familiar figure of the Westernized Chinese, but also by a Sinicized Westerner, a figure that has received relatively little critical attention in our field.

Wang Tao: Reformer and Litterateur

Wang Tao is perhaps most famous as a pioneer of modern journalism in China and a reform-minded intellectual, but he was also a celebrated writer of both fiction and nonfiction. Wang Tao is thus a central figure in modern Chinese political history and also of great importance for late-Qing literary studies[9] A native of Jiangsu, Wang originally trained as a classical scholar, but spent most of his career working with British missionaries, from whom he learned the journalistic profession. [10] Wang worked for eleven years as James Legge's (1815–1897) assistant in translating the Chinese classics. In 1867, he was invited by Legge to visit Scotland, and he traveled in the British Isles and Europe for over two years. These experiences made Wang both bilingual and bicultural, and he became at once an influential interpreter of the Chinese classical tradition to the West, and a key interpreter of the West to the late-Qing audience. Although Wang Tao favored reform and modernization in China, it is too simplistic to say that he was "pro-Western," for he was also critical of the West and warned of the dangers that Western imperialism posed to China.[11]

In 1870, Wang took up residence in Hong Kong where he worked as a journalist, eventually cofounding a Chinese daily on the model of Western newspapers. By 1884, he had returned to Shanghai where he became a regular contributor to the *Shen Bao* 申報, one of China's earliest modern newspapers. A prolific writer, Wang produced several volumes of travel writing, fiction, essays, poetry, diaries, and editorials. Beginning in 1884, some of Wang's fiction and selections from his travel accounts were serialized in the widely read illustrated newspaper *Dianshizhai's Pictorial.*[12]

As Rania Huntington has argued, Wang Tao's literary work occupies a "special space between journalism and entertainment fiction."[13] The short tales Wang published in the *Dianshizhai's Pictorial* simultaneously served as divertissements and as vehicles to introduce readers to new ideas, information about the West, and current events.[14] Many are based on Wang's own travels, and they often contain ethnographic asides, or comments on geography. "The Story of Mary" belongs to this "special space," for although it is patently fictional, it may have been inspired by Wang's acquaintances (Ho Kai and Yung Wing 容閎 [1828–1912] in particular; Yung Wing married American Mary Kellogg in 1875), and it drew on his own observations of courtship, romance and marriage in Europe.

"THE STORY OF MARY" AND THE DEBATE ON INTERNATIONAL MARRIAGE

"The Story of Mary" first appeared in the *Dianshizhai's Pictorial* and was later published in Wang's fiction collection, *Random Notes of a Recluse in Wusung* (*Songyin manlu* 淞隱漫錄; 1887), which was widely reprinted throughout the Qing and enjoyed a broad circulation. To give the outline of the plot in a nutshell: Mary is the young daughter of a London professor. She falls in love with a classmate, John, with whom she has a secret love affair. Mary's parents convince her, however, to marry not poor John, but a wealthy suitor, Simon. After the wedding, John reveals the affair to Simon, who is so distraught that he kills himself. Mary decides to leave her troubles behind by traveling alone to China. On the boat, she meets a Chinese scholar returning from studies in the West. They fall in love, and marry, settling in Shanghai. John hunts down the couple in China, and the story ends tragically.

The story should be considered against the backdrop of an emerging late-Qing discourse on the question of whether the Western woman could make a proper Chinese wife, a question at the center of controversy surrounding the issue of Chinese-Western intermarriage–or more specifically the marriages of Chinese overseas students with foreign women. Whereas sinologist Henry McAleavy once argued that representations of romance between Chinese men and Western women were more common in late-Qing literature than depictions of the opposite pairing because this idea was less controversial for Chinese male readers, I conversely argue that this gender/race formula was prevalent precisely because the idea *was* controversial, and hence a focus of cultural anxiety.[15]

As I have demonstrated elsewhere, the late-Qing controversy surrounding "international marriage" was initiated by the weddings of early pioneers like Yung Wing and American Mary Kellogg in 1875, and grew increasingly heated from the 1870s onward as the numbers of overseas students marrying abroad grew.[16] Due to the fact that the vast majority of overseas students were male, the controversy mainly focused on Chinese men taking foreign brides. Moreover, despite the fact that overseas students also married Japanese women, it was the marriages to Western women that aroused the most controversy. These marriages drew backlash because they were associated with Westernization as well as with conversion to Christianity, both signals of cultural disloyalty and deracination in the eyes of conservatives.

Late-Qing discourse on this issue produced a contradiction in terms between the categories of "Western" and "woman." If "Western" was increasingly associated with imperialist aggression and foreign domination in this era, "woman" conversely was viewed as the subordinate gender. In the figure of the "Western woman" (*xifu* 西婦 or *xinü* 西女), these contradictions were brought together—and not always with a Yin and Yang harmony. By the final years of the Qing dynasty (1644–1911), opponents of intermarriage among overseas students would carry the day with arguments that the Western woman was a dominant figure incapable of submitting to Chinese expectations of "wifely conduct" (*fudao* 婦道) and hence would lead her Chinese husband to "forget the nation" (*wangguo* 忘國), successfully prompting the court to ban such unions in 1910. In Wang Tao's time, however, the debates on this issue had yet to reach this fever pitch, and it was still possible to imagine that gender would trump national origins in this figure of the "Western woman." In other words, the Western wife's inherent femininity would enable her to conform to the Confucian gender ideology of "thrice following" (*sancong* 三從)—daughter follows father, wife follows husband, widow follows son—and thereby assimilate into the culture of her adopted country. To understand how this discourse emerged, it is necessary to first understand something about the construction of the figure of the "Western woman" in the writings of Chinese literati of the time.

OCCIDENTALISM AND THE "WESTERN WOMAN"

Wang Tao was in fact among the first Chinese writers to provide detailed ethnographic and fictional portraits of the "Western woman," with Mary probably his most full-fleshed Western female character. In the opening of this tale, Wang Tao goes to some lengths to establish Mary's otherness as a Western woman.[17] Wang's construction of Mary's Westernness, which is both central to her exotic appeal and a necessary precondition for the plot device of her miraculous transformation into a Chinese woman, can be considered a form of Occidentalism, by which I mean the stylized representation of the West as other to China.[18] As I have argued elsewhere, the representation of "woman" became integral to late-Qing Occidentalism, much as it has been to Western Orientalisms.[19] Although I do not have space to elaborate here, in brief, I have identified three basic elements of this discourse: the construction of the "Western woman" as binary opposite to the (traditional) "Chinese woman"; the use of "gender inversion" (the reversal of normative gender roles) as a central trope; and eroticization.

Wang Tao, who in fact was one of the leading architects of late-Qing Occidentalism, employs these three representational strategies. He portrays Mary as not only incredibly beautiful, but also highly intelligent, educated, forthright, outspoken, independent, mobile, and willing to freely pursue romantic (unchaste) love. Mary's exceptional mathematical talents, in particular, establish her exotic Westernness by associating her with "Western learning" (*xixue* 西學) and distinguishing her from the traditional heroine of classical Chinese literature, who is typically gifted in poetry and music.[20] In addition, there are several instances of gender inversion, a common trope in premodern Chinese literary and ethnographic representations of the foreign, throughout the narrative.

GENDER INVERSION AS A MARKER OF THE OTHER

The first instance of gender inversion emerges with Mary's proposal of marriage to the Chinese gentlemen, Feng, whom she meets on the ship. He is initially reluctant to accept on the grounds of both cultural and class difference, but Mary eventually convinces him. Then, when the couple decides to settle in Shanghai, Mary buys a house and provides financial support for the family. The trope of gender inversion is the most explicit in a scene where the couple encounters naval skirmishes during their travels on the coast. Mary suggests Feng join the government forces, saying that a "real man" (*da zhangfu* 大丈夫) should make his mark in frontier combat, and further offers to follow him to battle. Feng is simultaneously impressed and emasculated by Mary's bravery, sighing: "I am not even as worthy as a kerchief-wearing woman. In vain I sport this beard and these eyebrows [symbols of masculinity]. I will follow you to battle."[21] During an ensuing confrontation with pirates, Mary puts her mathematical skills to use and devises strategies that successfully defeat the enemy, thereby earning the respect of the troops and making the mark that a "real man" should. In this scene, "real man" becomes a floating signifier, finally attaching itself to the Western woman and diminishing Feng's masculinity in the process.

DOMESTICATING THE OTHER: ASSIMILATING TO CHINESENESS

If Wang Tao participated in the late-Qing construction of the "Western woman" as the Other, in the second half of this tale he turns the "Western woman/Chinese woman" dichotomy on its head as he narrates Mary's successful transformation into a homely wife who can "pass" for Chinese. The term "passing" commonly refers to the assumption of a racial, ethnic, religious, gender, class identity, or a sexual orientation that by implication is not "one's own." The discourse of passing presumes that one has a "true," original, pre-passing self: as the *Oxford English Dictionary* (OED) states, "passing (for)" is defined as "to be taken for, to be accepted, received, or held in repute as. Often with the implication of being *something else*" (my italics).[22] Passing thus foregrounds a disjuncture between an essential, given identity and an assumed or borrowed identity, a disjuncture between how one "looks" and what one "is," between the inside and the outside.

If Mary's education, independence, and forthright nature are hallmarks of her "Westernness," what is required to assimilate her to "Chineseness," to convert difference into identity? Before examining this question, it is first necessary to clarify what is meant when we employ the English term "Chinese," and to note how Wang Tao conceptualized "Chineseness." There are several Chinese phrases that have been used historically to express various forms of identity that are lumped together under the English term "Chinese," including *zhongguoren* 中國人, literally, "person of the Middle Kingdom"; *huaren* 華人, "person of China" (*Hua* 華); *tangren* 唐人, "person of the Tang [dynasty]"; and *Hanren* 漢人, "person of the Han [dynasty/civilization]." Historically, these terms have often been used interchangeably, but there are important distinctions among their connotations, particularly between *zhongguoren*, arguably the most inclusive of all these terms, and *hanren*, which had become by the Qing a narrow racial category denoting the Han Chinese ethnic majority. Although it is impossible to define these terms with any precision, the phrase *zhongguoren* is generally associated with a geopolitical identity, with residence in Chinese terrain, and with loyalty to the Chinese state; *huaren* with culture and Civilization (as in the dyad *hua/yi* 華/夷, "Chinese/barbarian"); and *tangren* and *hanren* with the notions of lineage and shared descent from a mythical ancestry.[23] The proliferation of these terms thus reveals the complicated entanglement of nation, culture, race, and descent in the conception of Chinese identity, a conception that fluctuated historically. In the "The Story of Mary" Wang Tao uses the two terms *zhongguoren* and *huaren* interchangeably to denote "Chinese," but never the terms *hanren* or *tangren*. He thus employs more inclusive and flexible notions of "Chineseness."

Although I do not have the space in this essay to elaborate on the substantial literature on the question of Chinese identity past and present, it is important to note a fundamental tension in Chinese intellectual history on the question of whether non-Chinese could become Chinese. The idea of mythical descent from a common ancestor has played a central role in defining Chineseness in the past century, as Prasenjit Duara and others have shown.[24] Yet, competing notions of Confucian culturalism also informed evolving notions of Chineseness, rooted in the centuries-old idea of *xianghua* 向化, literally, "turn toward civilization," by which non-Chinese could be assimilated or "transformed."[25] This ideology, which Pamela Kyle Crossley has dubbed "transformationalism," provided a non-descent based foundation for Chinese we-group membership.[26] As scholarship on the Qing dynasty has amply demonstrated, this ideology did not always work in practice, and many Chinese historically were resistant to the notion that non-Chinese could be fully "civilized."[27] Nonetheless, it played an important role in Chinese intellectual history, with education regarded as one of the primary mechanisms for this "transformation."[28]

"SOUNDING" CHINESE: MARY BECOMES A "NATIVE SPEAKER"

How does Mary forge a new identity? After their military adventures, the couple settles back in Shanghai, and Mary begins to refashion herself from an unconventional Western woman into a proper Chinese wife. This transformation begins with language, as Mary hires a tutor to teach her Chinese. Whereas Mary had engaged Feng as her Chinese teacher during her journey to China, now that she is a married woman, she hires a female tutor in proper deference to Confucian norms of gender segregation. Instead of teaching English and earning money as she had planned when she set out for China, Mary now spends her days at home learning Chinese.

Figure 1. "The Story of Mary (*Meili xiaozhuan*)," *Huitu houliaozhai zhiyi*, 1887.

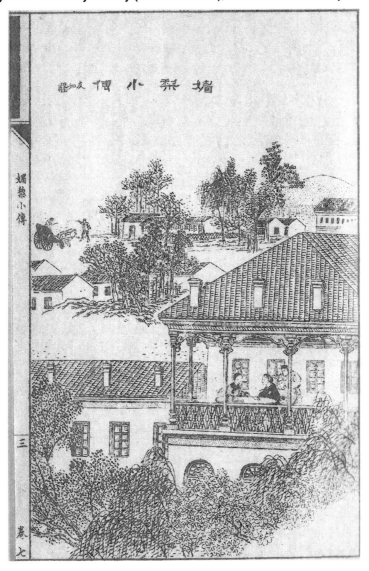

This pivotal scene of the narrative is illustrated in the *Dianshizhai's Pictorial*, which shows a picture of Mary seated across the table from her Chinese tutor engaged in study, with her husband looking approvingly over her shoulder (figure 1). The figures are seated on the veranda, properly ensconced in the domestic space. Mary and her Chinese tutor almost form mirror images of one another: although Mary wears a Western dress, it is plain and unadorned, and, in sharp contrast to other pictures of décolleté Western women in the *Dianshizhai's Pictorial*, her neckline is high and modest in the Chinese fashion; Mary's hair is swept into a low bun in the same style as her tutor. Just enough distinction between the two remains to indicate that one woman is Western and one Chinese. This scenario of tutelage represents both Mary's education in Chinese and the beginning of her "re-education" as a Chinese wife, as the theme of gender inversion has been replaced by idealized domesticity.[29]

Wang depicts language as a key first step in the process of Mary's domestication. As Wang writes:

> She engaged a female teacher to school her in letters (*wenzi* 文字). *Surprisingly*, she was able to wield a brush and learn calligraphy. She read widely of novels and anecdotal literature. She spoke language with a Chinese (*Hua*) accent, as fluently and mellifluously as an oriole trilling, and when listeners heard [Mary] from the next room, none could distinguish that she was a Western woman (my italics).[30]

I would like to distinguish here between Mary's ability to read and write Chinese and her ability to speak Chinese.[31] Mary's literacy in the Chinese language, and particularly her ability to write Chinese characters, marks her as civilized in Chinese terms—for literacy was central to Chinese high culture since antiquity, the written word possessing symbolic value lacking in the spoken language.[32] Based on this notion, Chinese political thinkers developed the belief that instruction in the written language, and by extension the classical Confucian cannon, was key to "civilizing" barbarians.[33] Mary's acquisition of this cultural capital

reflects her willingness to "submit to civilization." Wang Tao's use of
the word "surprisingly" here, expresses the notion that it is difficult,
even remarkable, for a Westerner to be able to write Chinese.[34] Mary's
mastery of the skill, therefore, signifies more than her linguistic talent
—it signifies her Sinicization.

If Mary's literacy in Chinese characters marks her as civilized, it
does not necessarily mark her as ethnically Chinese: after all, nonethnic
Chinese groups such as the Koreans also used the character system.
It is Mary's mastery of the spoken language, then, which she speaks
with a "Chinese accent" (*Huayin* 華音), that is more significant. As Ien
Ang notes in *On Not Speaking Chinese*, the ability to speak Chinese
is commonly regarded, among both Chinese and Westerners, as an
essential element of Chinese ethnic identity, even today.[35] Historically,
whereas the written language was associated with the universal notion
of civilization, the spoken language was more narrowly associated with
particularistic ethnic identities, not simply identity as a Han Chinese,
but more local, topolect-defined identities.[36] Wang never specifies which
"language" (*yanyu* 言語) it is that Mary speaks, but we might assume
from the story's setting in Shanghai that he means the Shanghainese
dialect of Wu. It is through her mastery of the spoken language that
Mary begins to erode the differences between herself and a local Chinese
woman as she becomes aurally indistinguishable from a native speaker.
At the same time, Mary's literacy in Chinese serves as an important class
marker, aligning her with ideals of gentry womanhood as evolving in the
Qing, which accorded a place for women as readers and participants in the
elite world of Chinese letters. Mary's choice of reading material, fiction
and anecdotal literature, is notable since the novel was long associated
with British women, but in China was a genre traditionally held in low
regard by elites, and fiction more broadly was considered less proper for
female readers than morally didactic texts on female virtue or refined
poetic works. Yet the late Qing was a time when novels and other fiction
gained prestige under Western influence and through the work of cross-
cultural mediators such as Wang Tao. By making his heroine versed

in fiction rather than poetry, Wang created a new model of femininity that merged both Chinese and Western characteristics, while perhaps promoting his own agenda with regard to raising the status of fictional literature in the Chinese cultural milieu.

"LOOKING" CHINESE: CULTURAL CROSS-DRESSING AND RACIAL PASSING

The second stage of Mary's transformation involves a change of clothing, like language an important marker of ethnic identity in the nineteenth century, both in China and the West. Following her mastery of the Chinese language, Mary "exchanged her [Western clothes] for Chinese dress in order to make herself into a Chinese woman."[37] In doing so, Wang writes, she appeared twice as seductive as before. The transformation is virtually complete, but for the fact that Mary still possesses several markers of her racial identity as a white woman. As the author tells us, only Mary's fair hair, blue eyes, and large feet "somewhat distinguished" her from a Chinese woman. Hence, she fashioned special embroidered shoes for herself, with pointed toes and rounded heels, drawing inspiration from Manchu "horse-hoof shoes," which enabled her to walk with a charming swaying gait and made her figure appear even more slender. "Her husband was delighted."[38]

This scene of ethnic cross-dressing parallels scenes of gender cross-dressing found in numerous classical tales, in particular in the work of Wang's precursor, Pu Songling 蒲松齡 (1640–1715). As Judith Zeitlin has demonstrated, in the Chinese literary tradition there were two branches of interpretation of female cross-dressing: the historiographic tradition, which treated cross-dressing as a dangerous and transgressive anomaly; and the romantic tradition, which treated female cross-dressers as virtuous and even heroic figures.[39] In the latter tradition, scenes of female cross-dressing are often lighthearted and mildly erotic, as a lovely woman is transformed into a pretty boy under her husband's gaze. The pleasure taken in transformation and illusion is the same here, with an ethnically cross-dressed Mary appearing doubly charming in her husband's eyes. As in many romantic stories of female cross-dressing, the pleasure is heightened by the imperfection of the illusion (as in pictures of women in male garb with tiny bound feet), which allows for the doubleness of woman-as-man, or, in this case, Westerner-as-Chinese.[40] (This doubleness was given visual representation in an unrelated item from the *Dianshizhai's Pictorial*, which depicted a boudoir scene of two Western women binding their feet [figure 2].)

Yet the act of cross-dressing is not simply a matter of playing dress-up; it carries with it the serious implications of boundary crossing, whether it be the boundary of gender or ethnicity. With clothing serving as symbols of social identity, the act of costuming allows the cross-dresser to assume the identity of the other. As Jean E. Howard has written in a study of cross-dressing and the theater in early modern England, "dress, as a highly regulated semiotic system, became a primary site where a struggle over the mutability of the social order was conducted."[41] Chou Hui-ling's study of the history of cross-dressing on and off the Chinese stage demonstrates that a similar situation pertained in late-Qing China.[42] Although these arguments focus on gender cross-dressing, Howard's point concerning dress as a semiotic system can also be extended to ethnic, racial, class, and other identities. Indeed, Pu Songling's *Liaozhai's Records of the Strange* (*Liaozhai Zhiyi* 聊齋誌異), first published in 1766, also contains several famous stories of animal spirits transformed into or passing as humans, and other variations on the theme of boundary-crossing through dress. Within these conventional frameworks, cross-dressing can thereby serve as a means of "trying on" or even permanently adopting a variety of other identities through the manipulation of sartorial codes.

In the context of the nineteenth century, when clothing was much more closely tied to ethnic or national identity than it is in our own age, ethnic cross-dressing, as a "struggle over the mutability of the social order," contested the notions of fixed cultural identities and ethnic essences, providing a means to assume the guise of another.[43]

Figure 2. "Western Women Bind Their Feet," *Dianshizhai huabao*, 1890.

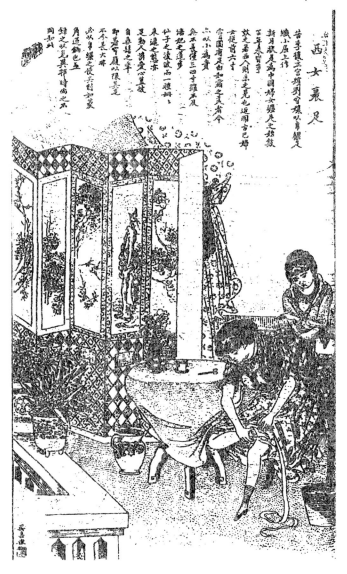

Christine Guth has written of the phenomenon of what she calls "cultural cross-dressing" in late-nineteenth-century Japan and America, including both Japanese who adopted Western dress and Westerners who donned Oriental dress. As Guth writes, these various practices of cultural cross-dressing raise "complex and challenging questions about the use of the body and its coverings to articulate social and ethnic differences."[44] Guth argues that in the context of Western imperialist ideology there was a general asymmetry regarding practices of cultural cross-dressing: that is, for an Asian to adopt Western dress was an act usually associated with embracing modernity and "civilized" behavior (though it could also be derided as ape-like mimicry), whereas for a Westerner to don Oriental dress was an act associated with a romantic retreat from modernity and with primitivism.[45] This asymmetry reflects the imbalance between the concepts of assimilation and "going native."[46] Sociologist Herbert Day Lamson noted in his study of 1920s Shanghai that Western expatriates virtually never adopted Chinese clothing, owing to the low-status associations of "going native."[47]

If the semiotics of dress within nineteenth-century Western imperialist ideology equated the image of the Oriental-in-Western-dress with civilization/modernization, and the image of the Westerner-in-Oriental-dress with "going native," Wang Tao's story complicates this association by representing Mary's ethnic cross-dressing as an element of her acculturation as a proper Chinese wife. In other words, he does not depict her adoption of Chinese costume as a rejection of modernity and a descent into primitivism, but as a gesture of Mary's identification with what she called the "most splendid" Chinese civilization.

The feet play an especially important role in Mary's ethnic cross-dressing, serving as the essential marker of Chinese femininity, for once Mary solves the problem of her feet she is able to pass for Chinese—her fair hair and blue eyes notwithstanding. As many historians have argued, bound feet became an important symbol of Han Chinese identity during the Qing, since Manchu women did not bind their feet.[48] Western women were similarly distinguished from Chinese women by their large and "natural" feet, a point on which missionaries fixated as a symbol of Chinese women's oppression relative to the West.[49] Bound feet signified not only ethnic, but also gender identity. Chou Hui-ling shows that one of the most famous Qing male actors of *dan* 旦 (female roles), Wei Changsheng (1744–1820) emphasized foot binding as a sign for "woman" in his performance style. Wei attached to his feet pieces of wood simulating women's bound feet in order to imitate a "feminine" walking gait.[50] Like Wei, Mary puts on her special shoes in order to both disguise her large, "natural" feet and to convincingly mimic a (Chinese) feminine gait.

If Mary's shoes are key to her ethnic crossing, these devices also draw our attention to the blurring of boundaries in this era: Mary after all takes inspiration for her special shoes from the Manchu fashion for "horse-hoof" shoes, a type of wooden platform shoe with a narrow platform stemming from the center of the sole that many believe was adopted by Manchu women during the Qing in order to mimic the "lotus shoes" worn by bound-footed Han Chinese women.[51] Producing a gait that resembled, yet remained distinct from, that induced by the tiny lotus shoes, the horse-hoof shoe at once subverted and reinforced the difference between Manchu and Han. Similarly, theatrical practice as exemplified by Wei Changsheng's false lotus shoes points to the blurring of the boundary between biological and performed femininity, and the production of gender as a realm of "play" for the consumption of Qing audiences. The figure of Mary in her platform shoes is thus emblematic of the third space of hybridity—neither Western nor Chinese, Manchu or Han, masculine or feminine—produced through the act of crossing.

Even more than Mary's change of dress, it is her performance of Chinese femininity that becomes central to her adoption of a new identity. If Mary's mastery of the Chinese language allowed her to "sound Chinese," her donning of Chinese costume allows her to "look Chinese." In her husband's eyes the transformation is complete; the disguise is so perfect

that none would guess the truth. He declares that he will now be able
to take her to his hometown in the north and tell his parents that he
had married a bride from South China (a region Wang Tao considered
"barbarian!"), "and none would be the wiser."[52] By way of her ethnic
cross-dressing, then, Mary effectively exchanges her English identity for
a new guise as a Chinese wife.

The ease with which Mary "passes" as Chinese suggests that the
boundary between a Western woman and a Chinese woman is permeable.
Feng's proposal of passing Mary off as a Southern Chinese woman,
displacing the difference of Westernness onto the regional difference
of Southern Chineseness implies that the distinction between Chinese
and Western is not absolute or binary, but rather part of a continuum—
such that with some slight of hand, "Southerner" (*nanren* 南人) can be
substituted for "Westerner" (*xiren* 西人).

Both cross-dressing and racial passing disrupt normative social categories of identity.[53] As in gender passing, racial/ethnic passing creates
what Marjorie Garber has called "category crisis": "a failure of definitional
distinction, a borderline that becomes permeable, that permits of border
crossings from one (apparently distinct) category to another."[54] Wang
Tao's tale of Mary's crossing from the category of "Western woman" (*xifu*
西婦) to "Chinese woman" (*Zhongguo nüzi* 中國女子) generates just
such a "category crisis." If the practice of gender impersonation (male-
female or female-male) in the traditional Chinese theater indicates that
gender roles are not necessarily mutually exclusive, Wang Tao's narrative
similarly suggests that Western and Chinese identities are not necessarily
oppositional categories. Elaine Ginsberg argues:

> Passing is about identities: their creation or imposition, their
> adoption or rejection, their accompanying rewards or penalties.
> Passing is also about the boundaries established between identity
> categories and about individual and cultural anxieties induced
> by boundary crossing. Finally, passing is about specularity: the
> visible and the invisible, the seen and the unseen.[55]

The notion of specularity is central to Mary's racial passing, as she simultaneously displays certain visual markers of Chinese identity while rendering invisible other markers of her Westernness, namely her feet. By manipulating these visual markers, Mary is able to affect her guise and cross undetected from one racial category to another.

Mary not only manages to "pass" for a Chinese woman, but to surpass Chinese women at their own game. When the couple travels to Hangzhou and other scenic spots, everyone marvels at Mary's exceptional beauty. When they invite famous courtesans to drink with them, none can compare with her loveliness: and "no one knew that she was a Western beauty."[56] Wang's fantasy of Mary's seamless metamorphosis into a Chinese woman, or at least a perfect copy of a Chinese woman, serves to interrogate the nature of identities, their creation or adoption, and their relation to the "seen and unseen." Wang Tao playfully represents race/ethnicity not as a fixed or immutable set of physical traits, but as something that is forged in a process of transformation or enactment. In Wang's fictional world, Mary's blue eyes and fair hair, as bodily markers of her racial difference, are rendered irrelevant in the face of her flawless performance of Chinese femininity. If theorists like Judith Butler have argued that "gender" is more performative than determined by the physical difference of sex, Wang Tao's story similarly prompts readers to consider the performative aspects of race and ethnicity beyond the differences manifest on the body.[57]

In this manner, like many other passing narratives, "The Story of Mary" disrupts the presumed naturalness of fixed identity categories.[58] Wang Tao does not entirely dismiss the notion of a "true self," however. In fact, Mary expresses some skepticism regarding her transformation. She tells her husband, in perfectly allusive classical Chinese, "to do it occasionally for amusement is one thing, but it would be difficult to imitate furrowed brows day after day."[59] The trope of "furrowed brows" is an allusion to the legendary beauty Xi Shi 西施 who was said to increase her charm by furrowing her brow. To "imitate furrowed brows" is to slavishly imitate, to adopt an affectation that is not true to one's nature. Mary thus sees an inherent falseness to her cross-dressing, which is fun as a game, but objectionable as a habit. To Mary, then, her "true self" is still an Englishwoman.

FROM BEWITCHING CREATURE TO FAITHFUL WIFE

Indeed, Mary's transformation is not destined to be permanent: for one day by chance she picks up an English newspaper and reads that her first lover John has arrived in China, planning, she suspects, to reunite with her. Instead of being moved by the individualistic romantic passion that first led to their secret trysts, Mary now allows duty to guide her actions. She thinks to herself, "I have now already found my better half. How could I go off with a scoundrel like you?"[60] This declaration contrasts sharply with Mary's attitude after her first marriage to Simon, when she still longed to see John. When John learns that Mary has married a Chinese man he is outraged. He stalks and kills her, symbolically reclaiming her from the Chinese husband. Before she dies, however, Mary reveals the moral transformation she has undergone on Chinese soil.

Aware of John's fury, Mary guesses his intent to kill both her and her new husband. She decides to kill him first, thereby taking vengeance for Simon's death and protecting Feng: "and then I will be able to face my husband in Hades," she thinks.[61] Spying John on her way to the theater with Feng one evening, Mary sends her husband back home on a pretext in order to keep him out of harm's way. Facing her former lover alone, Mary manages to shoot John as she is dying, simultaneously avenging her first husband and saving her second. Her heroic self-sacrifice serves as a means of making atonement to Simon for her unchaste behavior, both before marriage and later as a remarried widow. Whereas Mary had once been a woman of dubious sexual morals, by both English and Chinese standards of the time, Wang Tao now transforms her from the character type of the "bewitching creature" into "loyal wife."[62]

As in many classical tales, the ending supplies a resolution of the conflict between duty and individual desire. According to the traditional Confucian code of ethics, Mary's primary duty is to her first husband, whom she has wronged by her premarital affair and her second marriage. Through the act of revenge and Mary's own death, a rightful sense of order is restored. Mary's tragic death further implies that the interracial harmony depicted through her happy union with Feng is not to be, and the same might be said for Mary's life in the guise of a Chinese woman. American stories of boundary-crossing in the nineteenth century, including both miscegenation and passing narratives, often similarly ended in death, a punishment that restores order.[63] At the end of our tale, however, the West cannot fully reclaim Mary, for Feng buries her in China, giving her a final resting ground in her new home (and not alongside her English husband). Her epitaph reads: "The grave of a remarkable Englishwoman, Mary."[64] Mary therefore ends her life as both an Englishwoman and a Chinese wife.

Wang Tao's story thus raises the question: are these two identities compatible? On one hand, Mary's easy transformation into a passable Chinese wife through her acquisition of language and her ethnic cross-dressing suggests the performative nature of identity and the possibility of slipping between two identities—a type of ethnic code switching. On the other hand, Mary's tragic death and the final marking of her posthumous identity as an "Englishwoman" suggest that identity is fixed at birth and cannot be essentially altered. The performance of other identities is therefore nothing more than minstrelsy. Wang Tao leaves no final authorial commentary on the story, and the conclusion remains ambiguous.

CONCLUSION

The trope of passing in Wang Tao's "Story of Mary" prompts a reconsideration, in Ginsberg's words, of "the cultural logic that the physical body is the site of identic intelligibility," and opens a space for further reflection on the question of Chineseness beyond the limitations of racial descent.[65] Mary is not born Chinese, but *makes herself* Chinese. Hence, Chineseness appears as a matter of what Werner Sollors calls ethnicity as "consent" rather than "descent"—much in the same fashion as the pluralistic ideal of Americanness.[66] Playing with the idea that Chineseness is not only inherited, but also enacted, Wang's passing narrative disrupts the presumed boundary between Chinese and Western as mutually exclusive categories. In the third space of hybridity that ensues, new fluid identities emerge that are multiple and contingent, defying easy pigeonholing into ontological categories and notions of the essential self. In Wang Tao's own time, the fluid identity and third space of hybridity represented by Mary was perhaps only thinkable in Shanghai and other port cities that served as "meeting points" between East and West. Yet through this figure readers were able to imagine the multiplicity of possibilities and permutations enabled through the process of transculturation, viewed as a two-way street between China and the West, and released from the uneven power dynamic that structured most Sino-European encounters during this era.

For our own contemporary readings of this third space conjured by Wang's tale, the model of the Sinophone in many ways proves more useful conceptually than Chineseness for understanding the particular form of hybridity embodied in the figure of a Sinicized Westerner like Mary—one who in current parlance could be considered an "egg" (white on the outside, yellow on the inside). The Sinophone, as defined by Shu-mei Shih, is a "network of places of cultural production outside China and on the margins of China and Chineseness..."[67] It "disrupts the symbolic totality that is Chinese and instead projects the possibility of a new symbolization beyond reified Chinese and Chineseness."[68] Mary similarly works from the margins, producing her own Sinophone articulations as she participates in this linguistic and literary community, even as her ever-shifting and fluid identity calls into question the very notion of identic intelligibility. If Mary "becomes Chinese" through consent, she nonetheless refuses essentialist notions of such an identity. As Shih writes of the Sinophone: "the copy is never the original, but a form of translation."[69] Mary, after a fashion, represents a translation of Chinese femininity, with all the distortions, adaptations and incompleteness that translation entails: and therein lies her charm for Feng and for readers of Wang's fanciful tale.

By examining hybridity in the figure of a Sinicized Westerner and biculturalism as a two-way dynamic, my reading of Wang Tao's "Story of Mary" suggests the need to reconsider what asymmetries govern our general reluctance to critique the privileging of descent and blood ties in contemporary models of Chinese identity, even as we advocate multiculturalism and multiracialism in US society.[70] In this, do we not privilege American identity as the modern notion of consent, while relegating Chinese identity to the "old world" notion of descent? Do not our general presumptions regarding assimilation as a cultural process that flows in only one direction (toward the West) ironically reinforce notions of American soft-power superiority? Wang Tao's narrative of "passing for Chinese," with its delightful fictional heroine, Mary, provides much food for thought.

NOTES

1. An earlier discussion of Wang Tao's story was presented as "Can the Western Woman (*xifu*) Make a Proper Chinese Wife? The Ambivalent Discourse on Intermarriage during the Late Qing," at the China Gender Studies Workshop, Fairbank Center for East Asian Research, Harvard University. Thank you to the organizers and participants for their invaluable feedback. Thank you also to the anonymous reviewers of this volume.

2. Tao Wang, *Songyin Manlu* (Shanghai: Dianshizhai, 1887). It is difficult to pinpoint when exactly this story was written. It can be dated to sometime between the second half of 1884 and 1887. See *Zhongguo wenyan xiaoshuo zongmu tiyao*, 363.

3. Although critics like Marion Rust suggest that the "original" meaning of "passing" is to "pass for White," a search of the *Oxford English Dictionary* (OED) reveals that Joseph Addison used the term "pass for a Jew" as early as 1711.

4. Ho returned to Hong Kong from his studies in England with his new bride in 1882, during the time when Wang was in residence there, and the couple became quite prominent in society. Like Wang Tao's Mary, Alice was both well-educated and a woman of some means, suggesting her as a possible loose model or at least inspiration for Wang's heroine. See Paul A. Cohen, *Between Tradition and Modernity: Wang T'ao and Reform in Late Ch'ing China* (Cambridge, MA: Harvard University Press, 1974).

5. The theme of boundary-crossing was common in the genre of the Chinese classical tale, or "tale of the strange" (*chuanqi*), as Judith Zeitlin and others have demonstrated. Using this theme, authors like Pu Songling (who served as an important model for Wang) contested the boundaries between human and the supernatural, male and female, the real and the unreal. See Judith T. Zeitlin, *Historian of the Strange: Pu Songling and the Chinese Classical Tale* (Stanford: Stanford University Press, 1993).

6. In 1875, Yung Wing (1828–1912), the first Chinese student to graduate from Yale (1854), married American Mary Louise Kellogg (1851–1886), the daughter of a prominent Hartford, Connecticut family. See Emma J.Teng, *Eurasian: Mixed Identities in the United States, China, and Hong Kong, 1842-1943* (Berkeley: University of California Press, 2013).

7. On the audience for this pictorial and other newspapers in China, see Barbara Mittler, *A Newspaper for China? Power, Identity, and Change in Shanghai's News Media, 1872–1912* (Cambridge, MA: Harvard University Asia Center, 2004).

8. Homi Bhabha, comments at the symposium on Beyond US Multiculturalism? Asian Diasporas and New Transnational Cultures," sponsored by the Center for Bilingual/Bicultural Studies, MIT, October 2003.

9. Indeed, Henry McAleavy called Wang Tao one of the most representative Chinese writers of the 1870s and 1880s. Henry McAleavy, *Wang T'ao (1828?–1890) the Life and Writings of a Displaced Person. With a Translation of Mei-Li Hsiao Chuan, a Short Story by Wang T'ao* (London: China Society, 1953).

10. For more on Wang Tao, see Cohen, *Between Tradition and Modernity;* Rania Huntington, "The Weird in the Newspaper," in *Writing and Materiality in China: Essays in Honor of Patrick Hanan,* eds. Judith Zeitlin, Lydia H. Liu, and Ellen Widmer (Cambridge, MA: Harvard University Asia Center for Harvard-Yenching Institute, 2003), 341–96; Chi-fang Lee, "Wang T'ao and His Literary Writings," *Tamkang Review* 9 (1981): 267–85; Chi-fang Lee, "Wang T'ao (1828–1897): His Life, Thought, Scholarship, and Literary Acheivement" (PhD diss., University of Wisconsin-Madison, 1973); and Elizabeth Sinn, "Fugitive in Paradise: Wang Tao and Cultural Transformation in Late Nineteenth-Century Hong Kong," *Late Imperial China* 19 (1998): 56–81.

11. Wang was also sensitive to the mistreatment suffered by Chinese from arrogant Westerners, convinced of their civilizational superiority both at home and abroad. Wang had this to say in his diary about the Westerners in Shanghai: "When you look at the foreigners with their high noses and deep-set eyes, you can sense how crafty they are. They treat all Chinese very shabbily, and they make the house servants work like animals without the slightest pity. They despise people of education like ourselves and never bother to show us the least courtesy.... [because of China's poverty] Chinese gentlemen find they have no alternative to putting up with this contempt." Quoted in McAleavy, *Wang T'ao,* 6. Indeed, Paul Cohen called Wang Tao an "incipient" Chinese nationalist. See Cohen, *Between Tradition and Modernity.*

12. This publication, which Barbara Mittler has shown was aimed at both the male and female audiences, was an important vehicle for disseminating knowledge about the West, as well as the new hybrid culture of treaty-port Shanghai in the late Qing. As Barbara Mittler has argued, late-Qing

pictorials were aimed at a wide range of readers, including gentlemen, merchants, peasants, and women. Mittler, *A Newspaper for China*, 251. However, since Wang Tao's stories were written in classical Chinese, it is likely that the majority of his readers were educated men and elite women.

13. See Huntington, "The Weird in the Newspaper."
14. Several of the stories that Wang penned for the *Dianshizhai's Pictorial* in the late 1880s concerned relationships between Chinese scholars and Western women, some set in the West and some in China. See Emma J. Teng, "The West as a Kingdom of Women: Woman and Occidentalism in Wang Tao's Tales of Travel," in *Traditions of East Asian Travel*, ed. Joshua A. Fogel (London: Berghahn Books, 2006).
15. See Henry McAleavy, *That Chinese Woman: The Life of Sai-Chin-Hua, 1874–1936* (New York: Crowell, 1959).
16. See Teng, *Eurasian*. See Frank Dikötter, *The Discourse of Race in Modern China* (Stanford: Stanford University Press, 1992), 57–60.
17. The term "Western woman" (*xinü* or *xifu*), like the broader Qing term "Westerner" (*xiren*), homogenizes the various nationalities of the West, including Russians, Western Europeans, and North Americans (and sometimes Latin Americans). At the same time, it establishes a sharp distinction between Chinese and all Westerners. Despite the significant cultural differences between English, French, American, Russian, and other Western women (of which Qing writers like Wang Tao were not unaware), the frequent deployment of the term "*xifu*" in late-Qing sources meant that the construct of the "Western woman" took on a life of her own—primarily as a radically different figure from the "traditional Chinese woman." See Emma J. Teng, "The Construction of the 'Traditional Chinese Woman' in the Western Academy: A Critical Review," *Signs: Journal of Women in Culture and Society* 22 (1996): 115–151. This construct was produced in concert between Westerners in China, especially missionaries, and Chinese literati like Wang Tao, particularly those who had traveled to the West. See Susan Mann, *Precious Records: Women in China's Long Eighteenth Century* (Stanford: Stanford University Press, 1997), 8.
18. Late-Qing Occidentalism should be understood both within the context of a long tradition of representing "Barbarians" in the Chinese historiographic and literary genres, and within the context of Western claims to cultural superiority that were being introduced with increasing force into China at the time Wang Tao was writing.

19. For the details of my argument, see Teng, "The West as a Kingdom of Women." One important difference between late-Qing Occidentalism and contemporaneous Orientalisms arises from the fact that these modes of representation were produced within the context of uneven power relations between China and the West after the mid-nineteenth century. Hence, the image of a feminized West, as represented in Wang Tao's fiction, coexisted with late-Qing impressions of a masculinized, aggressive West.

20. See Wai-Yee Li, "Heroic Transformations: Women and National Trauma in Early Qing Literature," *Harvard Journal of Asiatic Studies* 59, no. 2 (December, 1999): 363–443.

21. See Wang Tao, *Hou Liaozhai Zhiyi Quanyi Xiangzhu* (Ha'erbin: Heilongjiang renmin chubanshe, 1988).

22. See the OED.

23. On the differences between various concepts of Chineseness, see David Yen-ho Wu, "The Construction of Chinese and Non-Chinese Identities," in *The Living Tree: The Changing Meaning of Being Chinese Today*, ed. Wei-ming Tu (Stanford: Stanford University Press, 1994); and Allen Chun, "Fuck Chineseness: On the Ambiguities of Ethnicity as Culture as Identity," *boundary 2* 23, no. 2 (1996): 111–138. On the concept of the Chinese *minzu*, see Joshua Fogel "Race and Class in Chinese Historiography," *Modern China* 3 (July, 1977): 346–375.

24. Prasenjit Duara, *Rescuing History from the Nation: Questioning Narratives of Modern China* (Chicago: University of Chicago Press, 1995).

25. On the historical assimilation of minorities in China, see Wu, "The Construction of Chinese."

26. Pamela Kyle Crossley, *A Translucent Mirror: History and Identity in Qing Imperial Ideology* (Berkeley: University of California Press, 1999).

27. See James A. Millward, *Beyond the Pass: Economy, Ethnicity, and Empire in Qing Central Asia, 1759–1864* (Stanford, CA: Stanford University Press, 1998); Emma J. Teng, *Taiwan's Imagined Geography: Chinese Colonial Travel Writing and Pictures, 1683–1895* (Cambridge, MA: Harvard University Asia Center, 2004); and Peter C. Perdue, "Erasing the Empire, Re-racing the Nation: Racialism and Culturalism in Imperial China," in *Imperial Formations*, eds. Ann Laura Stoler, Carole McGranahan, and Peter C. Perdue (Santa Fe, NM: School for Advanced Research Press, 2007), 141–169.

28. See Crossley, *A Translucent Mirror*.

29. This image forms a sharp contrast to a smaller picture of Mary in the background, which presents her in her Western guise. In a minuscule vignette, heroic Mary is represented riding alone in an open carriage on the streets, wearing a wasp-waisted Victorian dress and a hat, with a pistol in her hand, shooting the villain John. We thus have two images of Mary: Mary as a heroic Western woman, and Mary as a domestic Chinese wife, underscoring the remarkable nature of her crossing between these two identities. That the shooting scene, which represents the climax of the narrative, is greatly overshadowed by the more prominent picture of Mary's learning Chinese[ness] in the foreground suggests that the illustrator believed the latter would appear more novel or astonishing to readers. See Wang, *Songyin Manlu*.
30. See Wang, *Songyin Manlu*.
31. Wang presents a Sinocentric view of the Chinese language in this passage, calling the Chinese character system simply "letters/writing" (*wenzi*), and the spoken Chinese language simply "language" (*yanyu*). (Although not technically correct, I have employed the term "letters" as a translation for *wenzi* in order to capture the multiple meanings of the latter as "learning, literature, and written symbol.") By implication then, "to speak" and "to write" means to speak and write Chinese, the universal language of the civilized.
32. The knowledge of writing, which ancient myths held was given to the Chinese by the sage kings Fu Xi and Huang Di, distinguished those who were civilized from the barbarians, who had not been endowed with the teachings of the sage kings. As Mark Edward Lewis has demonstrated, since early Chinese history, writing and texts had become fundamental to cultural and state authority. See Mark E. Lewis, *Writing and Authority in Early China* (Albany: State University of New York Press, 1999).
33. See Emma J. Teng, "Taiwan as a Living Museum: Tropes of Anachronism in Late-Imperial Chinese Travel Writing," *The Harvard Journal of Asiatic Studies* 59, no.2 (1999): 445–484.
34. As Patrick Hanan has documented in his work on the missionary novels, due to the difficulty of mastering written Chinese, particularly classical Chinese, Western missionaries in China typically used Chinese "pundits" to aid them in translation and the composition of Chinese works. Wang Tao worked in this capacity for James Legge. See Patrick Hanan, "The Missionary Novels of Nineteenth-Century China," *Harvard Journal of Asiatic Studies* 60, no. 2 (2000): 413–444.

35. See Ien Ang, *On Not Speaking Chinese: Living Between Asia and the West* (London: Routledge, 2001), 23, 27, 50.
36. See, for example, Wu, "The Construction of Chinese"; and Victor H. Mair, "What Is a Chinese 'Dialect/Topolect'? Reflections on Some Key Sino-English Linguistic Terms," *Sino-Platonic Papers* (1991).
37. See Wang, *Hou Liaozhai Zhiyi.*
38. Ibid.
39. See Zeitlin, *Historian of the Strange.*
40. See illustrations in Zeitlin, *Historian of the Strange;* and Hui-ling Chou, "Striking Their Own Poses: The History of Cross-Dressing on the Chinese Stage," *The Drama Review* 41, no. 2 (Summer, 1997): 130–152.
41. See Jean E. Howard, "Cross-Dressing, the Theater, and Gender Struggle in Early Modern England," in *Crossing the Stage: Controversies on Cross-Dressing,* ed. Lesley Ferris (New York: Routledge, 1993), 20–46.
42. See Chou, "Striking Their Own Poses."
43. Like gender cross-dressing, ethnic cross-dressing encompasses a range of practices, including impersonation, masquerade, and crossing over.
44. See Christine M. E. Guth, "Charles Longfellow and Okakura Kakuzō: Cultural Cross-Dressing in the Colonial Context," *positions: east asia cultures critique* 8, no. 3 (Winter, 2000): 600.
45. Guth argues that individuals like Charles Longfellow and Okakura Kakuzo employed cultural cross-dressing to subversive ends. As she writes: "By donning exotic, often provocative, clothing from cultures other than their own, they expressed ideas about themselves, about their society, and ultimately about ethnic identity, in ways that simultaneously reinforced and subverted dominant colonial ideologies." See Guth, "Cultural Cross-Dressing," 607.
46. Guth, "Cultural Cross-Dressing." Although the adoption of Western-style clothing did not become widespread in China until after the founding of the new Republic in 1912, by the late nineteenth century a limited number of Chinese, particularly those like Yung Wing who traveled abroad, had already begun to engage in the practice of cultural cross-dressing, and by the fin-de-siecle, the streets of Shanghai were filled with young men and women dressed in foreign clothes. See Mittler, *A Newspaper for China,* 340. At the time Wang Tao wrote "The Story of Mary," however, cultural cross-dressing in China was still a "new" and unusual phenomenon, a phenomenon with strong connotations of crossing ethnic boundaries. Wang Tao himself made a strong point of wearing Chinese clothing when traveling abroad.

47. Herbert Day Lamson, "The American Community in Shanghai" (PhD dissertation, Harvard University, 1935).
48. See Dorothy Ko, "The Body as Attire: The Shifting Meanings of Foot-binding in Seventeenth-Century China," *Journal of Women's History* 8, no. 4 (Winter, 1997): 8; Dorothy Ko, *Every Step a Lotus: Shoes for Bound Feet* (Berkeley: University of California Press, 2001); Patricia Buckley Ebrey, *The Inner Quarters: Marriage and the Lives of Chinese Women in the Sung Period* (Berkeley: University of California Press, 1993); and Mann, *Precious Records*.
49. See Dorothy Ko, *Teachers of the Inner Chambers: Women and Culture in Seventeenth-Century China* (Stanford: Stanford University Press, 1994); and Hanan, "The Missionary Novels."
50. See Chou, "Striking Their Own Poses."
51. Mark C. Elliott, *The Manchu Way: The Eight Banners and Ethnic Identity in Late Imperial China* (Stanford: Stanford University Press, 2001), 247.
52. Feng's suggestion of deception indicates a conflict inherent in international marriage that has not been mentioned so far in the story. That is, the possibility that the marriage may not be acceptable to the parents. Yet this conflict is no different from that commonly found in classical tales involving "love marriages," whether to courtesans, ghosts, or fox-fairies. Arranged marriages were still the norm in China at the time.
53. Cross-dressing is intimately related to passing, but encompasses a wider range of practices.
54. See Marjorie B. Garber, *Vested Interests: Cross-Dressing and Cultural Anxiety* (New York: Routledge, 1992), 16.
55. See Elaine K. Ginsberg, "Introduction: The Politics of Passing," in *Passing and the Fictions of Identity*, ed. Elaine K. Ginsberg, (Durham: Duke University Press, 1996), 1–18.
56. Wang, *Hou Liaozhai Zhiyi*.
57. See Judith Butler, *Gender Trouble: Feminism and the Subversion of Identity* (New York: Routledge, 1990).
58. As Marion Rust has written of passing in British literature, the phenomenon ridicules "essentialist notions of a 'true' self preceding, and corrupted by, its subsequent enactments. In a sense, passing foregrounds what is between—between origin and enactment, body and gesture—calling into question all such fixed ways of determining identity." See Marion Rust, "The Subaltern as Imperialist: Speaking of Olaudah Equiano," in *Passing and the Fictions of Identity*, ed. Elaine Ginsburg (Durham: Duke University Press, 1996), 21–36.

59. Wang, *Hou Liaozhai Zhiyi.*
60. Ibid., 820.
61. Ibid.
62. On Confucian values and the limitations of Confucian gender ideology, see Ko, *Teachers of the Inner Chambers.*
63. See Gina Marchetti, *Romance and the "Yellow Peril": Race, Sex, and Discursive Strategies in Hollywood Fiction* (Berkeley: University of California Press, 1993); Werner Sollors, ed., *Interracialism: Black-White Intermarriage in American History, Literature, and Law* (Oxford: Oxford University Press, 2000); Ginsberg, *Passing,* and Gayle Freda Wald, *Crossing the Line: Racial Passing in Twentieth-Century U.S. Literature and Culture* (Durham, NC: Duke University Press, 2000).
64. Wang, *Hou Liaozhai Zhiyi.*
65. Ginsberg, *Passing.*
66. Sollors, *Interracialism.*
67. Shu-mei Shih, *Visuality and Identity: Sinophone Articulations Across the Pacific* (Berkeley: University of California Press, 2007).
68. Ibid., 35.
69. Ibid., 5.
70. For example, according to *Wikipedia*: "Chinese people are the various individuals or groups of people associated with China (or Greater China), either by reason of ancestry, heredity, ethnicity, nationality, citizenship, place of residence, or other affiliation." See https://en.wikipedia.org/wiki/Chinese_people. In contrast: "Americans are citizens of the United States of America. The country is home to people of many different national origins. As a result, Americans do not equate their nationality with ethnicity, but with citizenship and allegiance. Although citizens make up the majority of Americans, non-citizen residents, dual citizens, and expatriates may also claim an American identity." See https://en.wikipedia.org/wiki/Americans.

CHAPTER 8

LEARNING FROM EDITIONS

Nü yuhua (Female Jail Flower)
As Seen in Two Early Printings

Ellen Widmer

As the first twentieth-century novel by a woman writer, Wang Miaoru's 王妙如 *Nü yuhua* 女狱花 has received a fair amount of attention in scholarly circles.[1] The text is available in modern reprint,[2] but new insights about authorship and reception can be gleaned from two early editions. Neither has a copyright page. As a result, both pose problems in dating and interpretation. The two are somewhat difficult to access, so I shall first introduce them then discuss the insights that they yield.

1. Two Early Editions

A. Zhejiang Library edition.[3] Two copies. This is a self-published edition of 1904. It is almost certainly the first printed edition. Although no place of publication is indicated, the author herself, one of two prefacer/friends,[4] as well Wang's husband Luo Jingren 罗景仁 (the author of the colophon, identify themselves as Hangzhou natives. Given that the

Zhejiang Library is in Hangzhou, the chances are that this first edition was put together and distributed there, although the printing could have taken place elsewhere, presumably in Shanghai.

Both the cover illustration and the photograph of the author are of interest.[5] Beginning with the latter, the photograph seems to accord with observations in the prefaces by the two prefacer/friends and the colophon by the author's husband, Luo Jingren. Wang Miaoru is said to have married at twenty-three years old, but she died before the novel came out in 1904. Her poor health is not obvious from the picture, yet her high level of intelligence shines through. She looks to be someone who could have written *Nü yuhua*, said to be her favorite among the three texts attributed to her.[6] The reason Wang Miaoru's husband saw fit to incorporate this image into the text must be related to this statement by the author as quoted in his postface:

> My wife once said to me, "nowadays our women's world is backward in the extreme. I hate the fact that my body is weak and sickly. I cannot be like the Buddha and go down to hell to salvage all sentient beings. I can only use my poor pen and residual ink as a tool for awakening people to their [evil] ways. Revolution begins with radicalism and violence, but will eventually achieve harmony and peace. With just this one humble body I cannot hope [for a complete success] in bringing it about on my own. All I can do is to use this book to describe the origin and process of the revolution in detail, so that it is not just one [manifestation] of my bodily image, it represents a million images of revolutionaries like me] Miaoru.[7]"

Figure 3. Cover illustration of *Nü yuhua* (Zhejiang Library edition).

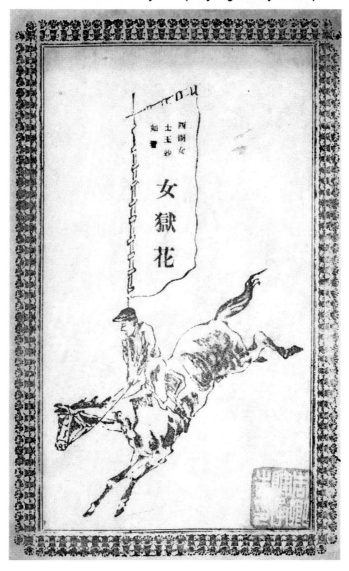

Figure 4. Photograph of Wang Miaoru.

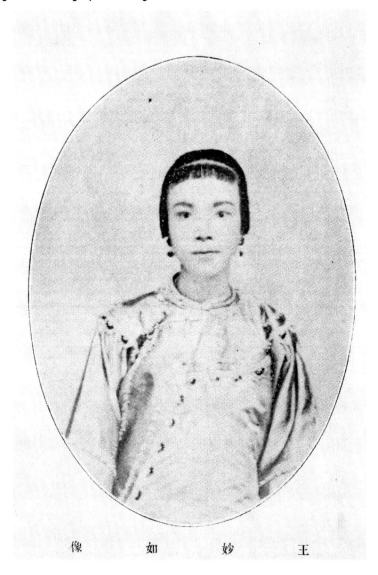

像　　如　　妙　　王

Buddhist imagery is also found on the final page of the text in the following words, when the husband of the second of two heroines says to her: "You have a big heart like a Bodhisattva who sacrifices herself for universal salvation and can salvage kind women directly and kind men indirectly from their experience of difficulty so that they end up on the golden lotus throne."[8] The Buddhist undertones to this reform-minded text are one easily overlooked aspect of the motivation behind it. The reforms proposed in the novel clearly do not emanate from a Christian point of view or from more secular reformist efforts. We should further note that the novel is quite pioneering in its inclusion of a photograph, for photographs were just appearing on the scene in China.[9] Most other novels of the time did not include them.

As for the cover illustration, it is telling in another way. Writing in his feminist publication *Nüjie zhong* 女界钟 (Women's Bell) in 1903, Jin Tianhe 金天翮 proclaimed: "[the woman leader I hope for] would stand before an embroidered battle flag and lead a revolutionary army of women. From her russet-and-white dappled horse, she would speak with elegant words to awaken women, now cloistered in the inner chambers, from their nightmare."[10] It is likely that the cover image bears some relationship to Jin's fiery rhetoric, for the woman, the flag, and the horse are all there. There is no indication of who drew the image, but it is fairly well drawn. Within the novel, Wang Miaoru shows her awareness of another text much cherished by feminists of this era, Herbert Spencer's "Women's Rights" (translated into Chinese in 1902),[11] since it is said to inspire one of the novel's heroines in chapter three. In concert with the reference to Spencer, this cover adds to the impression that Wang was well attuned to the feminist writings of her day.

Turning now to the specifics of the printing, this is moveable type with thirty-two lines per page and thirteen characters per line. The printing is not completely error free. For example, heroine Xuemei 雪梅 is referred to as Meixue 梅雪 on page 42. The modern reprint, which is drawn from this edition, corrects this and a number of similar errors. Except for the errors, the printing is elegantly done.

B. Nanjing Library edition. One copy. This is clearly a resetting of the text. It is a lithograph with thirty lines per page and twelve characters per line. And this time the title is not *Nü yuhua* but rather *Guige haojie tan* 闺阁豪杰谈 (Talk of a heroine from the inner chambers). A third title, *Honggui lei* 红闺泪 (Bitter tears from the inner chambers) appears at the head of the first chapter of this edition, but this is its only appearance. Bibliographies of late-Qing fiction sometimes mention *Honggui lei* as a third title, along with the other two,[12] but they do not reveal whether a book with this title ever circulated independently. Despite the two alternative titles, the novel is always known as *Nü yuhua*. One reason must be that the prefaces and postface are reprinted unchanged from the first edition. Since two of these three documents refer to the book as *Nü yuhua*, they establish this as the standard title.

In addition to raising a question about the title, the Nanjing Library edition raises at least one other question, this time about dating. It appears to be the product of a bookshop. A page at the end contains a list of publications by Shenheji shuju 沈鹤记书局, a Shanghai publisher that published mostly lithographs. The publications listed are predominantly works of fiction and drama.[13] However, the publication list is rather sloppy, much more so than the rest of the text, suggesting that it may be a later add-on of some kind. Shenheji shuju was active just before and during the Republic,[14] so it is quite likely that this edition came out later than 1904, perhaps a decade or so later. Because the prefaces and postface are reprinted intact, and because two out of these three documents are dated 1904, some bibliographers have assumed a publication date of 1904 for this edition, too.[15] However, the link to Shenheji shuju makes it likely that this edition was published sometime after 1904, and in Shanghai.

In addition to the name of the bookshop, two other names can be associated with this edition. Both are those of illustrators. The first is Zhu Dounan 朱斗南, who drew the cover illustration. He usually calls himself Maoyuan Zhu Dounan 茂源朱斗南, suggesting that he was from Suzhou.[16]

The cover illustration is a line drawing in red of a female martial artist with a sword in either hand. It is not in very good condition, but it conveys something of the revolutionary feeling of the text inside. As it happens, though, neither of the novel's two heroines fought with swords. Zhu Dounan worked in book production in Shanghai during the late Qing and early Republic. He has illustrations in several other works of fiction, three of which can be dated fairly accurately: *Xu Jin Ping Mei* 续金瓶梅 (Continuation of *Jin Ping Mei*) of 1912 or 1910,[17] and *Qingchao mingchen Lu gongan* 清朝名臣陆公安of 1910 or 1911 (Court cases of famous official Lu of the Qing Dynasty).[18] His *Tang gong chun Wu Zetian* 唐宫春武则天 (Wu Zetian in the spring palace of Tang) probably dates from around 1912.[19] He was associated with at least three other works of fiction.[20] He also illustrated or edited works outside the field of fiction, such as *Mudan ting bai wen ben gaikuang* 牡丹亭白文本概况 [Brief account of a vernacular version of *Peony Pavilion*] of 1908 and *Huitu Shiwu bencao* 绘图食物本草 (Illustrated pharmacopia of food) of 1916.[21] The fact that Zhu's other known works all came out after 1904 (between four and twelve years afterwards) is another reason to suppose that *Guige haojie tan* came out after 1904.

The other name is that of Xihua sheng 惜花生. This artist created a set of twelve illustrations, all of which were designed for *Guige haojie tan*. We know this from the words of the title that are printed on the outer margins of the illustrations. These are rather well done. To further identify this artist is not an easy matter. There are several known Xihua sheng's (or Xihua jushi's 惜花居士) who worked in Shanghai during the late Qing and early Republic. Among them are a writer, a translator, and a calligrapher.[22] These might all be the same person or they might all be different. Conceivably, not one of them is *Guige haojie tan*'s illustrator, or all or some might be our man.

Figure 5. Cover illustration of *Nü yuhua* (Shenheji shuju edition).

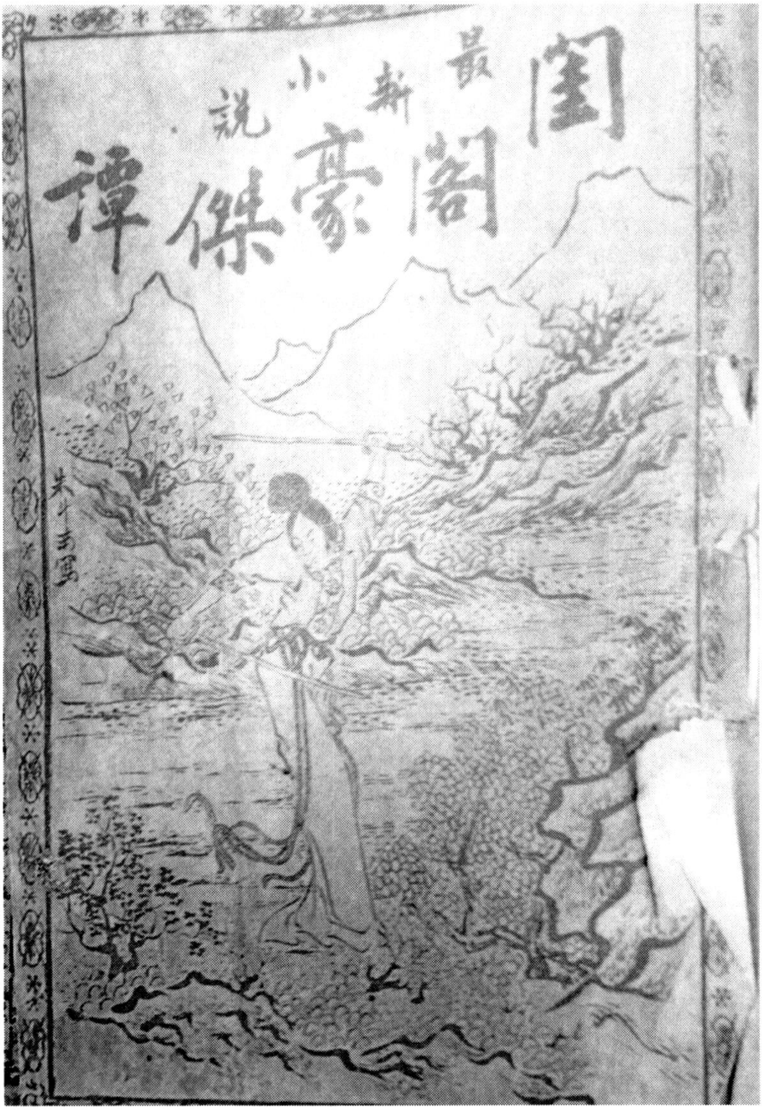

Not one of the three names just introduced—Shenheji shuju, Zhu Daonan, and Xihua sheng—is found in the edition in the Zhejiang Library or the modern reprint edition. It is only in the Nanjing Library edition that they are found.

Even though we cannot identify Xihua sheng, it is obvious that his set of twelve illustrations is meant to recapitulate the novel's twelve chapters. On a frame-by-frame basis, they retell the story but with a somewhat less radical emphasis than that of the printed version. The point will become clearer once we have looked at these illustrations in more detail.

The novel's central premise is that China has long suppressed its women and that change is desperately needed. Its construction is unusual in that one heroine (Sha Xuemei 沙雪梅) dominates the action during the first eight chapters, at which point a second heroine (Xu Pingquan 许平权) is introduced and eventually takes over.[23] Pingquan carries on Xuemei's work, but in a more peaceful way. There are two reasons for this arrangement. The first is that Sha Xuemei is basically an outlaw, who takes a combative approach to righting the balance between men and women. In contrast, Pingquan sees education, medicine, and novel writing as women's best hope for the future. At the same time, she respects Xuemei's contributions, holding that without them her own work could not have succeeded so well.

As we learn from the commentaries to chapters eight and nine, there is a second reason for the succession of heroines. It goes back to *Shuihu zhuan* 水浒传 (The water margin), a classic novel in which the first characters to appear are not the principal characters but subordinates, who slowly lead readers to the main characters. In addition to chapter-by-chapter commentary, *Nü yuhua* has many other trappings of traditional-style fiction, among them parallel couplets for chapter titles, old-fashioned stylistic markers, suspenseful chapter endings, and quick resolution of the suspense at the beginnings of the next chapters.

2. TWELVE ILLUSTRATIONS AND TWELVE CHAPTERS

We turn now to Xihua sheng's illustrations, each of which is keyed to one of the chapters. In four cases the caption on the illustration is an exact match with the title couplet; in six cases it consists of one of the two halves of the couplet; in two cases the chapter title and the captions are completely different.

CHAPTER ONE

Here the inscription replicates the full chapter title: "When men are honored and women demeaned, human rights are undermined; under a bright moon, the dreamscape is spectacular."

The dream comes up in the second half of this chapter. Xuemei is first introduced as a demon,[24] but the point is not developed. Her only unusual feature is that she has been trained in boxing by her father. Her parents have died by now, and she is exchanging boxing lessons for tutoring, since she wishes to educate herself in letters. We find her at her home one evening reading by a window. Suddenly, we are told, a young man walks into her room, and she follows him to a large house filled with men who are sitting in positions of authority and women who are kneeling subserviently. The young man takes a seat with the men and drags Xuemei into the subservient group of women. Xuemei thinks to herself that she has not done anything wrong. She stands up and starts to walk toward the men, planning to ask them what her crime was. They men yell at her to kneel. She persists in asking what her crime was. The men yell back that she has not done anything wrong, it is just that she is inferior. Enraged, she attacks the men, at which point the women rise. Then she wakes up and discovers that the whole thing had been a dream.

The illustration is a fair rendition of the most dramatic moment in this chapter.

Figure 6. Xihua sheng's illustration for chapter one of *Nü yuhua*.

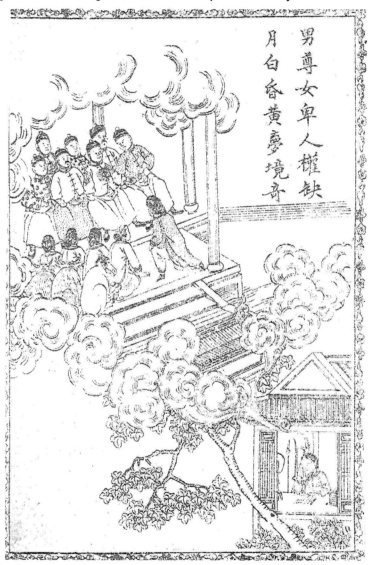

Chapter two

As with the first chapter, the inscription on the illustration is the full chapter title: "A bookworm and a heroic woman are engaged; with a flourish of words the young Confucian is chastised."

Xuemei's engagement is planned for the next spring by her own and her fiancé's families, but most of the chapter is taken up with an argument between the fiancé and his father. The fiancé is very conservative and wants only to study old-fashioned texts and pass additional examinations. (He is already a *xiucai*). However, his father thinks that the son puts too much stock in the examinations and that the old-fashioned texts he favors are worthless.

The illustration is a lot more placid than the chapter, in which the argument between father and son becomes quite heated, with each destroying the other's reading material.

Figure 7. Xihua sheng's illustration for chapter two of *Nü yuhua*.

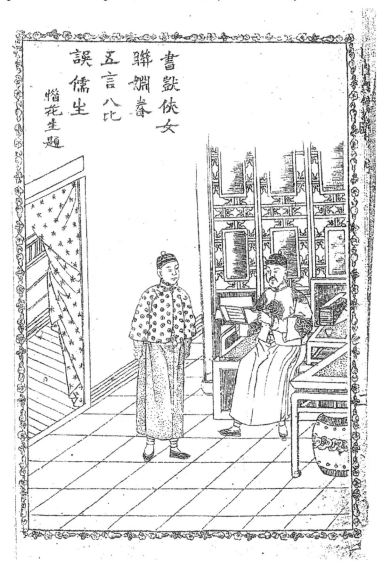

CHAPTER THREE

The caption replicates the second of the two couplets, thus "The heroic woman makes a great rumpus in the women's quarters."

The chapter tells us, first, that the fiancé's father has died of rage, which means that the wedding has to be postponed in order for the son to complete his mourning. Xuemei does not really want to marry, but she is talked into it by others. The first half of the chapter settles into a discussion of the husband's old-fashioned study filled with dreary old books, something that arouses Xuemei's contempt, although she does not give full expression to her feelings. As he reads, her husband falls so deeply asleep that she cannot inform him that she plans to spend a night away at a schoolmate's house. She returns home to find him in a fury. He invokes old-fashioned ideas of cloistering to insist that she should never have left home in the first place. At this point her eye falls on her copy of Spencer's "The Rights of Women," and she is jolted into remembering her dream of chapter one. She and the husband get into a harsh exchange, at the end of which he threatens to attack her. She parries, and with a loud "Aiya" he collapses.

The illustration shows the husband lying on the ground, with Xuemei standing on the sidelines. Xuemei looks calm, which is not how the chapter depicts her. Near at hand is a male servant looking anxious. In fact, no male servant appears in chapter three, though a maid comes on the scene at the beginning of chapter four, when the suspense at the end of the third chapter is resolved.

Figure 8. Xihua sheng's illustration for chapter three of *Nü yuhua*.

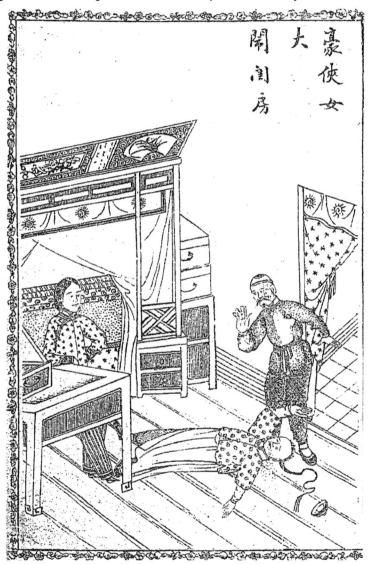

CHAPTER FOUR

The inscription on the illustration is again the full chapter title: "In the dark jail there is no daylight; a tidal wave emerges from deep within the world of women."

Being a well-trained boxer, Xuemei is strong enough to kill her husband with a single kick. Rather than implicate anyone, she tells the maid that she will turn herself in to the authorities. After she does so, the authorities are so outraged that there is talk of a death sentence, but clemency is granted on the grounds that she turned herself in. A cangue is fastened on her shoulders and she is sent to jail. Xuemei takes the opportunity to deliver a long tirade against centuries of male dominance. Everything from bound feet to inequalities in the marriage system comes up in her speech, which also contrasts China with the enlightened countries of Europe, where marriage is left to the young people to decide. At the end of the chapter Xuemei decides that nothing is to be gained by staying in jail. With her superhuman strength, she breaks the cangue then uses a boxing maneuver to exit her cell. Another boxing maneuver allows her to jump up to the eaves of the building. She is almost out of town when a group of pursuers catches up with her.

The illustration is drawn from the first paragraph of the chapter, when the cangue is put on. The official administering the punishment looks almost kindly, but the text describes him as harshly critical of her breaches of proper female decorum, not to mention the murder.

Figure 9. Xihua sheng's illustration for chapter four of *Nü yuhua*.

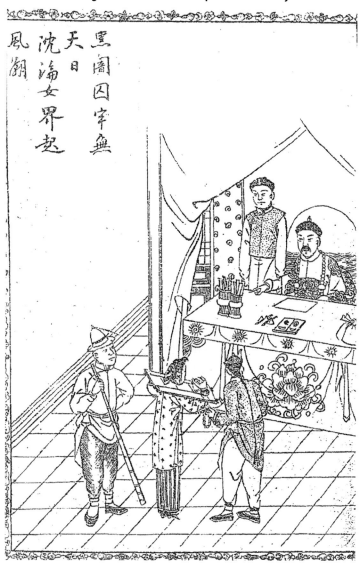

Chapter Five

Neither half of the title is reproduced in this caption. Instead the illustration substitutes "the female criminal in the depths of night jumps over the wall and escapes."

The chapter begins with Xuemei continuing her escape from prison. To elude her pursuers, she jumps from one rooftop to the next, until she reaches the city wall, then uses two more boxing maneuvers to leap up and over it. Finding herself out in the open she is overwhelmed by the spring scene. The vista of flowers and birds prompts a long internal monologue on how it is only in China that marriage takes place so unnaturally, with go-betweens and parental negotiations. She then stops by a tavern for some wine and food and is delighted to spot a feminist poem in good calligraphy on the wall. The poem is signed with the pen name Fobi 佛婢, or Buddhist Maiden. Xuemei regrets that she has no way to find this person. She walks some more and comes across a temple, deep in the mountains with the inscription "Hidden Tiger Palace" (Fuhu dian伏虎殿). She goes inside, where she observes a lion, some tigers, and a leopard. The lion does not attract much interest, but she is annoyed with one of the tigers for behaving aggressively toward the leopard, a female, who is treating him very respectfully. To punish him for his arrogance, she jumps on his back and begins pummeling him with her fists.

This time the illustration captures only the first few sentences of the chapter, the part that resolves the suspense at the end of chapter four.

Figure 10. Xihua sheng's illustration for chapter five of *Nü yuhua*.

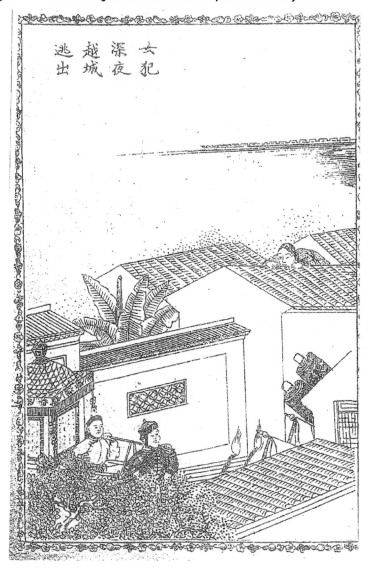

Chapter Six

The caption is the first half of the title: "the female citizen writes books to arouse the world."

With Xuemei atop his back and pounding away, the tiger is overwhelmed. He breaks free and disappears. Xuemei rests for a bit then proceeds on her way. At daybreak, a village comes into view. Because there is no inn, she looks for a house that might receive her and, when she finds one, knocks on the door. A maid ushers her into a living room, where a map of East Asia and pictures of four famous western women hang on the wall. Wen Dongren, the elegant lady of the house, soon appears. Xuemei is at first afraid to give her real name, but upon being treated respectfully is willing to reveal it. Dongren turns out to have heard of Xuemei's crime and arrest from an article in a newspaper which a friend had mailed to her. Next Xuemei observes a pile of books on a table along with evidence that Dongren is doing some writing. Xuemei and Dongren talk about how much men hate to see women read. It turns out that Dongren long ago decided never to marry, on the grounds that there is no such thing as a worthy man. Sadly, however, her previously bound feet have left her body in a weakened state. She cares about women's causes but cannot hope to make the kind of contribution that Xuemei is capable of. Xuemei's plan is to leave and work for the editor of the same women's newspaper that Dongren works for, but Dongren urges her to stay on. Xuemei reluctantly agrees. Soon she becomes seriously ill. She is treated by a doctor but is made more, not less ill by his prescriptions. In her delirium, she yells at Dongren, thinking that she is a man. Her lusty cries for vengeance include imagining men's severed heads piled as high as Mount Tai and a river of men's blood as immense as the Yellow River.

All that the illustration shows, however, is Xuemei (with bangs) chatting peacefully with Dongren. None of her murderous anger is portrayed.

Figure 11. Xihua sheng's illustration for chapter six of *Nü yuhua*.

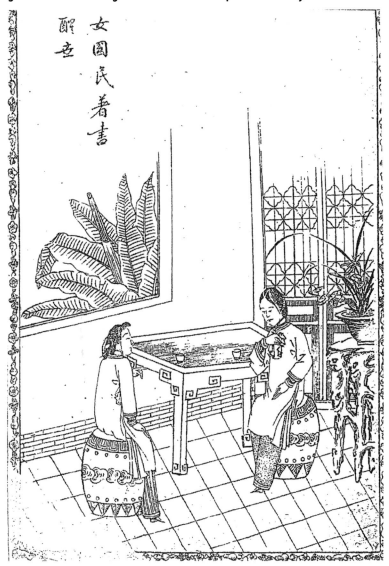

CHAPTER SEVEN

This is the second time that the inscription on the illustration diverges altogether from the chapter title. What the inscription says is "Xuemei is ill in Dongren's room."

In this chapter another doctor is called in to treat Xuemei, who is now at death's door. She is a neighbor, a woman specializing in Chinese medicine. Fortunately this second doctor prescribes the correct medicine and Xuemei recovers. Afterwards Xuemei and the woman doctor carry on a conversation about medical practice. The doctor, who sees herself as a kind of Bodhisattva, observes that women's bodies are different from men's, which means that one has to make a point of understanding them before one can diagnose and prescribe correctly. She further expresses the wish that she might someday go abroad and study Western medicine. After another month Xuemei has fully recovered and can finally move on. She and Dongren say a fond farewell. After a trip filled with adventures and misadventures, Xuemei arrives at a city gate. Inside, the city is beautiful. She finds an attractive guest house and has a nice dinner, including wine. As she eats and drinks she hears an appealing sound. What could it be?

The illustration focuses only on Xuemei's illness, most of which was already detailed in chapter six and does not reference any other events of the chapter.

Figure 12. Xihua sheng's illustration for chapter seven of *Nü yuhua*.

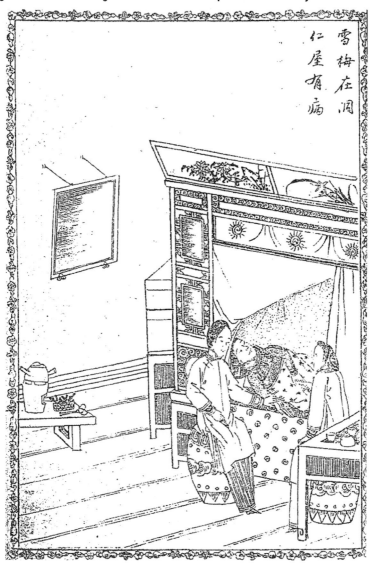

Chapter Eight

Once again the caption uses only half of the chapter title, in this case the first half, thus "the leaders of the two camps meet up in a guest house."

The sound turns out to be a recitation of the very poem Xuemei had encountered earlier, the one signed by Fobi. On further inspection, Xuemei finds out that its author has taken the room right next door. She turns out to be Xu Pingquan, the second heroine of the book. The two engage in a contentious debate about whether Xuemei's strategy of declaring war on men is superior, or whether something less violent might accomplish more. Many words are exchanged. The difference of opinion revolves around Xuemei's hatred of all men versus Pingquan's sense that Chinese men and women need to stick together. The two cannot agree, so Pingquan suggests they meet again the next day.

The illustration simply shows the two women meeting in their hotel and gives no hint of the wide divergence of opinion that develops between them.

Figure 13. Xihua sheng's illustration for chapter eight of *Nü yuhua*.

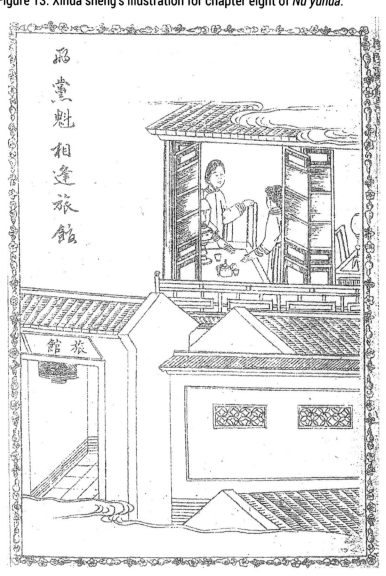

CHAPTER NINE

Again the caption is the same as the chapter title: "When the earth is
dark and heaven is obscured female learning arises. Lower the boats,
smash with an axe, seize men's power."

The next day's meeting never takes place. Xuemei tries to find Pingquan,
but she is not in. So she gets on a boat, with the goal of meeting the editor
of the women's newspaper that she and Wen Dongren had discussed
previously. She manages to meet this editor, Zhang Liujuan 张柳娟
and two of her friends. These three fill Xuemei in on the details of
Pingquan's background: her interest in Buddhism, particularly after
the patriotic suicide of her brother (out of despair at disadvantageous
treaties made by the Qing), and her strong commitment to educating
women. Pingquan is described as very well educated herself, thanks to
the support of her parents, who are no longer living. They had been
firm believers in serious education for women, and they held a dim view
of frivolous novels. Xuemei steps in to assist Zhang with a book that
Dongren had been working on but had to abandon because of her poor
health. Xuemei completes the project, and Zhang is satisfied with the
result. Called *Choushu* (仇书, The book of enemies), it will be published
in Zhang's magazine.

The tone of the four women's conversation is quite misandrist, but the
illustration makes the gathering look more like a genteel ladies' lunch.
The names of the four ladies at the lunch appear on the illustration,
but one name is wrong.[25]

Figure 14. Xihua sheng's illustration for chapter nine of *Nü yuhua*.

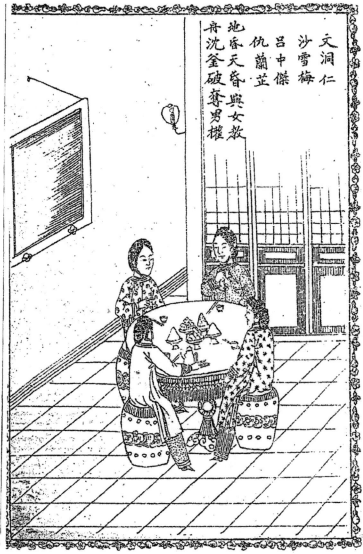

Chapter Ten

Once more the inscription on the illustration consists of only one half of the chapter title: "In an adventurous spirit they travel to Japan to study."

A good deal happens in this chapter. Pingquan tries to find Xuemei, who turns out to have left her room, as we already know. She then sets off to talk to Wen Dongren, who had previously invited her to visit. After their conversation, she resolves to go abroad to study. Her travel companion will be the woman doctor from next door, who correctly diagnosed and cured Xuemei's illness. They go to Japan and spend two years there—Pinguan in a regular school and the doctor in a medical school. During this time, their mutual friend Dongren dies of illness. Dongren's death reminds them of how fleeting life is, and they resolve to take a trip to Europe and America. They get as far as Paris. After visiting a great public library, they stop to buy a newspaper and learn that Xuemei, editor Zhang, and seventy of their friends have died after a failed insurrection, which leads them to self-immolate in a fire. The two travelers are much saddened by this development. The doctor decides to continue on to America and attend medical school there. She returns to China after a year and establishes a medical college. Her adventures will become the subject of another novel.

Pingquan heads directly back to China, with the aim of founding a school for girls. En route she encounters Huang Zongxiang 黃宗祥, a man whom she had previously met in Japan but did not remember well. He turns out to be good at listening to her laments about her dead friends and has a keen understanding of her moods.

This busy and not altogether happy chapter is represented in the illustration by its most hopeful moment, the impending trip of Pingquan and the doctor to Japan.

Figure 15. Xihua sheng's illustration for chapter ten of *Nü yuhua*.

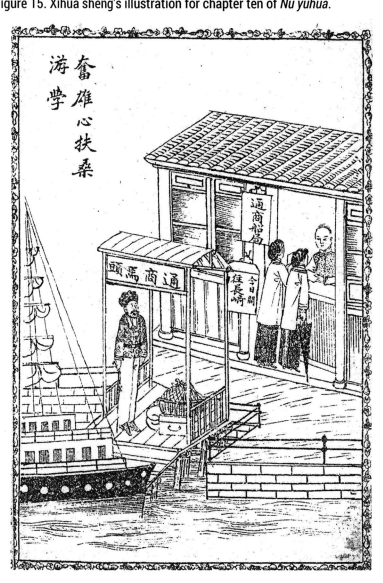

Chapter Eleven

This illustration takes the second half of the chapter title as its caption, "A speech at the opening of a school disrupts the order of things."

The topic of this chapter is the founding of a school for women in China. Pingquan and Huang Zongxiang discuss marriage but agree to postpone it until Pingquan can make her contribution to women's education. Being wealthy, Zongxiang will help supply money for her school, and he will live nearby, occupying himself by writing novels. She hires faculty, finds students, and sets up her school. Virtually the whole of the rest of the chapter is taken up with a strident speech she delivers to her students. It advises them to be independent. If they can make their own money, men will respect them, then men and women can become friends on an equal basis. Part of the speech draws on Xuemei's book, *Choushu*, which it assumes the students have read. We are told of its warnings against self-decoration: bracelets are like manacles, and earrings are like the signs clipped to criminals' ears to advertise their crimes. It further exhorts women to adopt the idea of exercise from Western countries and above all else to take education seriously. In sum, Pingquan argues, women do not have to attack men to claw back lost rights. Through education, making money, and other means they can win men's respect and lead better lives.

The illustration shows a handful of students listening to the speech, necessarily far fewer than the hundred that were enrolled in Pingquan's school. Another difference is that it gives no idea of the strident feminism of Pingquan's speech.

Figure 16. Xihua sheng's illustration for chapter eleven of *Nü yuhua*.

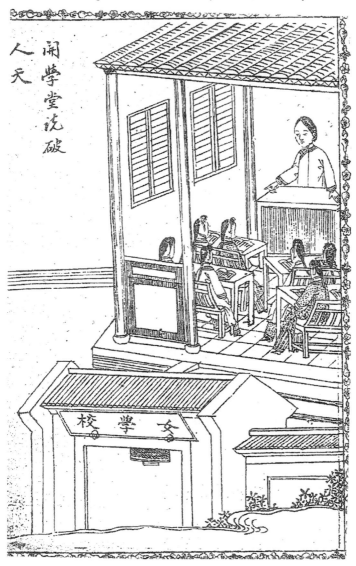

CHAPTER TWELVE

The final illustration takes its caption from the first half of the chapter title, "discussing how to improve pre-school education in Europe."

This chapter begins by noting that Pingquan has gone on to found a normal school and is reading application essays. The essays all focus on equalizing power between men and women. One might expect her to be happy at this development, but instead she sinks into a depression. She worries that her students' fierce attacks on men could profoundly disrupt family life and lead to the decline of humankind. She and Huang Zongxiang discuss these matters. They turn their attention to certain shortcomings in the European model of equality, among them that women still wear corsets and are not eligible to vote in elections. They then conduct a far-reaching discussion of the balance of power between men and women, even exploring the possibility that a new type of humanity might emerge someday, one in which the burdens of pregnancy and child rearing will not fall entirely on women. The action then fast forwards ten years. By now Pingquan has achieved her goal of furthering women's education, and the couple will finally marry. Each gives the other credit for a significant contribution to the advancement of Chinese women, the one through her educational efforts, the other through his progressive novels.

The illustration features an earnest conversation between a man and a woman, but there is a problem. Whereas the discussion in the text is explicitly between equals, the illustration is drawn in such a way that Huang Zongxiang looms over Xu Pingquan. It is very unlikely that Wang Miaoru would have approved an illustration of this kind.

Figure 17. Xihua sheng's illustration for chapter twelve of *Nü yuhua*.

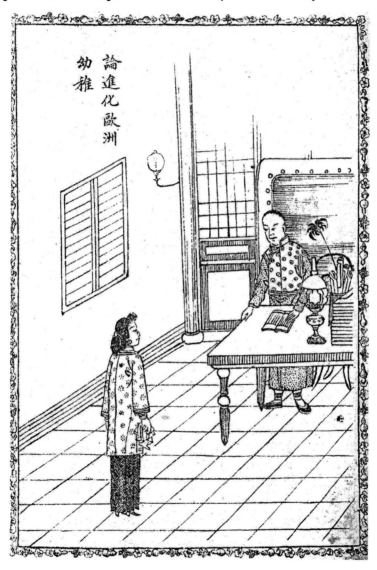

Discrepancies Between the Story and Xihua sheng's Illustrations

It is not just that this twelfth image fails to capture the idea of full equality between men and women. There are other ways in which the set of illustrations as a whole tells its own version of the story, one in which female violence is somewhat toned down. The first is its approach to Xuemei's intolerance of men. Although it is only once that she is pronounced a demon, she lives up to that billing in later chapters. This is not only because she kills her husband, a deed the illustrations do capture. It is also seen in her improbable jail break in chapter five, her fight with a tiger in that same chapter, and her delirious rant in chapter six, when she imagines mountains of severed heads and rivers of blood. It may even explain her grim, suicide-like death in chapter ten. None of these are depicted in the illustrations. What Xihua sheng depicts, instead, is a rather genteel lady who, after the initial act of murder, associates with other genteel ladies. The apparent gentility of all of his female characters masks the extent of the division between Xuemei and Pingquan. When the only discernible difference between them is one of hairstyle, the story changes significantly. Perhaps Xihua sheng was a little more conservative than Wang Miaoru, not quite accepting the idea that females could really equal males, and not fully acknowledging the depth of Xuemei's rage.

We have no way of knowing whether these differences were the result of conscious decision. Suggesting that they might have been is the fact that the story the illustrations tell is internally consistent, at least as far as the gentility of the women is concerned. The titles are another clue. Whereas the title *Nü yuhua* emphasizes Xuemei's time in jail and prioritizes her over Pingquan, both *Guige haojie tan* and *Hong guilei* mention the *gui*, or cloister, which would seem to prioritize Pingquan's non-violence, even though she herself is not cloistered. This evidence is far from conclusive. The case could be strengthened (or overturned) if we found out more about Xihua sheng.

It is important to remember that the text of the novel is itself somewhat ambivalent about Xuemei's violent feelings, first identifying with her causes, then acknowledging that her initiatives, while productive, are most valuable when they undergird Pingquan's program, then observing that too much hostility toward men on the part of women could have the unintended consequence of ending reproduction altogether. Pingquan's pious hope that the human race might die out and be replaced by a species in which men and women would be truly equal is too complex to express in a line drawing, but it may have inspired Xihua sheng's gentler approach to the contrast the novel explores. However, because of the cover illustration by Zhu Dounan, the edition as a whole cannot be accused of diluting the author's rhetoric. On the cover, Xuemei is properly belligerent and Pingquan is nowhere to be found.

CONCLUSION

Neither Zhu Dounan's cover nor Xihua sheng's pictorial retelling fully accords with Wang Miaoru's original *Nü yuhua*. Although the cover captures the martial artist spirit of the first eight chapters, there is never a moment when Xuemei fights with swords. And although Xihua sheng's set of illustrations grasps the more accommodating spirit of the final four chapters and their heroine Pingquan, it is not a balanced summation of alternatives as the novel poses them. Yet both the cover and the set of sketches have artistic appeal. Moreover, in embodying each side of *Nü yuhua*'s contrasting approaches, this pair of artists gets at the struggle that the print version aims to convey.

Returning now to the Zhejiang Library edition, we find that whereas its sketch and photograph draw readers closer to the author (both to her personal appearance and to a reference she might have made to Jin Tianhe), the illustrations in the Nanjing edition take them farther away. We cannot be certain that anyone at Shenheji shuju (or some other bookseller) deliberately orchestrated the Nanjing edition's package of slightly discordant elements, but it is very likely that neither Wang Miaoru nor Luo Jingren approved this edition.

Conceivably, Zhu Daonan had never read *Nü yuhua*. His cover captures Xuemei's swashbuckling spirit, but there is something rather generic in his depiction, and he has added swords. In contrast, we can be sure that Xihua sheng had read the novel. By suppressing Xuemei's demonic nature, enhancing her gentility, and eliminating distracting side-plots, he turns Wang Miaoru's clash between violent and peaceful approaches into a more cordial exchange of views. This may not have been Wang Miaoru's intention, but it is an informed diminution of the conflict she set down.

Notes

1. See for example Huang Jinzhu 黄锦珠, *Qingmo Minchu nü zuojia xiaoshuo yanjiu* 清末民初女作家小說研究 [Research on fiction of women writers of the late Qing and early Republic] (Taibei: Liren shuju, 2014), 97–102.

2. *Zhongguo jindai xiaoshuo daxi* 中国近代小说大系 [Compendium of China's early modern novels] (Nanchang: Baihua zhou wenyi chubanshe, 1993) vol. 64, 700–759.

3. Another copy can be found in the Shoudu Library in Beijing.

4. These are Cangsang jike 沧桑寄客 (叶女士) and Qiantang Yu Peilan 钱塘俞佩兰. (俞女士). The latter is the one who definitely came from Hangzhou.

5. These were both reprinted with the modern reprint edition.

6. See her husband's colophon. The others are *Xiao taohuayuan chuanqi* 小桃源传奇 [A drama, Small Peach Garden] and *Changhe ji shici* 唱和集诗词. [Collected poems].

7. See page 760 of *Nü yuhua*. 【妙如】尝对予曰：近日女界黑暗已至极点，自恨弱躯多病，不能如我佛释迦亲入地狱普救众生，只得以秃笔残墨为棒喝之具。虽然革命之事，先从激烈，后归平和，眇眇一身，难期圆满。惟此书立意将革命之事，源源本本历道其详，非但一我妙如之现影，实千百万我妙如之现影云. With thanks to Wai-yee Li for translation assistance.

8. See page 759 of *Nü yuhua*. 妹妹啊，你怀着菩萨心肠，舍身渡世，将直接之善女人，间接的善男子. 从火坑提到金莲座上。

9. Shengqing Wu, "A Paper Mirror: Autobiographical Moments in Modern Chinese Poetry," *The Journal of Chinese Literature and Culture* 3:2 (November 2016), 312–334.

10. 张女界之革命军，立与锦绣旗前，桃花马上，琅琅吐词，以唤醒深闺之妖梦者，必此人也。), *Zhonghua quanguo funü yundong lishi ziliao* 中华全国妇女运动历史资料 [Historical materials on the All-China Women's movement] (Beijing: Zhongguo funü chubanshe, 1981), 157.

11. This is a chapter from Herbert Spencer's *Social Statics*, 1851. See also Hu Ying, *Tales of Translation: Composing the New Woman in China, 1899–1918.* (Stanford: Stanford University Press), 2000, 190, and Mou Shixi-

ang 莫世祥, *Ma Junwu ji* 马君武集, 1900–1919 [Collected works of Ma Junwu] (Wuhan:Huazhong shifan daxue chubanshe), 1991, 16–27.

12. For example, see Tarumoto Teruo 樽本照雄, *Xinbian zengbu Qing mo Min chu xiaoshuo mulu* 新编增补清末民初小说目录 [Newly edited and supplemented index of novels from the late Qing and early Republic] (Jinan: Qilu shushe, 2002), 523.

13. Shenheji shuju is also known for publishing drum songs and other performance literature, as well as works on medicine, chess, and other topics. Titles in all of these categories can be accessed through Duxiu.

14. See Wang Qingyuan 王清原, Mou Renlong 牟仁隆, Han Xiduo 韩锡铎, *Xiaoshuo shufang lu* 小说书坊录 [Records of publishers of novels] (Beijing: Beijing tushuguan chubanshe, 2002), 156–158.

15. Jiangsu sheng shehui kexueyuan 江苏省社会科学院, *Zhongguo tongsu xiaoshuo zongmu tiyao* 中国通俗小说总目提要 [Annotated catalogue of Chinese popular fiction] (Beijing: Xinhua shudian, 1990), 906.

16. And probably distinguishing him from another man of the same name of a little earlier who was from Yangzhou.

17. Xi Bin 习斌, *Wanqing xijian xiaoshuo jingyan lu* 晚清稀见小说经眼录 [Records of rare late-Qing novels I have seen] (Shanghai: Shanghai yuandong chubanshe, 2012), 101–106.

18. Whereabouts unknown.

19. See *Zhongguo tongsu xiaoshuo zongmu tiyao*, 1255.

20. The undated *Sixu Jingu qiguan* 四续今古奇观 [Strange observations old and new, fourth sequel], on which see Xi Bin 习斌, *Wanqing xijian xiaoshuo jiancanglu* 晚清稀见小说鉴藏录 [Records of rare late-Qing novels I have collected] (Shanghai, Shanghai Yuandong chubanshe, 2013), 258. On other undated titles, see Xi Bin, *Wanqing xijian xiaoshuo jingyan lu* 清稀见小说经言录 [Records of rare late-Qing novels I have seen] Shanghai: Yuandong chubanshe, 2012, 105–106. Another is *Xinbian Wulin shazi* qiwen 新编武林杀子奇闻 [Newly edited Strange account of the murder of a child in Hangzhou].

21. See Liu Shuli 刘淑丽, *Mudanting jieshou shi yanjiu* 牡丹亭接受史研究 [Research on the history of the reception of *Peony Pavilion*) (Jinan: Qilu shushe , 2013), 18. See also Xue Qinglu 薛清录, *Quanguo zhongyi tushu lianhe mu lu* 全国中医图书联合目录, [Consolidated catalogue of books on Chinese medicine] (Beijing: Zhongyi guji chubanshe, 1991), 197.

22. Someone of this name wrote a novel called *E shaonian* 恶少年 [Evil youth] in 1909, on which see Tarumoto, 135. And the name comes up in *Shenbao* in 1888 as a calligrapher, on which see Qiao Xiaojun 乔晓

军, *Zhongguo meishujia renming cidian* [Dictionary of famous Chinese artists; second supplement] 中国美术家人名词典，补遗二编, 431. A Xihua jushi translated a novel by Ryder Haggard in 1900, under the title *Huayue xiangcheng ji* 花月香城记 [Account of flower moon fragrant city].Another person named Xihua jushi wrote a novel called *Zeng lu qiqing juan* 赠履奇情传 [An account of the strange feeling in giving a shoe] in 1906, on which see Tarumoto, 934.

23. The commentary to chapter six encourages us to see a third character, Wen Dongren 文洞仁, as a bridge between Xuemei and Pingquan.
24. See page 910 of 女狱花.
25. The illustration says that the lunch was attended by Wen Dongren, Sha Xuemei, Lü Zhongjie 吕中傑, and Chou Lanzhi 仇兰芷. These last two are friends of the newspaper editor Zhang Liujuan 张柳娟, a friend of Wen's. It is Zhang, not Wen, who attends the lunch.

CHAPTER 9

THE CHINESE GARDEN AS AN INTELLECTUAL ENTERPRISE

Jerome Silbergeld

These name plaques and paired inscriptions are a difficult undertaking.

—Jia Zhen, in *Dream of the Red Chamber*

You must search out the unconventional and make sure it is in accord with your own wishes. The trite and conventional should be totally eliminated.

—Ji Cheng, *The Craft of Gardens*[1]

In his essay "On the Conceptual Analysis of Gardens," James Elkins writes of the "strange" characteristics of the literature on gardens as "inspired" by the peculiar nature of gardens themselves and therefore as a bit unruly and fanciful when compared to the analytic literature on painting, architecture, and sculpture. Gardens in history, he observes, have yielded "a kind of wide-ranging freedom" in approaches taken by the critical literature; "writing on gardens is more heterogeneous, and its heterogeneity more central to a coherent account of its nature, than other branches of the fine arts."[2] In laying out his views, Elkins enumerates a variety of "ways of thinking about gardens," the gardens' prime characteristics gauged in terms of facilitated "viewing" of what lies within the garden but beyond its material surface, in its visual and textual reference. His seven numbered characteristics, and others not numbered but discussed, seem to hold as true of Chinese gardens as they do of their European counterparts: all gardens may be looked at as "representations of nature," and most may be looked at as "representations of history" or of painting or fiction; gardens are a "meeting-place of various disciplines," organized around "sets of polarities"; and they might also be considered as "open-ended sites of desire" that do "not represent anything" but instead embody a "psychic need."[3] More broadly, Elkins concludes that judging from the writings about them, "gardens are like mild soporifics, inducing a certain frame of mind or habit of thought, over which we have limited control...Gardens seem to break down conceptual boundaries, inducing a 'passive, contemplative experience'" (quoting Mark Francis and Randolph T. Hester), "not merely to stupefy the intellect, but to confound the senses" (here Elkins quotes Francesco Colonna), and they are (here he quotes Addison) "naturally apt to fill the Mind with Calmness and Tranquility, and to lay all its turbulent passions to rest." "But," asks Elkins incisively, "do they also lay *thought* to rest?"[4]

An overarching goal of the garden in China was to seem macrocosmic, all-inclusive, but this had to be accomplished as much by suggestion as by the physical reality of the garden. By stimulating the intellectual imagination to enlarge upon the material image, it made up for any material shortfall, encouraging the thoughtful, contemplative viewer to keep both eyes and mind wide open. Garden designers devised ways to confound the senses and confront viewers' expectations in order to trigger a radical comingling of the perceptual and conceptual, the seen and imagined, the visual and visionary. Both textual and visual reference were employed to engage the creative imagination in ways related to dreaming or fantasy, to interiority made to seem external. But in response to Elkins' important final question, Chinese gardens, while sometimes visually stupefying and not so unreasonably likened to the visual aesthetics of the European Baroque, by no means "laid thought to rest."[5]

* * *

While for the most part Western gardens tend to be regarded as external to and separate from built architecture, a variety of building types were integral to Chinese gardens, including the semi-open *xie* 榭, the well-known garden pavilion (*ting* 亭), and a two-storied *lou* 樓 which typically housed the owner's library on the upper floor, safe from flooding. Text entered the Chinese garden through name plaques (*bian e* 匾額) and paired couplets (*duilian* 對聯), inscribed in carved wooden plaques above and beside doorways, so that one entered a garden building to the accompaniment of literary text. Nothing reveals the poles of classical Chinese philosophy more clearly than the attitudes toward "names" held by early Confucian and Daoist literature. "Names" served as an instrument of regulation and measure of human order, extolled by Confucians, derogated by Daoists. In the *Analects*, Confucius famously made the "rectification" of names a first priority of statecraft, for "if names are not correct, language is not in accord with the truth of things. If language is not in accord with the truth of things, affairs cannot be carried on to success...," and downward things spiral with everything from rites to justice falling apart.[6] The equally famous and no less somber opening of the *Tao Te Ching* (*Daode jing* 道德經), with permanence and ephemerality as its subject, similarly called upon "names" to exemplify and make its point: "the name that can be named is not the eternal name." With the complex and unpredictable garden offering an unruly alternative to the controlling regularity of the Confucian urban order, one might expect the typical Chinese scholar recluse to have simply slipped behind his garden gate and to have left names, words, and books

—all his intellectual baggage—behind, so as not to let it get between him and his direct apprehension of nature. But gardens were the products of scholars, and scholars will be scholars. The life of the scholar is the life of the mind, of knowledge and imagination, of writing; and the garden, after all, was the cherished site of the scholar's studio, from which the scholar's brushed arts, both textual and visual, emerged. The Confucius of the *Analects* said that "a gentleman never competes" (*junzi wu suo zheng* 君子無所爭) but he wrote this because they did. "If they must," he said, "let it be at archery," but later scholar-gentlemen competed fiercely in scholarship and artistry, and this competition extended to providing names and couplets for the garden.[7]

Robert Harrist has linked the activity of naming to that of writing *about* the subject, beginning in the Northern Song period with the generation of Ouyang Xiu (1007–1072) when the naming game first becomes interesting: "What is perhaps more revealing than the names themselves are the things that pre-Song writers wrote, or rather, did not write, about the significance of site names in their gardens or landscape retreats."[8] Harrist writes that "there is no literary precedent for the Northern Song burst of writing addressed to the origins and meanings of names for studios, pavilions, ponds, and other sites associated with gardens. Scores of poems and essays on these themes appear in the literary collections of Ouyang Xiu, Su Shi [1036–1101], Qin Guan (1049–1100), and Chao Buzhi (1053–1110)."[9] A detailed overview of the development of artistic names over the later centuries and dynasties has yet to be undertaken by modern scholars (and will not be attempted here).

Ironically, our most articulate example of the name-giving process and all its attendant cultural behavior comes from fiction, from Cao Xueqin's (c. 1715–c. 1763) canonical *Dream of the Red Chamber / The Story of the Stone*, in the novel's seventeenth chapter, "The Grand View Garden Tests for Talent in Composing Couplets and Name Plaques" (Daguanyuan *shi cai ti dui e* 大觀園試才題對額). The tale is that of Baoyu ("Precious Jade" or "Precious Stone," born with a magic stone in his mouth) and his transit through the mortal realm. Baoyu, boy and stone, are set down together amidst fabulous wealth; his elder sister becomes a consort to the emperor, which is commemorated by the building of a fabulous garden. While fictive, the competitive nature of garden naming remains true to the values of the day.[10] In this chapter, Baoyu and his strict Confucian father—resentful of his son's wayward behavior and jealous of the youngster's extraordinary talent—are joined by the town's leading intellectuals to preview the sprawling new garden and suggest names for its many sites and buildings. The significance and challenge of naming garden sites was declared by the father, Jia Zheng, at the outset of the chapter: "These name plaques and paired inscriptions," he worried, "are a difficult undertaking....However magnificent the scene, if the pavilions and latticed chambers have no written inscriptions, it will seem to lack any interest; and though it be a scene of flowering willows, it will be wholly unable to display its beauty" (這匾額對聯一件難事 ....偌大景致, 若干亭榭, 无字標題, 也觉寥落无趣, 任有花柳山水, 也斷不能生色). It is interesting that in translating this simple passage, the most respected English-language version introduces an important garden feature not present in the original text, namely poetry: "All those prospects and pavilions—even the rocks and trees and flowers will seem somehow incomplete *without that touch of poetry which only the written word can lend a scene.*"[11] Perhaps as Elkins has suggested, in writing of the garden even the translator can become somewhat transfixed by his subject, envisioning rather than visioning the author's words; or perhaps in anticipating what most writers *would* write, he simply mentioned it on his own. Why the naming is so "difficult" is revealed in the details, and nowhere is the role of intellect in the Chinese garden made more evident. So, too, with the display of creativity that helps shape the "good" garden. With Jia Zheng's admonition and the challenging mechanics of Chinese regulated poetry in mind, let us join Baoyu as he, his father, and the invited guests undertake their garden tour and discuss the poetics of naming.

"I remember reading in some old book," said Baoyu, "that 'to recall old things is better than to invent new ones; and to recut an ancient text is better than to engrave a modern.' We ought, then, to choose something old but as this is not the garden's principal 'mountain' or its chief vista, strictly speaking there is no justification for having an inscription here at all – unless it is to be something that implies that this is merely a first step towards more important things ahead. I suggest we should call it 'Pathway to Mysteries' after the line in Chang Jian's poem about the mountain temple:

'A path winds upwards to mysterious places.'

A name like that would be more distinguished."

There was a chorus of praise from the literary gentlemen:

"Exactly right! Wonderful! Our young friend with his natural talent and youthful Imagination succeeds where we old pedants fail!"

Jia Zheng gave a deprecatory laugh:

"You mustn't flatter the boy! People of his age are adept at making a little knowledge go a long way. I only asked him as a joke, to see what he would say. We shall have to think of a better name later on."[12]

What stands out from this discussion and others is the question of *how* derivative versus *how* original a poem should be, a matter of constant critical consideration. Here, Baoyu has endorsed the "recutting of ancient texts," but the following passage demonstrates Baoyu is not above self-contradiction, and in the long run he saves his keenest endorsement not for mere knowledge of the poetic tradition but for truly creative artistry, as in this second example:

Over the center of the bridge there was a little pavilion, which Jia Zhen and the others entered and sat down in.

"Well, gentlemen," said Jia Zheng, "what are we going to call it?"

"Ouyang Xiu in his *Pavilion of the Old Drunkard* speaks of 'a pavilion poised above the water,'" said one of them. "What about 'Poised Pavilion?'"

"'Poised Pavilion' is good," said Jia Zheng, "but *this* pavilion was put here in order to dominate the water it stands over, and I think there ought to be some reference to water in its name. I seem to recollect that in that same essay you mention, Ouyang Xiu speaks of the water 'gushing between twin peaks.' Could we not use the word 'gushing' in some way?"

"Yes, yes!" said one of the literary gentlemen. "'Gushing Jade' would do splendidly."

Jia Zheng fondled his beard meditatively, then turned to Baoyu and asked him for *his* suggestion.

"I agreed with what you said just now, Father," said Baoyu, "but on second thoughts it seems to me that while it may have been alright for Ouyang Xiu to use 'gushing' in describing the source of the river Rang, it doesn't really suit the water round this pavilion. Then again, as this is a Separate Residence specially designed for the reception of a royal personage, it seems to me that something special is called for and that an expression taken from the *Drunkard's Pavilion* might seem a bit improper. I think that we ought find a rather more imaginative, less obvious sort of name."

"I hope you gentlemen are all taking this in," said Jia Zheng sarcastically. "You will observe that when we suggest something original we are recommended to prefer the old to something new. But when we *do* make use of an old text we are 'improper' and 'unimaginative'! – Well, carry on then! Let's have your suggestion!"

"I think 'Drenched Blossoms' would be more original and more tasteful than 'Gushing Jade.'"

Jia Zheng stroked his beard and nodded silently. The literary gentlemen could see that he was pleased and hastened to commend Baoyu's ability.

"That's the two words for the framed board on top," said Jia Zheng. "*Not* a very difficult task. But what about the seven-word lines for the sides?"

Baoyu glanced quickly around, seeking inspiration from the scene and presently came up with the following couplet:

> Three pole-thrust lengths of bankside willows green,
> One fragrant breath of bankside flowers sweet.

Jia Zheng nodded and a barely perceptible smile played over his features. The literary gentlemen redoubled their praises.[13]

* * *

If the scholarship about names and poetry in the garden is sparse, leaving considerable room for new research, even less has been written about garden design with any real specificity. As with all Chinese architecture, Chinese gardens have been almost constantly renewed and revised along with regular maintenance, meaning that even those gardens with the longest history are in good part modern. Despite the frequent appellation "Ming gardens," Ming being frequently regarded as the heyday of the Chinese urban garden, it hard to determine what today's older gardens must have looked like in Ming times. One might expect Ming or earlier paintings to help but mostly they do not. Like Elkins' Western writers about gardens, Chinese painters of the middle Ming-period in depicting actual gardens, readily succumbed to the garden's power to enchant, so that their paintings represent their own stimulated imagination and fail to establish an accurate record of gardens at that time. As a result, Jan Stuart has concluded that today, "it is unnecessary" or perhaps even impossible "to try to restore the physical properties" of those gardens using paintings from that period.[14] And yet, this separation between the garden and accounts of it in both text and image grew not from a sensory *conquest* of the intellect but, on the contrary, from painters who "emphasized the meaning of the garden not its appearance" and from garden owners who were "more concerned with the ideas in a garden than [its] physical attributes."[15] Textual reference—names and poetry attached to buildings and sites—was usually erudite in its reference to literature and history and strenuous in the demands it made on the knowledgeability of viewers. The garden design itself could be no less intellectually demanding in the way it engaged visitors' visual expectations, as established by years of viewing other gardens, to see if it could display a spark of insight with subtle but telling departures from or variation on the norms, unusual turns by a talented designer to be recognized by the discerning viewer. So in both text and image, the Chinese garden played heavily on the senses not to dull or displace the intellect but to activate it. Both text and image were called upon to help accomplish this, in ways that are far more challenging to today's mass audience than they were to elite viewers of the past. How this was achieved visually can be represented here by a few examples.

To begin with, most of China's urban gardens attempt to confound the senses through two strategies, fragmentations of space and confusions of scale. Beginning with a limited amount of space and the task of representing cosmic completeness, the strategy was usually to admit the limitation and further fragment the available space by means of walls which are then penetrated with window views ("leak windows") that suggest an endless sequence of such spaces. An example from Suzhou's Liu ("Lingering") Garden (figure 18) places the viewer in a darkened room that looks out through a square window into a lighted courtyard, from there through a round moon-gate into a dim courtyard with rockery, with a view past that through a six-sided window looking into another room, and beyond that room into a brightly lit corridor. Confusions of scale may be undertaken with rockery, where large composed stone sculptures and miniature table-top stones all represent mountains, full scale, and urge the viewer to visualize them on a grand scale.[16]

Figure 18. Fragmented space, Liu Garden, Suzhou.

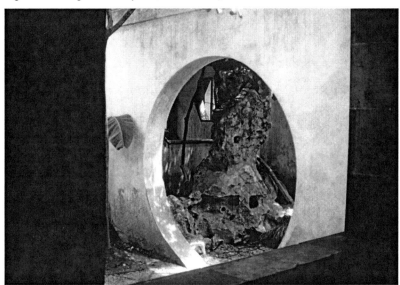

The same may be said of miniaturized tree plantings, *penzai* 盆栽 (bonsai in Japanese, now commonly used in English) and *penjing* 盆景(bonsai elaborated with miniature architecture and occasional figures), extended viewing of which serves to distort one's sense of proportions. Most gardens have a bonsai nursery, many containing specimens a century old or more. A related example from the Liu Garden juxtaposes a medium-sized pine tree with a potted pine, smaller but on the large end of the bonsai scale; these two are viewed alongside a design in the pebbled terrace that transforms these two pines into a two-dimensional image of the species (figure 19).

Figure 19. Confusion of scale, Yi Garden, Suzhou.

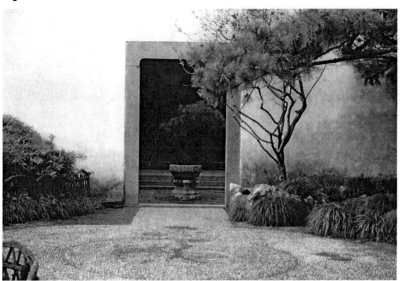

Similar to this, sliced marble (sometimes referred to as "dream stones" or Dali stones, from the primary site of their quarry in Yunnan province), are found throughout the garden buildings, inset into chair backs or the side arms of couches and suspended on the walls in frames like paintings, to which they refer (figure 20a). These stones invited the viewer to identify the painting they most resembled, and they were valued more the closer their chance patterns resembled specific painters' styles (figure 20b). In reverse, such small stones (both two- and three-dimensional) were often used for artistic inspiration in landscape painting (in all of these, the large writ small), as the garden was the primary site for studios from which so much of China's literature, calligraphy, and painting comes down to us. The intent and effect of such examples should be readily apparent, requiring viewers to *think*, to visit the files of visual memory for comparative examples.

Figure 20a. Dali marble with inscription, Zhuozheng Garden, Suzhou.

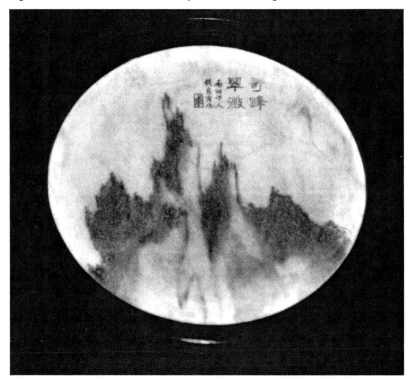

All of this is well known, transmitted in introductory books and scholarly articles alike. To utilize these strategies in working to achieve these ends is normal, conventional. More challenging examples take us to the heart of the matter, and perhaps they echo what Ji Cheng had in mind when he wrote in China's best-known traditional text on gardens, that "You must search out the unconventional and make sure it is in accord with your own wishes. The trite and conventional should be totally eliminated."[17]

This guidance implies that viewers already recognize the norms of garden design and the potential of garden design to channel a *dialogue about design*, referring to "trite and conventional" compositions by offering alternatives, and acknowledging the expected norms by violating them.

Figure 20b. Ma Shirong, 12th c., Landscape.

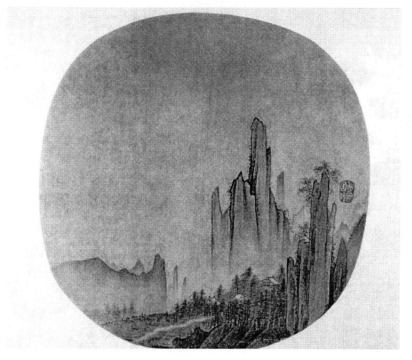

This fundamental topic has yet to be dealt with in the published literature, whether old or new, either in a general way or—far more importantly—with specific examples. A primary lesson comes from Suzhou's Liu Garden. Here, a lithic hierarchy begins with a raised dais made of low-grade "yellow stone"; next, a set of "bamboo-shoots" stones (hard pebbles in a softer matrix, shaped like baby bamboo shooting up from the soil) is elevated on this dais, scattered around the periphery; and the arrangement is capped by a dominant "Lake Tai" (*taihu* 太湖) limestone construction in the center. Stone representing the earth and being the focus of Daoist reverence, these stones represent more than an aesthetic arrangement (figure 21a). Loosely but directly they imitate a Buddhist temple's iconic altar setting (the paradisiacal Mt. Sumeru dais, with guardian figures at the four corners and the over-large Buddha figure in the center with flanking bodhisattvas). Here the stonework supplants sculpted Buddhist figures as objects of Daoist veneration (figure 21b).

Figure 21a. Stone altarpiece, Liu Garden, Suzhou.

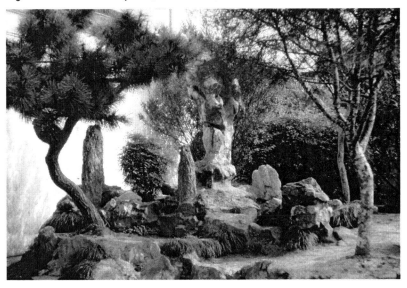

More simply, an elevated bridge at Suzhou's Huanxiu Garden was intended to represent the narrow, moss-covered and slippery stone bridge at Mount Tiantai, the crossing of which requires courage and cultivated discipline, and which leads at the far end past a stone obstacle to a Buddhist paradise[18] (figures 22a and 22b).

Figure 21b. Buddhist altar, Toshodaiji, Kyoto.

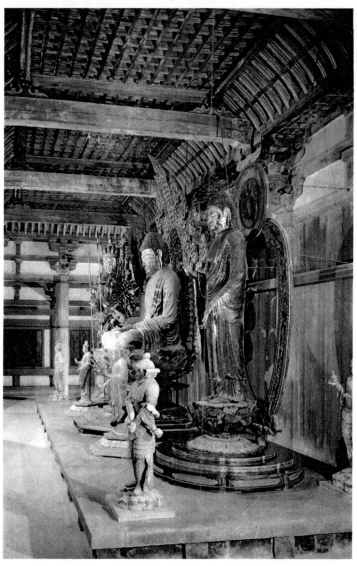

Figure 22a. The Tiantai Bridge, Huanxiu Garden, Suzhou.

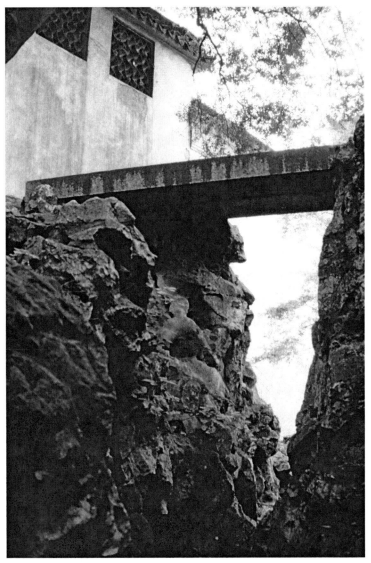

Figure 22b. Zhou Jichang, The Stone Bridge at Mt. Tiantai, ca. 1180, Freer Gallery of Art.

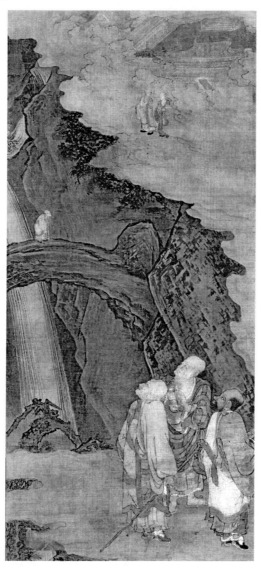

Figure 23. Ground plan of the Master of Nets Garden, with numbers for Figures 7 through 12 and arrows showing camera position and angle.

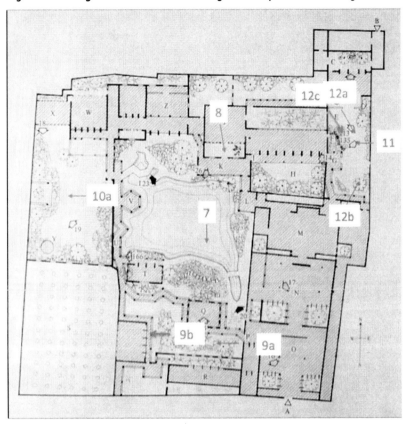

While Suzhou's Master of Fishing-Nets Garden (figure 23) is often "recognized as the finest example of the small scale garden,"[19] the names and couplets found there are not its strength. Its strength is visual. Much as site names and inscriptions engage the remembered body of extant poetry, garden designs engage the memory of other gardens, referring to and challenging expectations developed from the visitors' mentally archived viewing experiences. Like Suzhou's best-known gardens, the Fishing-Nets Garden has a history stretching back over many dynasties, claiming origins in the early Southern Song. Since then it has been reconstructed and renamed, bit by bit without cease, little of it documented but continuing to change right down to present day. Dating those textual and visual events is now difficult, but we know that the name Master of Fishing-Nets, Wang Shi Yuan 網師園, was not bestowed until the late eighteenth century.

In the garden, a sequence of critical design decisions began with the main viewing hall, a *xuan* 軒-type building—not the usual building type for a main hall and smaller than most—set back from the garden pond with a full wall of latticed windows facing the water. In a daring first act that defies expectations and looks like a well-planned surprise, which must have come with the owner's full collaboration if not fully from the owner himself, a two-story pile of rockery appears to have been unceremoniously dumped between the hall and the pond, thrust up so close to the windows as to entirely obstruct the view from within. On looking out, one sees little but rocks. The designer (or more likely the owner and his friends) came up with a name for this *xuan*, the Hillocks and Laurel Groves Hall, but it is the building's modern popular name that serves as a kind of saving grace: the Barrier of Clouds Hall. True, the barrier is stone and not mist but in this lies the literary conceit that nothing lasts, as the name-averse Daoists would have it, and that in time everything turns into its opposite, *yang* into *yin,* stone into water and clouds. The stones have been arranged so that one can climb through them, like Daoist immortals exploring the clouds, and those looking out the windows can imagine the entire hall with themselves in it floating aloft in the heavens -- an example in which name reformulates the image (figure 24).

Figure 24. The Hillocks and Laurel Groves Hall.

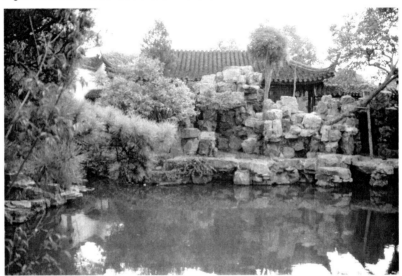

    With this, the best view of the pond is transferred across the water to an even smaller *xuan*, the Branch Beyond the Bamboo Hall 竹外一支軒. Here, then, as if by way of compensation for a good view spoiled at the main hall, comes a near-perfect garden view, seen through a moon gate and as calculated in its composition as if it were a painting. Since microcosmic completeness is the goal of the garden, the completeness of this view is a triumph, bringing together elements of darkness and light, near and far, dense and sparse, shallow and deep, round and straight, straight and crooked, water and stone, mineral and vegetable, evergreen vegetation and deciduous, and so forth, all carefully arranged in rhythmic *yin-yang* pairs and tightly framed (figure 25).

Figure 25. View from the Branch Beyond Bamboo Hall.

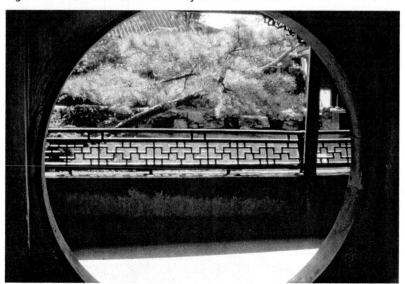

The transfer of prime view to the other side of the lake is a success, but the Barrier of Clouds Hall, buoyed by its serviceable name, is not really stripped of its primacy: the designer "makes up" for his deprivation of the usual view out the front windows with an unusually fine garden courtyard, long and narrow, to the rear—the south—providing full visual and physical access by latticed doors. Rocks, again, are the main feature, but here they are a series of high quality stones set well away from the building for good viewing. They are piled in a low, continuing ridge with enough small, interspersed laurel trees to provide shade for the entire length of the courtyard. It was for this backyard feature that the hall was formally named. The result is an exquisitely simple, elegant, and serene area of retreat. And as if to inform the visitor that he has indeed intended this "peripheral" courtyard as special, the designer offers a signal to those who can *see* what they are looking at: at the far end of the long courtyard and framed by it are located the garden's signature windows, three sets of fishing nets formed by wooden lattice (figures 26a and 26b).

Figure 26a. The Hillocks and Laurel Groves rear courtyard.

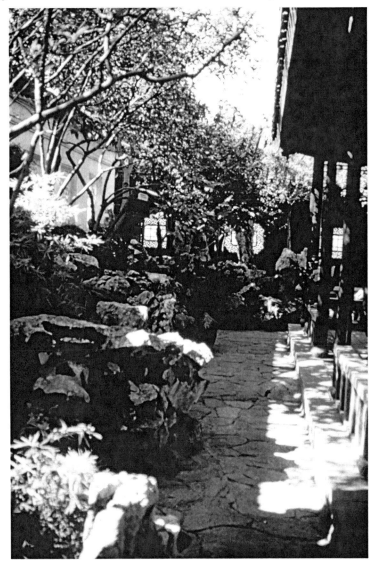

Figure 26b. Fishing Nets Lattice Window.

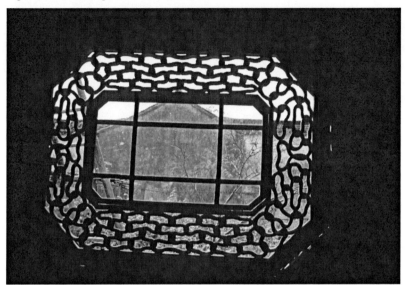

That rockery can by the sheer force of suggestion be turned into clouds constitutes an unexpected twist or reversal of meaning. But it depends on a recognition of the conventions that make it possible. Of course, many viewers might look at this setting without realizing the implications of the physical arrangement and the intellectual turn that these stones have taken. But an awareness of the possibility for such surprises transforms the normal "reading" of garden features into an anticipation of or active search for the unexpected. A similar reversal is enacted in the western courtyard of the Fishing-Nets garden, the Late Spring Courtyard, which features a pavilion-like building known as the Cold Stream Pavilion (Lengquan Ting 冷泉亭; figure 27a). Ordinarily, a pavilion is placed on the outskirts of the garden; looking toward it helps to locate the garden's intentionally appearing-and-disappearing pathways, while they are located so that looking from it provides a prime garden vista. Here, however, everything is confounded. This pavilion has been brought directly into the enclosed courtyard, cut in half and jammed up against a wall. Then the pavilion—the building from which to view the garden's stonework—is emptied of its observers, who are displaced by a large *taihu* rock, now brought indoors. The observers are repositioned, restricted to the outside, to venerate what now has become an enshrined stone. That such a radical departure from the norms of garden building can go unrecognized is demonstrated by the Metropolitan Museum's Astor Court, which claimed this courtyard as its model but whose builders (from Suzhou) failed to include the stone; only years later was a portable potted stone introduced *into* the pavilion (figure 27b).

This subject, which might be categorized as visual irony, has not to my knowledge been written about, but once the game is joined the garden abounds in slowly disclosed surprises. Two final examples can be found in another of the Fishing-Nets Garden's courtyards. Libraries were traditionally located on a second story to guard against possible flood damage, especially in Suzhou with its high water table. To its protective elevation was added the conceit of having to earn one's way upward through scholarship. This is driven home when one enters the "Five Sacred Mountains Studio" and seeks a stairway to the library chamber above, for there is none! It is only by persistence or accident that one eventually discovers an entryway that is not indoors but out, concealed as a tight passageway through the two-story rockery jammed against the side wall of the building—in what should be called the Library Courtyard but isn't (that is around the corner; figure 28).

Figure 27a. The Cold Stream Pavilion, Master of Nets Garden, Suzhou.

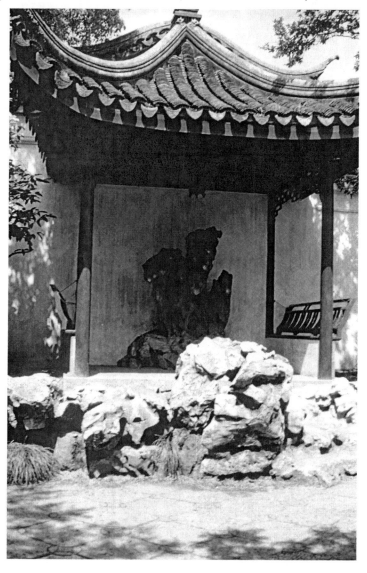

Figure 27b. The Astor Court, Metropolitan Museum of Art.

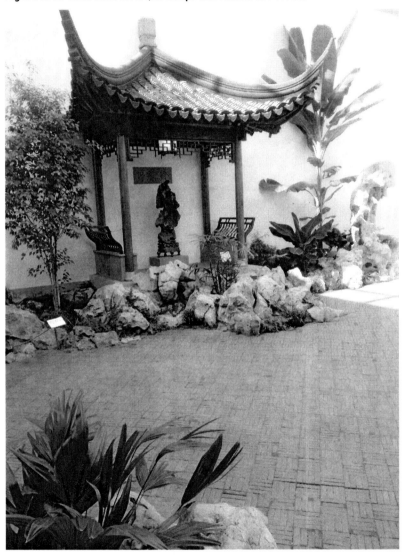

Figure 28. Entryway to the Five Sacred Mountains Studio Library.

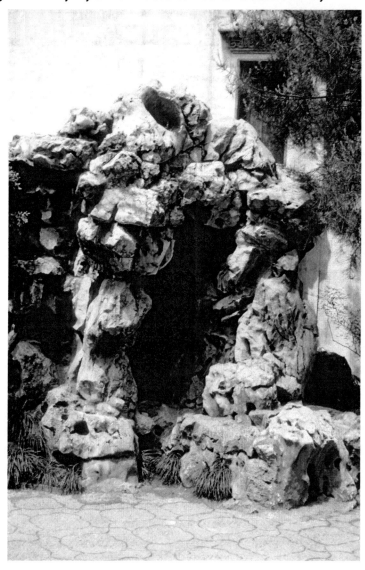

In this courtyard is something even more unusual if not unique: the entire east wall is not painted the usual limestone white but jet black (figure 29a).

Figure 29a. Black Wall in the Five Sacred Mountains Studio Courtyard.

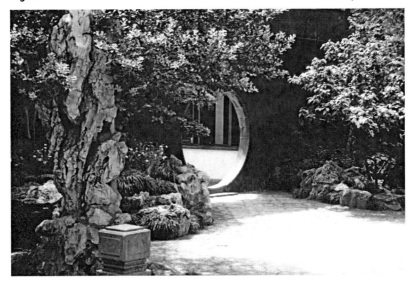

Even if one notices this, its purpose lies undiscovered until one stands in the right place looking in the right direction to notice that the entire moon gate leading to the courtyard beyond turns white from the sunlit wall in the courtyard beyond. With that, it looks like a full moon lighting up the night sky. That this is not merely the visitor's imagination but there by intent receives confirmation from the cassia or cinnamon plant planted next to the gate, the traditional symbol of the moon, silhouetted against the bright disk as if in a painting (figure 29b).

Figure 29b. Black Wall and Cassia Tree in the Five Sacred Mountains Studio Courtyard.

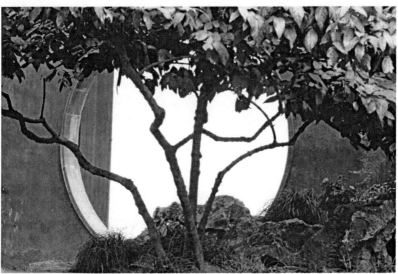

Once again, this has to be *noticed* by the visitor, as there are no other cues in the garden and no guiding literature that decodes this or other examples (as was the case with the Barrier of Clouds Hall, the Branch Apart from Bamboo Hall, and the Cold Springs Pavilion). Viewers have to fend for themselves and participate, look intensely, and perhaps return repeatedly to the site before seeing what they are looking at. Not only that, but the garden staff also needs to notice. In recent years the black wall has disappeared from the garden, not torn down but simply repainted like the other walls, *white*, now giving the visitor a recent ruin to gaze upon and a little more history to ponder in the thinking man's garden (figure 29c).

Figure 29c. The Black Wall Painted White in the Five Sacred Mountains Studio Courtyard.

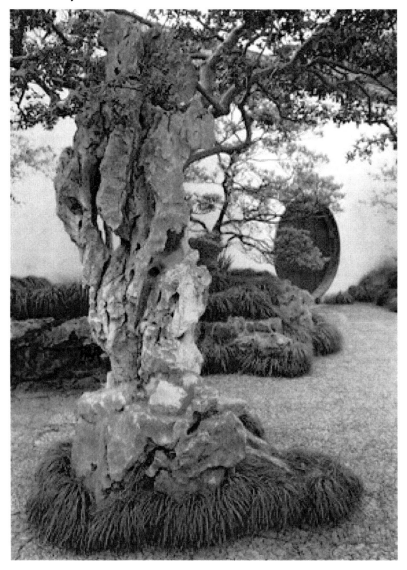

* * *

The generic language of "*the* Chinese garden"—the gardens' diversity excluded from the generalized singular—is well known.[20] The role of its basic elements—rocks and water, plants, and architecture—has been well articulated. The essential nature of Chinese garden design, its miniaturization, "borrowed scenery," and related efforts to "make more from less," has been written about many times over. But it is only in the study of particulars, rarely undertaken, that the greater creativity of a garden's design is revealed, and it is there that we can see an internal dialogue about aesthetic standards taking place. Such specific examples bear the mark of a high art, sophisticated and in open consultation with itself, just as much of "later" Chinese painting (meaning, chiefly, post-Song) has been applauded for being a self-conscious art, an art of scholarly paintings engaged with and *about* their own history, a sophisticated "art-historical art."[21] In the examples chosen here, departures from the ordinary are to garden composition as puns are to language, revealing an unanticipated level of design possibilities; their intent is to further complicate the visual situation, and to generate surprise and pleasure, at least among those who recognize what they are up to. The surprise comes at the very point where it manifests their designer's creativity. It is at that specific point that they stimulate the visitor's own intellect, reward knowledge and alertness, and arouse the appetite for more.

NOTES

1. Ji Cheng, trans. Alison Hardie, *The Craft of Gardens* (preface dated 1631) (New Haven and London: Yale University Press, 1988), 65.
2. James Elkins, "On the Conceptual Analysis of Gardens," *Journal of Garden History*, 13.4 (October–December 1993), 189.
3. Elkins, 190–191.
4. Ibid., 197.
5. Edward Schafer uses "baroque" for the choice stones collected by Chinese "petromaniacs": "There is no question about the bizarreness of the most celebrated specimens of this group. Du Wan, and other writers as well, repeatedly describe choice examples in such terms as '*odd*' (*yi* 異), '*singular*' (奇), and '*fantastic*' (怪)." Edward H. Schafer, *Tu Wan's Stone Catalogue of Cloudy Forest: A Commentary and Synopsis* (Berkeley and Los Angeles: University of California Press, 1961), 8–9.
6. *The Chinese Classics: Volume I: The Confucian Analects, The Great Learning, The Doctrine of the Mean*, trans. James Legge (Hong Kong: Hong Kong University Press, 1960), 263–264, slightly modified.
7. Cf. Legge, 157.
8. Robert Harrist, "Site Names and their Meanings in the Garden of Solitary Enjoyment," *The Journal of Garden History*, 13:4 (October–December 1993), 202.
9. Harrist, 202.
10. Chen Congzhou on *Red Chamber's* garden: "Here fiction is perfectly mixed with fact. Call something fictitious and yet it may be based on a prototype the author has seen or even touched. Call something real and yet it may have been enlivened by the author's imagination. That is why the book has such fascination for and appeal to the reader." Chen Congzhou, *On Chinese Gardens* (Shanghai: Tongji University Press, 1984), 28.
11. Cao Xueqin, trans. David Hawkes, *The Story of the Stone, Volume I, The Golden Days* (Harmondsworth: Penguin, 1973), 324–325 (my italics).
12. Hawkes, *Stone*, 328.
13. Ibid., 329–330. For more on garden names, see Richard Strassberg, "The Necessity of Names in Chinese Gardens," and "Appendix A: Names in Liu Fang Yuan," in T. June Li, ed., *Another World Lies Beyond: Creating Liu Fang Yuan, the Huntington's Chinese Garden* (San Marino: Huntington Library, 2009), 42–51, 105–112 (the Appendix illustrates, translates,

and gives the poetic references for each name plaque in this modern garden); Craig Clunas, *Fruitful Sites: Garden Culture in Ming Dynasty China*
(London: Reaktion Books, 1996), 144ff. and throughout.

14. Jan Stuart, "Ming Dynasty Gardens Reconstructed in Words and
    Images," *Journal of Garden History*, 10.3 (July–September 1990), 171.
    There is a logical conundrum here: if we were to be left with no reliable
    visual document of the middle Ming garden, on what reliable basis can
    we show that to be the case?

15. Stuart, 171.

16. That most large garden stones, even if free-standing, are composite
    structures and so, not merely a "found art" is frequently overlooked. I
    would argue that both garden stones and, frequently, table-top scholar's
    rocks should be recognized as integral and important to the history
    of Chinese sculpture from Ming times on, if not from Song. On gar-
    den stones, see especially Schafer, *Tu Wan's Stone Catalogue*; John Hay,
    Kernels of Energy, Bones of Earth: The Rock in Chinese Art (New York:
    China Institute in America), 1985; Robert Mowry, *Worlds Within Worlds:
    The Richard Rosenblum Collection of Chinese Scholars' Rocks* (Cambridge:
    Harvard University Art Museums, 1997).

17. See note 1. Ji's garden text, nevertheless, is quite conservative itself and
    does not describe any *specific* unorthodox departures, like those that
    occupy the remaining part of this short study.

18. See Wen Fong, *The Lohans and a Bridge to Heaven*. Freer Gallery of
    Art Occasional Papers 3, no. 1 (Washington, D.C.: Smithsonian Institu-
    tion, 1958); Wen Fong, "Sacred and Humanistic: *Five Hundred Lohans*
    at Daitokuji," in Wen Fong, *Art as History: Calligraphy and Painting as
    One* (Princeton: P. Y. and Kinmay W. Fong Center for East Asian Art,
    Department of Art and Archaeology, and Princeton University Press,
    2014), 215–270.

19. Chen Congzhou, 6.

20. That most modern study has been (unnecessarily) limited to the Yangzi
    delta region and the royal gardens of Beijing is emphasized in my article,
    "Beyond Suzhou: Region and Memory in the Gardens of Sichuan." *Art
    Bulletin*, 86.2 (June 2004), 207–227.

21. Cf. Max Loehr, "Some Fundamental Issues in the History of Chinese
    Painting," *Journal of Asian Studies*, 23.2 (February 1964), 238: In the Ming,
    "Chinese painting thus contemplated itself, became itself art-history. As
    a consequence, it was no longer painting pure and simple but a kind of
    humanistic discipline, an art blended with learning; it was painting about

painting, allusive, commentatorial, and increasingly abstract because its content was thought."

CHAPTER 10

FOTUDENG'S SPELL PRACTICE AND THE DHĀRAṆĪ RECITATION RITUAL

Koichi Shinohara

Huijiao's 慧皎 (497–554) *Biographies of Eminent Monks* (*Gaoseng zhuan* 高僧傳), compiled around A.D. 530, tells many stories of spell practice attributed to early monastic leaders.[1] Spell practice is also described in considerable detail in a number of translated sūtras and collections of dhāraṇīs. These sūtras and collections name individual spells, transcribe them phonetically in Chinese characters, explain their origins and benefits, and prescribe proper rituals for reciting them. They often mention tangible signs that confirm the success of recitation and guarantee desired outcomes. In this essay, I examine briefly how reading the accounts of spell practice in these two very different types of sources side by side might shed light on spell practice in early Chinese Buddhism. [2]

Spell practices described in these two roughly contemporary sources are similar in many regards, yet there are also significant differences. They appear to be rooted in a common culture of spell practice that was also varied and included many different practices. They also present spell practices with different emphases. The intended audience of dhāraṇī instructions, for example, was ritual practitioners. These instructions describe in detail the specific steps that practitioners must follow. The spells they present may be used for a variety of purposes and on different occasions. These instructions also include standardized descriptions of the signs that confirm the ritual's success, most strikingly visions of deities that appear miraculously at the climactic point of the ritual, before the desired outcomes are actually realized. These instructions, furthermore, often promise successful attainment of desired goals in general terms without describing what they are. The emphasis is on describing the signs rather than the eventual outcome.

Huijiao's stories situate the practice in specific contexts. They specify the problems the monks solved by reciting spells. The ritual's efficacy in these stories is confirmed by the actual realization of the desired goals themselves, observed by many who were present, rather than by miraculous signs, such as visions of deities. What is miraculous in these stories is the outcome; they may or may not have been accompanied by other unusual signs.

Both types of accounts highlight the attainment and demonstration of supernatural knowledge through spell practice.[3] Yet, over the long run one area of important difference was the relationship between spell recitation and image worship. Huijiao's accounts of spell practice do not involve images. Earlier dhāraṇī instructions do not necessarily require images, but the practice of reciting dhāraṇīs to an image quickly became a dominant pattern of dhāraṇī rituals, provoking a further rich and varied evolution.

I begin this brief and exploratory investigation with the well-known biography of Fotudeng 佛圖澄 (232–348), a foreign monk who became an influential figure at the Later Zhao court of Shi Le 石勒 (r. 319–333) and Shi Hu 石虎 (r. 333–334) and played a vitally important role in establishing early Chinese Buddhist community.[4] I first review several stories describing Fotudeng's use of spells, and then situate these stories in the larger context by examining stories in Huijiao's collection that attribute similar practices to other monks.[5] These examples would show that many other monks used spells in similar ways. I then turn to a dhāraṇī instruction in *The Supernatural spells of Great Dhāraṇīs Taught by the Seven Buddhas and Eight Bodhisattvas.*[6]

SPELL PRACTICE AND SUPERNATURAL KNOWLEDGE IN HUIJIAO'S BIOGRAPHY OF FOTUDENG

References to Spell Practice
In the introductory section of the biography, Fotudeng is described as being skilled in reciting spells (*shenzhou* 神咒); he was also capable of employing demonic beings (*guiwu* 鬼物).[7] He mixed sesame oil and rouge (*yanchi* 胭脂) and smeared it on his palm; events more than 1,000 *li* 里 away appeared clearly in his palm as if he was facing them at the site where they occurred.[8] He could also make others see them after going through proper purification. Additionally, he listened to the sound of bells and could always predict future events correctly.[9] Fotudeng used spells to secure supernatural knowledge. But he also used them in a variety of different ways.

Sometimes Fotudeng is described as a great healer. He cured a chronic illness that no one could cure. He brought Shi Hu's son Bin 斌 back to life by saying a spell over a tooth pick,[10] but knew that the illness of one of the crown prince Shi Sui's 石邃 two sons was incurable.[11] When the moats of the city dried up, Fotudeng went to the source, sat on a bench, burned incense, and recited spells. After three days a small dragon appeared, and water came in abundance.[12] In another story, after a long drought, Shi Hu ordered Fotudeng to pray for rain, two white dragons descended to the shrine and a heavy rain came.[13]

In some stories, he seemed actively to affect an expected outcome through ritual practice. Of the disciple sent to the Western Regions Fotudeng said, "In my palm I see that the incense-buying disciple is in a certain place and at the point of death at the hands of brigands."[14] He burnt incense and said prayers. Later the disciple returned and confirmed this account.[15] He also miraculously knew of a fire in Youzhou; after sprinkling wine, he said, "A rescue has been effected."[16] The fire had been contained.[17]

Fotudeng's Supernatural knowledge

Above all, Huijiao's biography emphasizes Fotudeng's supernatural knowledge and his ability to predict future events, framing the many stores of his success at Later Zhao ruler Shi Le's court around this theme. Wishing to spread the teaching, Fotudeng first visited the ruler's general Guo Heilüe 郭黑略, who then brought Fotudeng to Shi Le's attention. Guo Heilüe had taken the Five Precepts and become Fotudeng's disciple. Since then Guo Heilüe always predicted the outcome of battles correctly. Shi Le questioned him, and Guo Heilüe spoke of a monk with exceptional skills who had predicted that Shi Le would conquer China and that he, the monk Fotudeng, would become Shi Le's teacher. Guo Heilüe's predictions were all Fotudeng's words. Shi Le, calling this a gift from heaven, summoned Fotudeng and asked him about the efficacy of the Buddha's teaching. Knowing that Shi Le would not understand profound doctrines, Fotudeng enacted a miracle; when he filled his begging bowl with water, burnt incense, and recited a spell, a blue lotus flower, in brilliant color, appeared. She Le was persuaded.[18] The demonstration of supernatural knowledge and enacting a miraculous vision are presented as strategies for securing the patronage of the ruler.

Even though in this important story Fotudeng demonstrates his powers with a miraculous vision, in most stories told in the biography, the efficacy of his powers is demonstrated by the predicted outcome. The reliability of Fotudeng's supernatural knowledge is unambiguously and dramatically confirmed by the predicted outcome revealed later.

In many stories Fotudeng predicted or knew of the outcomes of battles before they became publicly known. Duan Bo's 段波 massive army attacked and Shi Le was frightened. Fotudeng told him that judging from the chiming of the temple bell, the leader of the enemy would be captured on the next day at dawn, and indeed soldiers ambushed the enemy leader and captured him.[19] When Liu Yao 劉曜 usurped the throne and his son, sent to attack Shi Le, was defeated, Fotudeng told his disciples that Liu Yao's son was captured even before the news arrived.[20] Three years later Liu Yao himself attacked Loyang, and his army was completely routed. Fotudeng "smeared something on his palm and looked at it. He saw a man being bound in a great crowd and being tied about the elbows with a red silken cord."[21] It was at that time that Yao was captured alive.[22] Later, Fotudeng knew of the plight of Guo Heilüe, who had fallen into an ambush, and spoke to his disciples about his escape.[23] He repeatedly told Shi Hu about the futility of attacking Yan 燕.[24]

Some stories illustrate Fotudeng's supernatural knowledge around other similar themes. People at Fangtou 坊頭 were about to attack Shi Le's camp. Fotudeng knew of this beforehand and told Guo Heilüe to warn Shi Le.[25] Fotudeng often warned of threatening rebellions.[26] Fotudeng predicted Huan Wen's 桓溫 invasion.[27] He warned of a disturbance involving two young boys and a Xianbei slave.[28]

Some stories tell of a personal threat to Fotudeng.[29] He exposed Shi Le's trick to test him.[30] In another passage Fotudeng is said to have known the content of a conversation between his disciples who were away; these disciples discussed their master.[31]

Fotudeng knew of other kinds of hidden things. He knew of the ancient Aśoka image in Linzi 臨淄 and identified its location.[32] While in the capital he spoke of the distant fire in Youzhou 幽州 and appeared to have extinguished it by sprinkling wine over it.[33]

Fotudeng demonstrates his knowledge of the past lives of others. Facing the grave threat of the invading Eastern Jin army, Shi Hu expressed his anger at the Buddha's failure to protect him. Fotudeng then explained that in a previous life Shi Hu as a merchant hosted a large feast at a temple in Jibin 罽賓; an arhat predicted then that in later lives Shi Hu would first be reborn as a chicken and then as a king in China. This prediction was realized, demonstrating the efficacy of donating to the monastic community.[34]

Fotudeng predicted the death of Shi Le and She Hu's usurpation[35]; he also predicted his own death and the death of Shi Hu.[36]

OTHER BIOGRAPHIES IN HUIJIAO'S COLLECTION

Spell practice
Several biographies in Huijiao's collection explicitly note that their subjects engaged in spell practice. Dharmakṣema 曇無讖 (385–433) understood spells well and was known as a great spell master in India.[37] Once in a mountain he recited a spell on a piece of rock and opened a spring for the king.[38] At one time, Dharmakṣema told Juqu Mengsun that demons had entered villages, predicting a major epidemic. Mengsun did not believe him. Dharmakṣema then magically let him see the demons. Mengsun was alarmed. Dharmakṣema then recited spells for three days, and then told Mengsun that the demons had left. At the border, hundreds of escaping demons were seen.[39]

Guṇabhadra 求那跋陀羅 (394–468) was learned in a wide range of fields, including the art of spells. He built a temple to the west of the Phoenix Pavilion at the boundary of Moling 秣陵 District. The sound of doors opening was heard every night at midnight, but no one was seen. Monks were often troubled by bad dreams. Guṇabhadra burned incense, recited spells, and spoke to the demons, ordering them either to become protective deities of the temple or to leave. Dozens of monks and laypeople then had the same dream; thousands of demons carrying baggage were seen to leave in the dream. The temple was then pacified.[40]

There was a drought in 462. Prayers were offered to mountain and river deities to no effect for several months. The Emperor Xiaowu 孝武 (r. 453–464) requested Guṇabhadra to perform a rain ritual, saying that if the ritual failed, he would not grant him an audience again. Guṇabhadra fasted and recited scriptures and secret spells, and in the late afternoon the next day, clouds gathered in the northwest direction, and as the sun set, a violent wind rose and heavy clouds appeared. The rain continued for several days.[41]

The biography of Ratnamati is appended to Guṇabhadra's biography; in this biography Ratnamati is said to have practiced spells and was able to see the past events in peoples' lives by smearing unguent in his palms, in a manner somewhat similar to Fotudeng's practice.

Zhu Fakuang 竺法曠 (327–402) was skilled in spells and traveled in villages performing healing. Someone who had the ability to see demons reported that dozens of demons stood guard around Fakuang all the time.[42] Another monk Zhu Daolin 竺道隣 produced an Amitābha image. Fakuang gathered supporters and built a large hall for it. They cut down trees and a drought followed. Fakuang then recited a spell to cause water to arrive.[43]

Beidu 杯度 (?–?)[44] and Huifen 慧芬 (407–485)[45] are said to have been skilled in spells and to have performed healing.[46] Many entries in the *Biographies of Eminent Monks* collection indicate that their subjects recited spells for a variety of purposes, such as healing,[47] bringing about rain,[48] and taming animals.[49]

These passages suggest that subjects of the biographies in Huijiao's collection shared a common culture of spell practice. Some monks, particularly the Indian monks Dharmakṣema and Guṇabhadra, were known for their successes in spell recitation. Many Chinese monks were also known for their skill in this art. Like Fotudeng, these monks used spells for healing and for causing rainfall.

Supernatural knowledge

Stories of supernatural knowledge similar to those emphasized in Fotudeng's biography also appear in other biographies in Huijiao's collection. Kumārajīva's 鳩摩羅什 biography, for example, tells that taken hostage by Cavalry General Lü Guang 呂光, Kumārajīva warned him repeatedly of dangers in the immediate future. Lü Guang, disregarding Kumārajīva's warning, rested his army at the foot of mountain and lost thousands in the flood caused by heavy rain during the night. Lü Guang later became the ruler of Later Liang, and Kumārajīva's biography reports in some detail how Kumārajīva predicted rebellions and an impending military disaster for him.[50]

Dharmakṣema's biography concludes with the following story. Dharmakṣema insisted on travelling to the West in search of a manuscript that preserved the latter part of the *Nirvāṇa sūtra*. Juqu Mengsun 沮渠蒙遜 (r. 401–433), his patron, made a public display of offering provisions and valuable gifts to him, but secretly planned to kill him. Dharmakṣema spoke of his impending death to his community, and eventually was killed by the assassin sent by Juqu Mengsun.[51]

In these stories from biographies of foreign "translator" monks, as in many stories in Fotudeng's biography, an ambivalent relationship with the secular ruler frames the subject's demonstration of supernatural knowledge. Another biography, set in the south and from a much later period, is similarly framed as a story of a monk who was favored by a ruler.

Fayuan 法願 (415–487) was born in a family that worshipped a local deity, and he himself had studied music and dance and was very skilled in a variety of worldly arts and physiognomy. Once seeing the reflection of his face in a mirror, he said that he would be given an audience with the emperor. Fayuan then came to the capital city and made his living by reading people's physiognomy. Before they achieved their fame, Zong

Ke 宗殼 and Shen Qingzhi 沈慶微 consulted him, and Fayuan correctly foretold that Zong would become the Regional Inspector of Three Regions and that Shen would achieve a status as high as that of the Three Dukes.

Emperor Taizu 太祖 of Song heard about him and put him to a test, letting him read the physiognomy of a prisoner, serving in forced labor at a metal factory, and a handsome slave, both dressed in courtly robes and crown. Fayuan pointed at the prisoner and warned him of dangers, telling him that as soon as he stepped down from the stairs of the palace he would be placed in shackles and chains. Fayuan told the slave that though he was born with a lowly status, he briefly had escaped it. The emperor was impressed and allowed Fayuan to stay in the rear quarter of the palace.

It was after this incident that Fayuan sought permission and became a monk. When Emperor Xiaowu assumed the throne, Zong Ke was assigned to serve as the Regional Inspector of Guangzhou 廣州. Zong Ke took Fayuan with him and honored him as his master of the Five Precepts. When Liu Yixuan 劉義宣 rebelled, Zong Ke consulted Fayuan, who predicted a dire outcome and urged him to change his plan. Fayuan's prediction proved correct. When Zong Ke was reassigned to serve as the Regional Inspector of Yuzhou 豫州, he again took Fayuan with him. Prince of Jingling 竟陵王 rebelled, and Fayuan advised Zong Ke correctly again.[52] The biography also reports that Fayuan mysteriously predicted the demise of the Song dynasty.[53]

The resemblance of this biography to Fotudeng's biography is notable. Fotudeng predicted that Shi Le would become the ruler; Fayuan predicted brilliant careers for Zong Ke and Shen Qingzhi. As She Le subjected Fotudeng to a test before accepting him, Taizu tested Fayuan. Both monks maintained an affiliation with an important figure in the government, a general or a high-ranking official. And both Fotudeng and Fayuan provided valuable political or military advice to the ruler.

A variety of stories of remarkable knowledge appear in other biographies in Huijiao's collection. Many monks are said to have been able to

predict future events. Buddhabhadra 佛馱跋陀羅 (359–429) predicted
dangers in ocean travelling[54] and the arrival of five vessels from India.[55]
Fan Cai 范材 and She Gong 涉公 are explicitly said to have been able
to predict future events.[56]

Many are said to have predicted their own unexpected deaths,
explaining them as consequences of their karmic conditions.[57] As noted
earlier, Dharmakṣema knew the ruler Mengsun's plot to kill him beforehand.[58] A remarkable story is attributed to An Shigao 安世高 (?–?); in a
previous life, he was a renouncer who predicted that he would be killed
by a youth for a karmic debt he owed him from a yet earlier birth (T.
2059: 50.323b14–24). Others simply spoke of their approaching death.[59]
Tanshi 曇始 (?–?), like Fotudeng, predicted the death of a ruler.[60]

Other biographies mention diverse kinds of supernatural knowledge.
Buddhayaśas 佛陀耶舍 (?–?) could tell that the tiger he and his teacher
encountered in a field had eaten its fill and therefore they did not need
to fear it.[61] While residing elsewhere Yu Fakai 于法開 (?–?) knew the
progress of Zhi Dun's 支遁 (314–366) lecture and instructed his disciple
on how to debate him.[62] Travelling with his disciples, Shi Daoan was
caught in a storm, and when they reached an inhabited house, he could
tell the name of the unknown host.[63] On his way to a layman's residence
for a meal Zhu Senglang 竺僧朗 (?–?) told his companions that someone
was stealing their robes; he could also predict the number of visitors to
his temple one day before they came.[64] Zhu Fahui 竺法慧 (?–?) often
told his disciple Fazhao 法照 that the disciple had broken a leg of a
chicken in a past life and that he would suffer from it. This prediction
was fulfilled when someone unexpectedly threw Fazhao to the ground
and permanently damaged his leg. Fahui also knew the approaching
death of a man who ploughed the field.[65]

Huijiao's biographies of Fotudeng and other monks who practiced
spells mention a variety of settings in which they recited spells, yet
supernatural knowledge, forms of omniscience, appear to have been of

particular interest. Monks often displayed their extraordinary knowledge to royal patrons.

I now turn to a brief examination to a dhāraṇī instruction. Many of the issues mentioned in the account of spell practice in Huijiao's biographies also appear in this instruction.

SPELL PRACTICE IN A DHĀRAṆĪ COLLECTION

A distinctive kind of spell practice, recitation of dhāraṇīs, was popular around the time Fotudeng's biography developed. A significant body of early instructions for dhāraṇī recitation is preserved. In this tradition, the term *shenzhou*, or "supernatural spell," was often used synonymously with dhāraṇī. As noted earlier, spells are often designated as *shenzhou* in the biographies of Fotudeng and others in Huijiao's collection. Biographies in Huijiao's collection typically mention spell practices without spelling out the ritual in detail. Dhāraṇī instructions spell out the rituals in greater detail. The spell practice in Huijiao's biographies and dhāraṇī instructions show significant similarities and appear to have belonged to a common culture of spell practice, but they were also distinct.

In order to illustrate this relationship, I now turn to an early Chinese dhāraṇī collection, in four fascicles, called *The Supernatural Spells of Great Dhāraṇīs Taught by the Seven Buddhas and Eight Bodhisattvas.*[66] This work, from the fourth to the fifth century, was later incorporated into another work in ten fascicles from the first half of the sixth century, *Miscellaneous Collection of Dhāraṇīs.*[67] This later and much larger work, attributed to the Liang period (502–557),[68] is roughly contemporary to Huijiao's biographical collection. Together these collections point to a growing tradition of dhāraṇī practices.

The entries in the *Seven Buddhas and Eight Bodhisattvas* dhāraṇīs are presented according to a more or less fixed formula. Each dhāraṇī, attributed to the first seven Buddhas of this World Age of the Wise and the Eight Bodhisattvas, is said to have a much longer cosmic history, having been taught by an astronomically large number of past Buddhas in earlier world ages. Each dhāraṇī is given a name. After reciting the dhāraṇī a fixed number of times, the practitioner is instructed to take yellow or five-colored strings and make a certain number of knots. These appear to refer to the preparation of amulets to be worn on one's body.

Some passages describe the extraordinary worldly powers of the dhāraṇī. Other passages promise advances in a more distinctly Buddhist path toward salvation. For our present discussion we might note that many of the dhāraṇī practices described in these collections explicitly mention acquiring different forms of supernatural knowledge. The entry on the dhāraṇī taught by bodhisattva Mahāsthāmaprāpta 大勢至菩薩, for example, mentions that those who practice it will acquire knowledge into past lives and will be able to see up to myriads of past births freely without any obstructions, just as one clearly sees a mango fruit in one's palm.[69] The entry on the dhāraṇī taught by Ruler of the Heaven of Those who Delight in Creation (hualetian 化樂天王) mentions in addition to the knowledge of 400 past births; knowledge of 400 future births; knowledge of what is in other people's minds; knowledge of astronomy, geography, and magical diagrams; and records of prognostications.[70]

Fotudeng and other early Chinese Buddhist monks frequently engaged in spell practice. As examined above, among its various benefits, the attaining of supernatural knowledge and consequent ability to predict future events received a great deal of attention. In reading the repeated references to Fotudeng's supernatural knowledge in Huijiao's biography, we need to take into account this connection between spell recitation and supernatural knowledge that is also so important in dhāraṇī instructions.

Some passages in the dhāraṇī instructions explicitly address military assistance from supernatural beings. At a time when a kingdom is threatened by neighboring powers, if the king recites the dhāraṇī taught by bodhisattva Jiutuo 救脫 facing the direction from which enemies invade, the eight divisions of supernatural beings will rain down sand and stones, a dark wind will blow with thunder and lightning.[71]Similarly, when the king recites the dhāraṇī of the past Buddha Kanakamuni, gods Brahmā, Śakra, and the Four Heavenly Kings are said to rain down swords and a black wind makes the sun and the moon invisible, while demons suck vitality from the enemies.[72] Though Fotudeng's biography does mention resorting to such assistance only obliquely, for example, in the account of the prayers Fotudeng and other monks offered at the time when general Guo Heilüe was in danger,[73] Fotudeng's role as an adviser to rulers constantly engaged in battles suggests that practices such as these, described in the dhāraṇī texts, might have been a part of his repertoire.

The account of Fotudeng's magical demonstration, or "techniques of the Way" (daoshu 道術), at his first audience with Shi Le[74] shares a common ground with dhāraṇī practice, which frequently involves visions, typically of the Buddhas and other deities appearing in front of the practitioner. Some passages speak of the deities appearing on the seat of a lotus flower: Maheśvara for example is said to appear in front of a worldly king who has recited the dhāraṇī twenty-one times and sits in silence; in a liminal state, between dreaming and being awake, he will see the deity in space, sitting on the seat of a white lotus; a ray of bright light touches the king's body; as soon as the light touches the king, the king will be purified and enter into a samādhi; his mind is delighted, and for that reason, all his wishes will be fulfilled.[75] The vision Fotudeng presented to Shi Le is described more modestly, without mentioning a deity. But it also involved the recitation of a dhāraṇī and the appearance of lotus flowers and extraordinary light.

CONCLUDING THOUGHTS

Significant differences between the dhāraṇī instruction and the accounts of spell recitation in Huijiao's biographical collection are also to be noted. In Huijiao's account spells are not affiliated with named deities, for example.[76] One particularly consequential difference appears to have been the incorporation of image worship into dhāraṇī practice.

The stories of spell practice in Huijiao's collection generally do not include references to images.[77] This is particularly noteworthy since Huijiao gave a prominent place to images in his collection (in the "merit making," or *xingfu*興福 section).[78] Stories of miraculous images attributed to Indian king Aśoka are reproduced. In Huijiao's account of contemporary Chinese Buddhism both spell recitation and image worship were considered important, but these two types of Buddhist practice had little to do with each other.

Images do not play a role in spell practices attributed to the Buddhas in the *Seven Buddhas and Eight Bodhisattvas*. These rituals culminate in visions. But spell recitation became closely connected with image worship early in the evolution of dhāraṇī practice. Images are mentioned twice in the instructions attributed to Bodhisattvas in the *Seven Buddhas and Eight Bodhisattvas*. In the *Miscellaneous Collection of Dhāraṇīs*, roughly contemporary to Huijiao's collection, there appears a carefully spelled out ritual of the spell that is to be recited in front of an image.[79] The image became the site of miraculous signs that confirm the success of recitation, emitting light, shaking, and speaking in a loud voice.

The tradition of spell practice documented in dhāraṇī instructions appears to have originally emerged as a part of the common and widely shared culture of spell practice also glimpsed in Huijiao's biographical collection. One shared preoccupation of the spell culture was the attainment of supernatural knowledge. The tradition of dhāraṇī recitation came to incorporate image worship at a time relatively early in its evolution. A rich and varied evolution of a distinct ritual tradition, later known as Esoteric Buddhism, followed that innovation.

NOTES

1. Chinese Buddhist canonical texts are identified by the numbers assigned to them in the *Taishō Shinshū Daizōkyō* 大正新修大蔵経 (Ed. Takakusu Junjirō, et al., 100 vols., Tokyo, 1924–32).] For the date of Huijiao's biographical collection, I follow Makita Tairyō's suggestion in "*Kōsōden no seirits* 高僧伝の成立," part 2, *Tōhō gakuhō* 東方学報 (Kyoto), 44 (1973), 103–104.

2. Spells occupy a very important place in early Chinese Buddhist and Daoist literature. Michel Strickmann discussed early Chinese Buddhist and Daoist spell practice extensively, for example in *Chinese Magical Medicine* (edited by Bernard Faure, Stanford: Stanford University Press, 2002); *Mantra et mandarin: le bouddhisme tantrique en Chine* (Paris: Editions Gallimard, 1996). Among more recent studies of dhāraṇī practice are Paul Copp, *The Body Incantatory: Spells and the Ritual Imagination in Medieval Chinese Buddhism* (New York: Columbia University Press, 2014); "Mantra and Dhāraṇī in the Religious Traditions of Asia," *Bulletin of the School of Oriental and African Studies*, 77 (2014): 1–194; Ronald Davidson, "Studies in Dhāraṇī Literature I: Revisiting the Meaning of the Term Dhāraṇī," *Journal of Indian Philosophy* 32 (2004): 1–30; Koichi Shinohara, *Spells, Images, and Maṇḍalas: Tracing the Evolution of Esoteric Buddhist Rituals* (New York: Columbia University Press, 2014).

3. Such demonstration helped secure lay patronage. The story of Srīgupta that appears in several sources spells out the relationship between the Buddha's omniscience and lay patronage in considerable detail. I discussed this story in "Taking a Meal at a Lay Supporter's Residence," *Buddhist Monasticism in East Asia* (London and New York: Routledge, 2010), 22–24.

4. Fotudeng's biography was translated with an informative introduction by Arthur Wright, "Fo-t'u-teng: A Biography," *Harvard Journal of Asiatic Studies* 11, nos. 3,4 (December 1948): 321–371. The article is now reprinted in Arthur Wright, *Studies in Chinese Buddhism*, edited by Robert M. Somers (New Haven and London: Yale University Press, 1999), 14–68.

5. The focus of my exploration is Huijiao's biographies of Fotudeng and other monks in his collection, and their presentation of spell practices, rather than the historical life of Fotudeng. Fotudeng lived in the third and

fourth century, centuries before the appearance of Huijiao's sixth-century biography. The biographical tradition of Fotudeng would have gradually evolved over this long period. Wright briefly discusses the sources of Huijiao's biography of Fotudeng, *Studies in Chinese Buddhism*, 41–43.

6. T.1332.
7. M. Strickmann discusses Buddhist and Daoist demonology extensively, see *Chinese Magical Medicine*, 38–88.
8. The short biography of Baoyi 寶意 or Ratnamati relates that Ratnamati was skilled in spells and smeared unguent on his palm to see people's past (T. 2059: 50.345a18).
9. T. 2059: 50.383a18–19 [Wright, 3]. Fotudeng based his prediction of the capture of the enemy leader Duan Bo on the chiming of temple bells, T. 2059: 50.384a21 [Wright, 11]. He also predicted Shi Le's death by the sound of a bell, 384b27–c1 [Wright, 17].
10. T. 2059: 50.384b21–24 [Wright, 16].
11. T. 2059: 50.384c17–21 [Wright, 20].
12. T. 2059: 50.384a1–12 [Wright, 9].
13. T. 2059: 50.385b12–15 [Wright, 27].
14. Wright, *Chinese Buddhism*, p. 57.
15. T. 2059: 50.385b18–22 [Wright, 29].
16. Wright, *Chinese Buddhism*, p. 62.
17. T. 2059: 50.386b3–6 [Wright, 37].
18. T. 2059: 50.383b25–c10 [Wright, 4].
19. T. 2059: 50.384a20–25 [Wright, 11].
20. T. 2059: 50.384a26–b3 [Wright, 12].
21. Wright, *Studies in Chinese Buddhism*, 51.
22. T. 2059: 50.384b3–15 [Wright, 13].
23. T. 2059: 50.385a1–10 [Wright, 22].
24. T. 2059: 50.385b25–27 [Wright, 31].
25. T. 2059: 50.383c17–19 [Wright, 6].
26. Shi Cong 石葱 384b17–20 [Wright, 15]; Shi Sui 石邃 384c21–385a1 [Wright, 21]; Shi Xuan 石宣 386b8–c2 [Wright, 38].
27. T. 2059: 50.385c22–24 [Wright, 33].
28. T. 2059: 50.384a12–20 [Wright, 10].
29. T. 2059: 50.383c23–384a1 [Wright, 8]; 384c21–385a1 [Wright, 21].
30. T. 2059: 50.383c19–23 [Wright, 7].
31. T. 2059: 50.384c8–16 [Wright, 19].
32. T. 2059: 50.23–25 [Wright, 30].
33. T. 2059: 50.386b4–8 [Wright, 37].

34. T. 2059: 50.385a21–6 [Wright, 24].
35. T. 2059: 50.384b26–c1 [Wright, 17].
36. T. 2059: 50.386c2–27 [Wright, 39–40]. Fotudeng also knew that mad man Hemp Tunic would be brought to the capital from Wei District two hundred *li* away and instructed that he not be put to death (T. 2059: 50.385c25–29 [Wright, 34]).
37. T. 2059: 50.336a5–6.
38. T. 2059: 50.336a6–9.
39. T. 2059: 50.336b8–13.
40. T. 2059: 50.344c22–28.
41. T. 2059: 50.344c29–345a7.
42. T. 2059: 50.356c28–257a3.
43. T. 2059: 50.357a3–4.
44. T. 2059: 50.392a2.
45. T. 2059: 50.416c2.
46. Huitong 慧通 (T. 2059: 50.398c7) and Daofa 道法 (–474, T. 2059: 50.399b7) are also said to have used spells frequently.
47. Kumārajīva (T. 2059: 50.332c24–27); Guṇavarman (T. 2059: 50.340b17–18); Zhu Fakuang (T. 2059: 50.356c28–257a2); Shiyue 耆域 (?–?; 388b4–16); Heluojie 訶羅竭 (d., 298, T. 2059: 50.389a6–11); Puming 普明 (?–?; T. 2059: 50.407b14–18); Huifen (T. 2059: 50.416c2–3)
48. Guṇabhadra (344c29–345a7); Zhu Fakuang 竺法曠 (T. 2059: 50.357a3–4); She Gong (T. 2059: 50.389c3–6); Tanchao 曇超 (419–492, T. 2059: 50.400a12–b2), Zhu Senggai 竺曇蓋 and Zhu Sengfa 竺僧法, T. 2059: 50.406c17–19). Tanchao's biography tells an elaborate story about a dragon.
49. Faxian 法顯 (T. 2059: 50.339? –420?, 338a1–5); Sengliang 僧亮 (T. 2059: 50.411a12–15).
50. T. 2059: 50. 331c8–25.
51. T. 2059: 336c11–17.
52. T. 2059: 417a2–17.
53. T. 2059: 418a28.
54. T. 2059: 50.334c24–335a3.
55. T. 2059: 50.335s21–b18.
56. T. 2059: 50.389b5–8; 23–24.
57. Jinyuan 帛遠, or Fazu 法祖, T. 2059: 50.327a24–b7.
58. T. 2059: 50.336c11–16.
59. Daoan (T. 2059: 50.353c9–11); Daoli 道立 (T. 2059: 50.356b21–24); Sengrou 僧柔 (431–494) (T. 2059: 50.378c21–24) Zhu Fodiao 竺佛調 (?–?)

(T. 2059: 50.388a1–5); Baozhi 保誌 (418–514) (T. 2059: 50.394c26–280); Puheng 普恒 (402–479)(T. 2059: 50.399b23–25).

60. T. 2059: 50.392b23–c6.
61. T. 2059: 50.333c21–24.
62. T. 2059: 50.350a28–b4.
63. T. 2059: 50.352a15–21.
64. T. 2059: 50.354b2–4; 22–25.
65. T. 2059: 50.389a22–29.
66. T.1332. The version of this work reproduced in the Taisho collection dates it to Eastern Jin (317–420; T. 1332: 21.536b10).
67. T.1336.
68. T. 1336: 21.580c15.
69. T. 1332: 21.540b8–10; 538c17548b25–26.
70. T. 1332: 21.549b2–12; 550c29.
71. T. 1332: 21.539c6-8.
72. T. 1332: 21.537c1–4.
73. Passage 22, 385a4.
74. T.2049: 50.383c7–8.
75. T. 1332: 21.550b4–9; also 548c6.
76. One intriguing exception appears in the biography of Faxian; this monk left the Southern capital Jinling in 475 and returned with "Avalokiteśvara's spell for expiation of sins" from Khotan (T. 2059: 50.411c3–4). A text with a similar title was translated in 490 (T. 2145: 55.13b24). See Yoshikawa, Tadao and Funayama, Tōru, Kōsōden 高僧伝 (Tokyo: Iwanami, 2010), IV, 292n8. The Avalokiteśvara cult appears to have played an important role in the evolution of dhāraṇī practice in India and early dhāraṇīs were often affiliated with this deity. This reference in Faxian's biography may thus reflect a larger development in spell practice gradually leading toward what became a popular practice in Esoteric Buddhism in India and Central Asia.
77. An Amitāyus image is mentioned in Zhu Fakuang's biography but the image does not appear to have been a part of his spell practice (T. 2059: 50.357a3–7).
78. T. 2059: 50.409–413.
79. Shinohara, Spells, Images, and Maṇḍalas, 11–13.

CHAPTER 11

THE NOT-SO-LONG
ARM OF THE LAW

MONASTICS AND THE ROYAL COURT

Phyllis Granoff

INTRODUCTION: CONTEMPT FOR THE COURT

Courts of law and those who run them fare scarcely better than do
doctors in classical Sanskrit literature.[1] To be sure, prescriptive texts
provide high-minded descriptions of the chief judge who is to decide
a case, the king who is to pronounce the punishment, and the various
officers of the court. Thus, the *Bṛhaspati Smṛti*, which probably belongs
to the 5th or 6th century CE, declares that the court of law in which
learned Brahmins sit is equivalent to the sacred area on which a sacrifice
is performed (verse 1,1.59).[2] Those who hear law cases are to be dedicated
to the truth, without anger or greed, knowledgeable in the *śāstras*, or
learned texts, which include the *dharmaśāstras*, or law books, and of
impeccable conduct. (verse 1,1.62). No one who is unfamiliar with local
customs, who denies the authority of the Vedas and is ignorant of the

learned texts, who is crazy, angry, or greedy for money should be allowed to take part in a case (1,1.64).

We know from Sanskrit literature that at least in the popular imagination, actual court proceedings did not in any way measure up to this ideal.[3] Perhaps the most famous description of a court room is the one in the play *Mṛcchakaṭikā, The Little Clay Cart,* ascribed to someone named Śūdraka. We know nothing of Śūdraka and there has been considerable debate about the date of the drama; scholarly opinion now places it in the 5th century CE.[4] The impoverished merchant Cārudatta, the play's hero, is accused of the murder of the woman he loves, the courtesan Vasantasenā. She is, of course, not even dead, but the wicked Śakāra, the king's brother-in-law, did indeed attempt to strangle her. He is convinced that he has killed her and decides to put the blame on the noble Cārudatta. There is no doubt about Śakāra's being unfit to speak in a court of law; he is greedy, full of anger, definitely on the crazy side, and he knows nothing of high culture. Throughout the play, his references to literature and learned treatises are all mangled and reveal his thoroughgoing lack of knowledge of any texts whatsoever. The judge is aware that Śakāra is not a suitable plaintiff; he attempts to shoo him away but Śakāra threatens him and the judge caves in. Śakāra is not the only one who has come to the court whose presence there makes a mockery of the ideals of the *Bṛhaspati Smṛti.* Brought there to hear the charges against him, Cārudatta has no illusions about what is facing him. Here is what he says (9.14):[5]

Just look at this glorious court room!

A veritable ocean swarming with savage beasts! The greedy ministers are sunk in worry as if drowning in its waters, while the messengers scurrying to and fro are like conch shells bobbing on its waves. Mighty whales and crocodiles, the cages for confining the prisoners, cluster in the distance, while closer lurk these dangerous beasts, the elephants that will trample to death the accused, and horses that will lead them to their place of execution. And what a deafening clamor there is; one could easily mistake the shouts of the petitioners for the screeching of predatory gulls, while the law clerks are as venomous as sea serpents. Proper legal procedure, the shore that the ocean should never breach, has been battered and smashed to bits. Such is this king's court.

Cārudatta's opinion that law courts are corrupt and lawyers greedy was an opinion not uncommonly held, if we are to judge from comments in a wide range of texts. The Pali *Petavatthu* reserves an entry for a hungry ghost who was a dishonest judge, a *kūṭavinicchayika*. When it came time to pass judgement truthfully, he let honesty fall by the wayside and pursued a dishonest course. [6] Many texts suggest that this was the norm for ordinary judges.

The 5th-century Buddhist monk Buddhaghosa in his commentary to the *Samyuttanikāya* tells the story of the Buddha in a previous birth. As a young prince, not yet even able to talk, the Bodhisattva was nonetheless able to tell when a court proceeding was dishonest. One day, the story goes, the king was seated in the court with the child on his lap. The case concerned property. The *Bṛhaspati Smṛti* tells us that two types of cases come before the court: disputes about property and cases of violence (1,12.3). Cārudatta's case was a murder case; in Buddhaghosa's commentary the case was clearly a property dispute, although no specific details are given. The ministers decide the case incorrectly; they give the disputed goods not to their rightful owner, but to someone who has no right to them. The Bodhisattva makes a noise which indicates his displeasure at the verdict. The king demands that the ministers uncover the source of the Bodhisattva's displeasure, and they determine that they must have made an error in their judgment. But they have a difficult time believing that the baby Bodhisattva understood what was happening, and so as a test they repeat their incorrect verdict. The Bodhisattva makes the same noise of displeasure. The king realizes that the baby has indeed understood, and he resolves to take greater care in deciding cases. The child has been true to his name; he is called Vipassī, which means that one who examines things carefully and does not make hasty decisions. [7]

In the *Dīghanikāya*, the child Vipassī always sits on the king's lap when he delivers a verdict. It is in fact the child who decides the case.[8]

The reason behind the failure of the king's ministers to decide a case correctly is not made explicit in the story of Vipassī. Another text suggests that incorrect verdicts at the king's court were the result of the rampant corruption of which Cārudatta was a victim in *The Little Clay Cart*. Thus in the *Samyuttanikāya Aḍḍakaraṇasutta*, King Pasenadi tells the Buddha that he is utterly disgusted with his role as presiding judge. One day, seated in the court, he explains, he saw how supposedly distinguished kṣatriyas, Brahmins, and householders, filled with lust, driven by their desire for worldly pleasures, deliberately lied and gave out the wrong verdict; they did so even though they themselves were already wealthy, possessing much gold and silver and abundant stores of grain. [9] In his commentary, Buddhaghosa explains further: seated in the court the king saw how the ministers had taken bribes and deliberately thrown a case. He thought to himself, "If this is what they do, right in front of my eyes, though I am lord of this whole earth, what will they do when I am not present?... I've had enough of sitting in the same place with these liars and bribe-takers." The king turns the responsibility of serving as presiding judge over to his army chief and renounces his duties at the court. [10] The Buddha agrees with the king's decision and roundly condemns in general the addiction to sense pleasures; like fish caught in the fisherman's net, people addicted to pleasures come to a sorry end indeed.

The *Bhaddasāla jātaka* tells a similar story about one Bandhula, the head of the army of the king of Kosala. One day a crowd of petitioners outside the royal court, having been deprived of their rightful property by the corrupt court, raised a hue and cry when they saw Bandhula. They told him about the wrongful verdict, and he hastened to the court, where he undid the verdict and gave the just pronouncement, handing the property in question to its rightful owners. The people were delighted and praised Bandhula. The king, on learning what had happened, dismissed the magistrates and put Bandhula in charge of the courts. This would not have been an entirely unprecedented appointment. In a description of the legal process that was current among the Licchavis, Buddhaghosa, commenting on the *Mahāparinibbāna Sutta,* describes a system of checks and balances to ensure that a just verdict was reached. First, the magistrates make a decision, and if the accused is deemed guilty, then the case goes before judges. They offer their verdict, and if it is once more against the accused, then the case is turned over to men learned in the sacred texts. The last person who passes judgment before the case reaches the throne is the head of the army.[11] In a similar passage commenting on the *Mahāgosiṅgasutta,* Buddhaghosa describes the process of moving from a small village unit to a county court if a decision cannot be reached; from there, the case goes to a superior judge, and from him to the leader of the army in the absence of a decision. Finally, the case comes before the king. The king has the final say; his words cannot be disputed. Similarly, the commentary tells us, the Buddha is the last resort in questions of the meaning of the dhamma. [12]

Returning to the reluctant king, after Bandhula was appointed all the verdicts were just, but the former magistrates, deprived of their income from bribes, slandered Bandhula and told the king that he was after the throne. The king had Bandhula and all his children killed.[13]

The stories of King Pasenadi and his army commander Bandhula tell us both that courts were commonly corrupt and that it took a truly exceptional individual to conduct them properly. King Pasenadi clearly felt that he was not up to the task. The army captain Bandhula seemed up to the task, but he too eventually could not escape the corruption and fell victim to the machinations of the dishonest court officers. In fact, if we recall the story of the Buddha as the baby Vipassī, we are left with the impression that it was only the Buddha who was capable of judging disputes. In his comments on the *Cūḷasīhanādasutta* in the *Majjhimanikāya, Mūlapaṇṇāsa,* Buddhaghosa again likens the Enlightened and adult Buddha as a teacher to a judge at court, who has to settle a disagreement between contending parties with conflicting views. As the *sutta* opens, the Buddha proclaims to his monks that only those who follow his doctrine deserve to be called true renunciants; those who follow other doctrines do not deserve to be called true monks. He then describes a hypothetical situation in which followers of other teachers might come forward and say the same thing of their teachers: "Only those who follow our teacher's doctrine deserve to be called true monks; those who do not follow our teacher's doctrine do not deserve to be called true monks." How is the dispute to be resolved? The Buddha asks the monks question after question. Buddhaghosa explains what the Buddha is doing: he is acting just like a judge in a court of law, resolving a dispute by a process of careful questioning. [14]

Buddhaghosa's comments, likening a religious dispute to a disagreement in a court of law, are not entirely surprising. The language of the court proceedings in a text like the *Bṛhaspati Smṛti* with which I began is indeed remarkably close to the language of the philosophical debate. The *Bṛhaspati Smṛti* tells us that once the defendant has been summoned to the court of law, the plaintiff, the *vādī* is to set out his position (*pakṣa*). It is to be flawless, contain a clear statement of what he wishes to prove (*sapratijñā*), and must be substantiated by references to the texts and through valid means of proof (*pramāṇāgamasaṃyuktam*; 1,2.5). Furthermore, the reasoning of the plaintiff cannot contain a flaw and must be acceptable. That is, it cannot be *aprasiddha* or *sadoṣa* (1,2.8). The king should not permit a plaint that is impossible to prove (*asādhya*) or that leads to conflict (*viruddha*; 1,2.8).

To anyone familiar with the language of debate in Indian philosophy, all these terms are immediately recognizable. They are all terms used to describe the debaters and the requirements of an argument in a standard philosophical debate; the debater, also called a *vādī*, must have a clear proposition that he wishes to prove (*pratijñā*), and the reason he adduces to prove his position cannot contain any logical fallacy (*doṣa*). The reason that the debater uses also must be acceptable to both parties; it cannot be unestablished (*aprasiddha*). The proposition in a debate cannot be incapable of proof (*asādhya*), and it cannot be contradicted by other means of knowledge (*viruddha*).

While the precise definitions of these problems to be avoided in statements in the court of law and in arguments in a philosophical debate will necessarily differ, the shared terminology is striking. Debates in Indian philosophical texts in which there are learned judges who pass judgment on the validity of the arguments and pronounce a verdict as to which party is correct are the mirror image of the law court with its contending parties and judges. In medieval texts, both philosophical debates and law cases take place in the court of the king. Buddhaghosa's comments, in which contending religious groups are likened to the plaintiff and defendant in a law case, and the Buddha is likened to the examining judge, highlight this strong parallel between a philosophical debate and a court case.

The observation that the court of the king was both a court of law and an arena for philosophical debate and that similar rules governed them both does not imply, however, universal royal jurisdiction over either matters of religion or members of any recognized religious order. The *Bṛhaspati Smṛti* also tells us that there was a clear division between members of religious orders and ordinary citizens when it came to testifying or bringing a complaint before the royal judge (1,1.74-5). Even in cases of violence and property disputes, the clear prerogative of the royal law court, members of a religious order were to be judged according to the rules of their order and by members of their own order and not in the royal court. Ascetics who were feared for their ability to employ spells and their power to curse were also not to be judged by the king (1,1.76).[15]

When we turn to the writings of the monastic groups, we see that they too were leery of the royal court, if for different reasons. In one often-cited story, the Pali Buddhist *vinaya* clearly indicates that Buddhist monastics have no place filing claims in the king's court. The problem in doing so does not seem to be associated with the general sentiment expressed in other Buddhist texts such as the ones cited here, namely that court proceedings are corrupt and judges easily bribed. It lies elsewhere: in a fear of inciting public disapproval, regardless of the whether a complaint made to the court was legitimate or false, and regardless of whether the verdict was just or unjust. If the *Bṛhaspati Smṛti* is afraid of the powers of the renunciants, the renunciant community is even more afraid of the powers of the state, the police, and the local populace on whom they depend for support. Jain monastic rules accord with what we see in the Buddhist *vinaya*. Whether a monk is ultimately convicted of a crime or not, appearing at court can have disastrous consequences not only for the individual monk directly involved but also for the entire Jain monastic community. For both Buddhists and Jains in these stories, what is at stake is nothing less than the reputation of the religion and its practitioners. In what follows, I examine a few stories from the monastic rules of both groups.

MONKS AND NUNS IN A COURT OF LAW AND THE COURT OF PUBLIC OPINION

In the Pali *vinaya*, the Buddhist nun Thullanandā was often in trouble.[16] Most of her indiscretions were settled within the monastic community, but there was one case in which she resorted to the outside court. Thullanandā has a dispute with a layman over a storage shed that the layman's father had donated to the nuns. When the donor died, the impious son sought to reclaim what his father had given. Not one to give up, Thullanandā took the layman to court. The judges asked her, "Noble one, is there anyone who can vouch for the fact that the shed was given to the nuns?" Thullanandā replied, "Have you ever heard or seen that a gift being given requires a witness?"[17] The judges had to admit that they had not and they decided the case in favor of the nuns: the shed was theirs. At this the layman, having been defeated in the court case, was annoyed, angry, furious in fact. He loudly railed against the nuns, shouting that they had stolen his shed. Not one to let things go, Thullanandā complained again to the court. The judges fined the layman.

But he was also not one to let things go, and this time he enlisted a rival sect, the Ājīvikas, in his fight against the nuns. He told them to shout abuse at the nuns. For this Thullanandā had him arrested. [18]Now the local people got involved. It was their turn to be annoyed, angry, furious in fact. "See how these nuns first stole this man's shed. Then they had him fined, and when that was not enough they had him arrested. This time they'll have him killed altogether." This finally roused the rest of the nuns. They too worried, "What will that litigious Thullanandā do next?" The Buddha learned of the events and asked, "Is it true that Thullanandā brought a case to the court?" When he was told that it was indeed true, he had harsh words to say about Thullanandā and any nun —and here the commentator Buddhaghosa adds "or monk"—who brings a case before the court. In explaining why, the Buddha repeated a phrase that appears frequently in the *vinaya*: such behavior will not lead to new converts, nor will it please those who are already favorably inclined towards the Buddhist teachings. [19]

If we look closely at this short passage, we see that the nuns are not bothered by Thullanandā's court case until the local populace is aroused and speaks against the nuns as a group. It does not matter that Thullanandā was in the right and the layman was in the wrong; local sympathy is with the layman, and the nuns now risk losing the active support or at least tolerance of the locals. This is the real problem with going to court: you cannot predict the response of the local people, who are less concerned with the right or wrong of a case and more concerned with protecting one of their own.

The prohibition concerning taking a case to court also occurs in the Sanskrit *Mahāsaṃghika Vinaya*, where it similarly reaches a head when the laity get involved. There Sthūlanandā quarrels with naked non-Buddhist nuns whose lodging is adjacent to that of the Buddhist nuns. The wall that separates their lodgings has fallen down, and Sthūlanandā demands that they repair it; the very sight of the naked nuns is an offense to the modesty of the Buddhist nuns. After an angry exchange in which Sthūlanandā calls them shameless and they return the insults, Sthūlanandā goes to court.[20] The judges are not entirely unbiased; they are described as *śraddhā* and *prasannā*, believers in the Buddha and his doctrine and favorably inclined towards the Buddha and the Buddhist doctrine. They pronounce in favor of the Buddhist nuns, but the hapless non -Buddhist nuns are unable to reconstruct the wall. It is the rainy season and the wall falls down as soon as they rebuild it. Desperate, the non- Buddhist nuns complain to the Buddhist lay community. The laity then reports this to the head nun, Mahāprajāpati, who informs the Buddha, provoking the rule that a nun or monk is not to quarrel with anyone and must not take a case to court.[21]

An interesting exception to these stories, in which the Buddha himself convenes a kind of mixed court involving both monks and the king, is to be found in a *Jātaka*, the *Nigrodhamigajātaka,* which is the story of the Buddha in a past birth as a deer named Nigrodha. As the story begins we meet a young girl, daughter of a wealthy merchant, who is eager to renounce the world and enter the Buddhist community of nuns. She is the only child of her parents, and they deny her request. She decides that she will wait until she is married and then seek the permission of her husband. The opportunity presents itself when on a festival day her husband questions why she has not put on jewelry and fancy clothes like other women who are going out to enjoy the festivities. She replies with a long account of the impurity of the body. He is convinced of her desire to renounce and hands her over to some nuns, who belong to the faction of the Buddhist schismatic Devadatta. The new nun does not realize that she was pregnant when she became a nun. As the signs of her pregnancy become obvious, the nuns seek the advice of Devadatta. He is not Omniscient, since he is not the Buddha, and he is also devoid of compassion. Unable to discern if she became pregnant before or after she joined the nuns, he roughly demands that she be thrown out of the community. The pregnant nun asks the other nuns to take her to the Buddha, under whom it had been her intention to renounce in the first place. The Buddha in his wisdom knows for sure that she had become pregnant while she was still a householder, but he is nonetheless troubled. His worry is that followers of other teachers (*titthiya*) will slander him, saying that the Buddha accepted a pregnant nun whom Devadatta had cast out. And so the Buddha convenes a court to deliver a verdict about the pregnant nun: did she violate her chastity as a nun or was she already pregnant when she entered the order. Although this seems to be a question about monastic behavior and violation of the monastic rules, the court is not simply a monastic court. The court consists of the king, two monks named Mahāanāthapiṇḍika and Cūlaanāthapiṇḍika, the lay disciple Visākhā, and a number of members of leading families. When everyone has gathered, the Buddha summons Upāli, the monk known for his scrupulous adherence to the principles in the *vinaya*. Upāli, he demands, is to determine the truth about this nun. Upāli asks Visākhā to examine the nun. Visākhā does so and determines that the nun had become pregnant before she renounced, while she was still a householder and living as wife to her husband. Visākhā informs Upāli, and in front of all those assembled Upāli pronounces that the nun is without fault.[22]

What is interesting about this case is that the Buddha, afraid of public opinion and the potential damage to his reputation from the slander of his competitors, convenes a court that is not completely a monastic court, in order to pass judgment on whether or not a nun has violated the monastic rules. The king is present, as in a state court, and the determination is made by a lay Buddhist woman. Based on her findings, the final verdict is delivered by a monk. This is an unusual case in which a nun's appearing in court serves to prevent harm from coming to the Buddha and his followers. Nonetheless, like the stories of Thullanandā, this story describes an environment in which the Buddha and his monks must be ever vigilant to protect the Buddhist community from negative publicity and maintain popular support. And by and large that is done by seeing to it that monks and nuns stay out of court.

Jain monastic rules share a similar anxiety over losing lay support; if anything, they are even more solicitous of preserving the good name of the monastic community and avoiding anything that might upset the local community. As in the Buddhist case, the local community can be Jains who might be turned off and leave the fold, and non-Jains, who in any case are suspicious of or hostile to the monks. [23] Punishments in the Jain monastic rules are listed according to the gravity of the offense, and the offense is rated as increasingly serious the greater possibility it offers for the monastic community as a whole to be criticized, ostracized, or even banished altogether. The following examples show that as in the Buddhist case it is not necessarily the mere act of going to court that is the problem for the Jain monk; what is at issue is the reaction of the local people, and a negative reaction can happen whether the monk wins or loses the case. My examples come from a Śvetāmbara Jain text of rules for the monastics, the *Bṛhatkalpabhāṣya*. The *Bhāṣya* by Saṅghadāsa in Prakrit has been dated to the 6th century CE. The Sanskrit commentary was begun by Malayagiri in the 12th century and completed by his disciple Kṣemakīrti. [24]

Some of the hypothetical situations in the *Bṛhatkalpabhāṣya* are complicated, and this one is no exception. Without asking permission, a monk carts off some branches and grass for thatching a roof from a householder's home. The problem is that to begin with the grass and sticks did not belong to the householder, whom we will refer to as householder A. Householder A had stolen the material from someone else; we will call the rightful owner householder B. The monk is seen carrying off the stuff either by householder B or the police. He is asked where he got it all. The monk is caught. If the monk tells the police that he got it from householder A, who, we recall, had in fact stolen it, then householder A will be seized as the thief that he is, taken forcibly to the court, tried, convicted, and punished. This is clearly not good; the monk will have been responsible for the bodily harm that the thief-householder incurs as a punishment. And we can imagine, as in the case of the Buddhist nun Thullanandā, householder A's family and friends will also not be happy at the outcome. But suppose then that the monk refuses to answer the question and is himself taken for the thief and dragged to court.

This is also not good. The locals now may become totally disillusioned with all the Jain monks as a whole, "See how those monks steal from others!", they might say. The monk is given the severest punishment by his fellow monks if the locals are so outraged that they expel the Jain monks from their midst.[25]

In another even more complicated example, a monk runs into trouble after he has accepted a piece of cloth from a female householder.[26] The point of the various troubles that befall him is to illustrate that it is necessary for a monk to ask the lady donor why she is giving him the donation before he accepts it. He should only accept the donation if she replies that she is giving him the donation because it is meritorious to make donations to a monk.[27] This monk in our hypothetical mess fails to ask and just accepts the cloth. The scenario is complicated by whether or not her husband was home when his wife made the gift, but the problems in either case are the same, and here I summarize the long discussion. The monk is in trouble whether or not the woman has nefarious motives; either way he becomes an object of suspicion. I begin with the case where the woman does actually want something from the monk.

The monk who does not ask the lady donor why she is giving him something is potentially in trouble because the very next day the woman might show up at his lodgings. She might ask him to have sex with her, or perhaps to tell her fortune and predict whether she will have a son; or perhaps she might seek some potion to make her husband in thrall to her. The monk is to tell her that ascetics do not have sex; that he does not know how to tell the future, and that he does not have any potions. If at that point she asks for the return of the cloth she had given him, he is to give it back. But what if he has cut the cloth up to use as a covering for his bowl, for example? Well, then he is to give her the pieces. But she might refuse to accept the pieces and demand the whole cloth. The next step is to the court. If the disgruntled woman takes the monk to court, then the Sanskrit commentary explains what he is to say. [28] The monk is to tell the officers of the court, "Suppose the owner of a tree sold the tree and the purchaser paid the price demanded, cut down the tree, and carted it off. Now suppose again that the seller regretted the sale and said to the buyer, 'Take back your money and give me back my tree, exactly as it was.' And suppose the buyer responded, 'I cut that tree into small pieces. How can I give you back your tree in one piece?' Now suppose again that the two, arguing in this way were to take their case to the king's court. Now tell me, officers, would you make the purchaser give back the tree? And if you would make him give back the tree, you could only make him give back the wood that he had cut the tree into and not the original tree in its uncut form.'" The monk wins the case.

The text continues. It could also be that the monk simply no longer has the cloth. He might have given it to a guest or it might have gotten burnt in a fire. The monk is to tell the woman the truth about what became of the cloth. If she nonetheless persists in insisting that he return it and goes to the court, he will win the case because as the Sanskrit commentary explains, once something is given the original owner has no further claim to it.[29]

But as in the case of the Buddhist nun Thullanandā, winning the case will not solve the monk's problems. And here the second possibility, that the woman had no ulterior motive when she gave the gift, and the first one, that she did, converge. There is still her husband and the local community to worry about. The husband of the woman might well be suspicious of the conduct of the Jain monk with his wife. If the husband is present and the monk does not directly ask the woman why she is giving him the cloth, the husband might think she is giving it to him because she wants something from him—sex, a love potion, a prediction of the future, or perhaps because she has already had a relationship with this particular monk. If he is a Jain, his suspicion of his wife and the monk will cause him to lose his faith in all the monks and to renounce being a Jain. If the husband is away, then when he returns he will learn from the elders that his wife had given the monk a cloth without his asking why and again he will suspect her. The in-laws will also suspect the woman and the monk. The result is that the husband and his relatives might abandon their belief in Jainism, cease supporting the monks with alms, and even harbor deep hatred of Jain monks as a whole.[30]

And this of course is the real problem, loss of support from the lay community. Although a court appearance is embedded in the discussion, it is irrelevant to the outcome for the monks. For the Jain monks the problem is not so much going to court, but what people think and say about the monk and his dealings with secular society. Win or lose at court, the fear is that the monk will be caught in a web of suspicion that casts a shadow over the entire monastic community.

The Jain monastic rules in the *Bṛhatkalpabhāṣya* suggest that there may be another advantage to monks and nuns if their cases are handled within the monastic community and not by the state court. The Jain and Buddhist monastic rules differ from the way in which the state treats some crimes, for example, cases of rape. In fact, the Jain rules explicitly state that they treat the victim of a rape differently from the way in which she would be treated by the state court. Buddhist rules accord with the Jain monastic rules. I turn now to examine this striking case in which monastic rules are at variance with the law around them.[31]

RAPE AND ITS VICTIMS

The discussion on the treatment of rape in the state court and by the Jain monastic community begins with *Bṛhatkalpabhāṣya* 2280. The verse first introduces the case of two householders and how they fare in the royal court. It is the beginning of the rainy season. A woman, having recently dyed her clothing, takes a pot and goes out to fetch water. Worried that the dye might run, she removes her clothing and takes shelter in a temple. But the temple is not empty; a young man has had the same idea and taken shelter from the rain there. Seeing the naked woman, he becomes aroused and takes her by force. They are discovered by others. The commentary explains that we are to imagine the same scenario, but this time with a monk and a nun; first, however, the text deals with the householders.

In the next verse we learn what happens to the male householder. He is seized by the police, tied up with his hands behind his back and taken at once to court. Without delay, the court officers begin the questioning and the man confesses. Verse 2282 explains the reaction of the young woman's family. They need convincing that the young woman was at fault and so the court officers persuade them of her guilt by means of the parable of the horse and the mare. Imagine, they say, a horse and a mare tied up in the courtyard, for example the court of the king. As long as the mare is well caparisoned, the horse cannot touch her. But as soon as they remove the armor-like coverings from the mare, the horse rushes to cover her. Similarly, they say, if the woman had not been naked, she would not have been raped. Their verdict is that she alone is guilty; the rapist is not guilty. This, the Jain text tells us in verse 2284, is the way the case goes in the king's court. But for the Jains, both are guilty, and the man is even more guilty than the woman since men are stronger and more is required of them. The monk should have controlled his sexual desire.

The topic of rape recurs many verses later, when a nun, for some reason not fully protected by her robes, is raped and made pregnant by a householder (4132). The first thing the rules state is that she is not to be expelled from the community of nuns. This is not so much an act of compassion towards the victim as it is a gesture to protect the Jain monastic community. Expelled, she might harbor resentment and hate the monks and even lay the blame on one of them! The monks have a choice about what to do with the rapist; if they are able, they should chastise him themselves. Otherwise they can turn him over to some householders or to the police (4133). The pregnant nun is cared for, either in the monastic lodgings or in the home of some lay people. She is not to be punished as long as she took no pleasure in the act or in her pregnancy or in her newborn child. Nonetheless, just to please outsiders and conform to their notions of what a raped woman deserves, they are to assign the blameless nun some kind of light punishment (4142-3). Again, it is not a question of guilt, but of protecting the community from public censure, in this case, from accusations that they are deviant in that they do not punish the victim of a rape. The Pali *Vinaya* has an account of the rape of the nun Uppalavaṇṇā. Similar to the Jain rules, Uppalavaṇṇā is not found to have committed any offence because she found no pleasure in the act.[32]

The treatment of rape is not really at variance with other discussions that either advise against taking a case to court or illustrate the pitfalls of doing so. Treating the raped nun with sensitivity and kindness keeps her within the fold and prevents her from slandering the monks or otherwise doing damage to their reputation. I close with a few concluding comments.

CONCLUSION: THE PAST AND THE PRESENT

Buddhist and Jain monastics have nothing to gain by going to court in the passages that I have examined in this paper. The court that matters to them is the court of public opinion, which seems in fact to be unconnected with the verdict of the law court. Indeed, the locals in these stories seem quick to find reasons to condemn the monks and nuns, and there is a constant fear of providing them with ammunition. In every case, the security and prosperity of the group take precedence over any simple legal right or wrong. The Buddhist rule that prohibits monks and nuns from taking a case to court has as its object the protection of the larger unit, the Buddhist monastic community as a whole and thus the very survival of Buddhism. The Jain rules perhaps regard the court itself with less fear, describing as they do how monks outsmart the officers of the court with their clever sermons, but the verses and commentary make clear that winning at law is irrelevant; what is important is avoiding behavior that leads to suspicion and sanction. Thus, even if going to court does not in and of itself threaten the security of the Jain community, it certainly can do nothing to help it.

I believe that the concern for the community over individual rights and wrongs that we see in these stories from the monastic rules has a parallel in the way that law was regarded in the larger society around them. There is a rule in the *Bṛhaspati Smṛti* that the king or chief judge is to reject hearing a case that might lead to a disturbance in the capital city or the kingdom. This is in fact the definition of the plaint that leads to conflict, mentioned earlier (1,2.13) and that is not to be permitted in the king's court. As a final comment, I would like to suggest that the strong desire to protect the community at large that we see in these texts may have had a longer life than has been noticed. I would suggest, for example, that it is even embedded in the Indian constitution. One of the most dramatic law cases over religious practice in the courts today is the case over animal sacrifice. Those in favor of sacrifice argue that any court ban on the practice would impinge on religious freedom. Those opposed to the practice reject this argument and refer to article 25 of the Constitution of India, which restricts freedom of religion when public order, morality, and health are at stake. [33] What this shares with the examples in the texts on monastic regulations is the idea that the need to protect a common good takes precedence over all other concerns. This is not the only case in which assumptions so prevalent in early and medieval law texts, whether Brahmanical, Jain, or Buddhist, seem to resurface in contemporary guises. In discussions of hate speech and the recent banning of Wendy Doniger's book *The Hindus, An Alternative History*, scholars have argued that statute 295A of the Indian penal code, which makes criminal speech that insults religious feelings, is a colonial intrusion into Indian law.[34] In fact, among the categories of prohibited (and therefore punishable) speech across the different religious groups in medieval India is speech that leads to hurt, dissension, and violence. The hurt that speech incurs can be emotional as well as physical. *Dharmaśāstra* texts explicitly forbid speech that defames either religion or the crown. [35] Any type of speech that is in any way abusive of another is prohibited, whether or not it is true. The overriding concern in these rules as in the stories examined here is to maintain the harmony of the larger group.

NOTES

1. Phyllis Granoff, "The Buddha as the greatest Healer: The Complexities of a Comparison", *Journal Asiatique* 299. 1 (2011): 5–22. The literature on law in pre-modern India is vast. The standard reference remains P.V.Kane, *History of Dharmaśāstra*, 5 vols, Poona: BORI, 1962-75. Another pioneering work is Robert Lingat, *The Classical Law of India*, trans J.D.M. Derrett (Berkeley: University of California Press, 1973). Among more recent work are important articles, monographs and translations by Donald R. Davis, Patrick Olivelle and David Brick.

2. *Bṛhaspati Smṛti*, GRETIL, http://gretil.sub.uni-goettingen.de/gretil/1_sanskr/6_sastra/4_dharma/smrti/brhasppu.htm verse 1,1.59, accessed July 15, 2016. Julius Jolly, trans., *The Minor Law Books* Oxford: Clarendon Press: Sacred Books of the East, vol. 33, 1889), 1.11. See also online http://www.sacred-texts.com/hin/sbe33/sbe3358.htm accessed July 16, 2016. The date of the text is given in the introduction, which also remarks that court procedure described in the *Bṛhaspati Smṛti* is very close to what appears in the *Mṛcchakaṭikā* that I discuss later. For an excellent overview of *Dharmaśāstra* texts, see Patrick Olivelle, "Dharmaśāstra: a textual history," in *Hinduism and Law: An Introduction*, eds. Timothy Lubin, Donald Davis, Jayanth K. Krishnan (Cambridge: Cambridge University Press, 2010), 28–58. Olivelle's discussion of the *Bṛhaspati Smṛti* is on pp. 49–50.

3. While my examples come from early medieval literature, the negative opinion of courts and judges would persist throughout history. In the 17th century Nīlakaṇṭha Dīkṣita would begin his satire, *Kalividambana*, with biting verses about the court and judges. V.Raghavan, "Kalividambana: A Satire on the Present Age", *Sahitya Akademi*, 13.2 (June 1970): 76–86.

4. On this see Diwakar Acharya, introduction, *The Little Clay Cart* (New York: New York University Press, 2009).

5. This improves upon my translation in my article "Justice and Anxiety: False Accusations in Indian Literature", *Rivista degli Studi Orientali* 83 (2010): 384–385.

6. *Petavatthu,Cūḷavaggo*,   9.   *kūṭavinicchayikapetavatthuvaṇṇanā*;   see www.tipitika.org, accessed August 7, 2016.

7. *Samyuttanikāya, nidānasaṃyutta, 4, Vipassīsuttavaṇṇanā*; see www.tipitika.org, accessed July 2, 2016.

8. *Dīghanikāya, Mahāpadānasutta, Vipassīsamaññā,* paragraph 41; see www.tipitika.org, accessed July 10, 2016.

9. *Samyuttanikāya, Sagāthāvagga, Kosalasaṃyutta* 7, *Aḍḍakaraṇasutta,* accessed July 2, 2016.

10. *Samyuttanikāya, Sagāthāvagga, Kosalasaṃyutta* 7, *Aḍḍakaraṇasuttavaṇṇanā,* accessed July 2, 2016.

11. *Mahāparinibbānasuttavaṇṇanā* Pali Tipitika, www.tipitika.org, accessed August 2, 2016.

12. *Papañcasūdanī, Mahāgosiṅgasuttavaṇṇanā,* ed. J.H. Woods and D. Kosambi (London: Pali Text Society, 1979) vol. 2, 252.

13. *Bhaddasāla jātaka,* 465, *Jātaka aṭṭhakathā, 4, dvādasanipāta* Pali Tipitika www.tipitika.org, accessed July 19, 2016.

14. *Majjhimanikāya, Mūlapaṇṇāsa, Sīhanādavaggo, 2, Cūḷasīhanādasuttavaṇṇanā,* accessed June 25, 2016. Idāni bhikkhūnampi ekā niṭṭhā, titthiyānampi ekā niṭṭhāti dvīsu aṭṭakārakesu viya ṭhitesu bhagavā anuyogavattaṃ dassento sā panāvuso, niṭṭhā sarāgassa, udāhu vītarāgassātiādimāha. Tattha yasmā rāgarattādīnaṃ niṭṭhā nāma natthi. Yadi siyā, soṇasiṅgālādīnampi siyāti imaṃ dosaṃ passantānaṃ titthiyānaṃ "vītarāgassa āvuso sā niṭṭhā"tiādinā nayena byākaraṇaṃ dassitaṃ.

15. This is in contrast to the stray reference in the *Arthaśāstra* 1.19.29, where it is stated that the king examines cases concerning the gods (devatā), hermitages (āśramas), Brahmins (śrotriyas), and heretical religious orders (pāṣaṇḍas).

16. For a discussion of stories about Thullanandā, see Reiko Ohnuma, "Bad Nun: Thullanandā in Pāli Canonical and Commentarial Sources", *Journal of Buddhist Ethics* 20 (2013): 18–66. On pages 53–55, Ohnuma argues that Thullanandā here is sticking up for the rights of women against more powerful males and that this is her offense. I offer here a different reading. Ohnuma translates the term *ussayavādikā* as "speaking with envy". The gloss appended to the text defines it as *aḍḍakārikā,* "bringing a case to court". In this case *vādi* is a technical term, meaning a plaintiff. *Ussaya* would then be an intensifier. Thullanandā is simply too litigious or too eager to go to court. Gregory Schopen has written a number of articles dealing with nuns in the *vinaya.* See for example "On Incompetent Monks and Able Urbane Nuns in a Buddhist Monastic Code", *Journal of Indian Philosophy* 38 (2010): 107-131. This and several other articles have been reprinted in *Buddhist Nuns, Monks, and Other Worldly*

Matters, (Honolulu: University of Hawaii Press 2014). Not surprisingly Thullanandā figures in many of the stories he discusses.

17. This is how I take the line "api nāyyo [api nvayyā (syā.), api nāyyo (ka.)] tumhehi diṭṭhaṃ vā sutaṃ vā sakkhiṃ ṭhapayitvā dānaṃ diyyamāna"nti." Ohnuma takes it to mean that Thullanandā is reminding the magistrates that they themselves knew full well that the shed had been given to the nuns. In my interpretation the nuns do not need any proof; proof of a gift is not required.

18. Verbal assault is a ground for suing someone in the *Manudharmaśāstra. The Law Code of Manu: A New Translation by Patrick Olivelle* (Oxford: Oxford World Classics, 2004), 143–144.

19. *Pācittiyapāḷi, 8. Adhikaraṇasamathā, 2. Saṅghādisesakaṇḍam (Bhikkunīvibhaṅgo), 1 Paṭhamasaṅghādisesasikkhāpadam,* paragraphs 678–680 and commentary on the same section, www. tipitika.org, accessed July 15, 2016. Andrew Huxley, "Pāli Buddhist Law in Southeast Asia," 167-182 in *Buddhism and Law: An Introduction,* edited by Rebecca Redwood French and Mark A. Nathan (Cambridge, Eng.: Cambridge University Press, 2014) seems to have misinterpreted this passage as approving of Thullanandā's behavior. The only exception is if Thullanandā appears in the court not of her own volition but is dragged there and has no choice but to present her case. In the *Mūlasarvāstivādavinaya,* an exception is made if the nuns are impoverished. See Gregory Schopen, *Buddhist Monks and Business Matters* (Honolulu: University of Hawai'i Press, 2004), , "The Good Monk and His Money in a Buddhist Monasticism of " the Mahāyāna Period", 1–19, originally published in *The Eastern Buddhist,* n.s. 32.1(2000): 85–105.

20. She calls them *ahrīka,* which is the derogatory term Arcaṭa uses for the Jains in the *Hetubinduṭīkā,* section 26, GRETIL from the edition by Pandit S.Sanghavi and Muni Shri Jinavijayaji (Baroda: Oriental Institute, 1949; Gaekwad's Oriental Series CXIII) http://gretil.sub.uni-goettingen. de/gretil/1_sanskr/6_sastra/3_phil/buddh/arhebt_u.htm, accessed July 24, 2016.

21. Taisho 1425, vol. 22, 518a16–17 . Akira Hirawkawa, trans., *Monastic Disciple for the Buddhist Nuns, An English Translation of the Chinese Text of the Mahāsāṃghika Bhikṣuṇī-Vinaya* (Patna: Kashi Prasad Jayaswal Research Institute, 1999), 138–142. The Sanskrit fragment glosses *utsayavādā vihareyā* with *kalahaṃ kareyam* "quarrel". Gustav Roth *Bhikṣuṇī Vinaya* (Patna: K.P. Jayaswal Research Institute, 1970),

139, GRETIL http://gretil.sub.uni-goettingen.de/gretil/1_sanskr/4_rellit/
buddh/bhivin_u.htm, accessed July 21, 2016.
22. *Nigrodhamigajātaka. Khuddakanikāya, Ekanipāta,* Pāli Tipitika, http://
www.tipitaka.org/romn/, accessed May 29, 2017.
23. I have written in detail about the concerns of the Jain *vinaya,* "Protecting
the Faith: Exploring the Concerns of Jain Monastic Rules", in press, in a
volume on Jain law edited by Peter Flügel.
24. Citations are from Guru Shri Chaturvijaya and his Shishya Punyavi-
jaya, eds. *Bṛhat Kalpa Sutra and the Original Niryukti of Sthavir Arya
Bhadrabahu Swami,* (Bhavnagar: Shri Atmananda Sabha, 1932).
25. *Bṛhatkalpabhāṣya* 2039–2044.
26. Ibid., 2792–2813.
27. Ibid., 2808–2809.
28. Ibid., 2803.
29. Ibid., 2804.
30. Ibid., 2798–2799.
31. I have discussed this material in my paper "Protecting the Faith" from
which I take this section.
32. *Vinaya,Pārājikakaṇḍam, vinītavatthu,* paragraph 68, www.tipitika.org
accessed July 18, 2016.
33. Daniela Berti, "Animal Sacrifice on Trial. Moral Reforms and Religious
Freedom in Himachal Pradesh", paper delivered at Yale University, 2016.
This restriction to religious freedom is not unique to the Indian constitution, as I was reminded by Gilles Tarabout at the workshop on Entan-
glements of Law and Religion in South Asia that took place at Yale University, April 28, 2017 and for which this paper was initially prepared.
34. Rupa Viswanath, "Roundtable on Outrage, Scholarship, and the Law in
India: Economies of Offense: Hatred, Speech, and Violence in India",
Journal of the American Academy of Religion 84 (2016): 352–363.
35. For examples and a general discussion of types of forbidden speech,
see the two articles by Collette Caillat, "The Rules Concerning Speech
(Bhāsā) in the Āyāranga- and Dasaveyāliya-Suttas", in *Aspects of Jainol-
ogy III, Pt. Dalsukh Bhai Malvania Felicitation Volume 1* (Varanasi: P.V.
Research Institute, 1991), 1–15; "Prohibited Speech and *Subhāsita* in the
Theravāda Tradition," *Indologia Taurinensia* 12 (1984): 61–73.

Chapter 12

Who Guards the Buddha-Word?

The Saṃgha's Precarious Position in Matters of Scriptural Authority

Tanya Storch

Beginning with the Jin dynasty (265–420) and continuing through the entire Nanbeichao period (420–581), the Chinese saṃgha was continually losing its political independence from the government, with its prerogatives granted during the Latter Han period (25–220) being revoked or threatened by the state's expanding control over the Buddhist community's inner affairs. One of the prerogatives lost during that period was control over verifying the authenticity of the Buddhist scriptural canon. In the late third through the late fifth centuries, the saṃgha searched for its own criteria of authenticity, finding it in the authority of a translator, exegete, and head of the saṃgha. But in the sixth and seventh centuries, both in the southern and northern territories, imperial authority began actively presenting itself as the ultimate guardian of the Buddhist canon.

THE HISTORICAL WEAKNESS OF THE CHINESE SAṂGHA

Even before Shi Dao'an 釋道安 (312–385) formulated proper principles for the Chinese saṃgha's organization and behavior,[1] its political independence was challenged by imperial power. In 340, the regent of Emperor Cheng of Eastern Jin (317–420) passed a decree forcing monks to bow to secular authorities, in effect canceling old privileges which allowed monks to remain standing in front of secular authorities—accorded to them because of their religious beliefs.[2]

This decree was a turning point in the history of the saṃgha in China and the beginning of a difficult power-dance between the Buddhist community and the state, which continues to this day. As history has shown, the political position of the saṃgha in China has been marked by persistent weakness despite the significant and widespread influence of Buddhism in all areas of Chinese society. In this respect, the Chinese saṃgha differs dramatically from that of such countries as Thailand, where historically (though less so in recent times) the Buddhist community enjoyed a good degree of political control over not only its own affairs but also affairs of state and the monarch's family.[3] Throughout Thailand's history, the Buddhist clergy always selected the head of its community. This *saṃgharāja* governed with little or no intervention from the government and regularly influenced state policy. There are known cases of the saṃgha's successful resistance against monarchs who failed to respect its authority properly, resulting in the monarch's temporary or permanent loss of political power.[4]

In China, the saṃgha seems to have enjoyed a degree of independence from state control only at the very beginning of its long history, specifically when it was small and mainly contained among the foreign population. As the edict of 340 and measures taken in the following centuries demonstrate, as soon as this religious institution had become socially visible due to the inclusion of ethnic Chinese, especially Chinese of aristocratic origin, the question of its subordination to imperial institutions became urgent. Privileges granted to Buddhist clergy during the Han dynasty disappeared one by one, and eventually the saṃgha was brought under the total control of the state. Government officials exercised control over monks (and over nuns, after the female saṃgha had evolved) in ways far more intrusive and severe than they did over regular citizens. For instance, according to the Tang and Song dynasties' criminal laws, the punishments for theft and destruction of property by monks were significantly harsher than those applied to lay people because, as members of the saṃgha, they had taken vows against stealing and violence.[5]

Originally, monks were granted rights to leave the monastery daily to beg for food, proselytize and perform conversions in public, initiate new monks without government permission, and build altars and monasteries in the wilderness. Most of these rights disappeared during the Nanbeichao period, when the influence of Buddhism in China grew rapidly and when Buddhists seemed to have an opportunity to build a strong and politically influential community. It was during this time that the saṃgha also sought to establish its control over the Buddhist scriptural canon and its right to serve as the sole guarantor of the authenticity of the Buddha's words.

THE SAṂGHA'S EARLY ATTEMPTS TO ORGANIZE A CANON OF SACRED SCRIPTURES

The saṃgha's earliest attempts to organize its own scriptural canon were made soon after the Luoyang translation center had produced a sizable number of texts. There is evidence that Zhu Shixing 朱士行, who lived in the Wei kingdom during the Three Kingdoms period (220–265), produced the earliest account of Chinese Buddhist translations.[6]

Although Shixing was not known to have translated Buddhist texts himself, his knowledge of the early Chinese translations was clearly enough to make him realize that the essential Mahāyāna scriptures were missing. In preparation for his westward trip with the purpose of obtaining the missing texts, he made a list of all available translations made during the Latter Han period (25–220).

In the following century, translators and exegetes made attempts to organize a canon of texts associated with Buddhist teachings. We know that Zhu Fahu 竺法護 (ca. 233–310), a famous translator from Dunhuang, compiled a subject list of translated scriptures which either he translated or were done under his guidance. This early critical bibliography of Buddhist scriptures was known as the *Zhu Fahu lu* 竺法護錄 (Zhu Fahu's Catalog).[7] The time of its compilation is from the end of the third century through the first decade of the fourth century.[8] To borrow Stefano Zacchetti's term, we must conclude that we are dealing here with a situation where a translator of scriptures served as a parameter of the canon, that is, he personally decided which scriptures constituted the authentic words of the Buddha.[9]

The next attempt at drawing boundaries for the authentic Buddhist doctrine in China was made by Zhi Mindu 支敏度, who was well known for his exegetic activities in Jiankang, the capital of the Eastern Jin dynasty (317–420). Mindu composed the *Jinglun doulu* 經論都錄 (A Comprehensive Catalog of Scriptures and Commentaries), which included Buddhist translations along with commentaries by distinguished Chinese Buddhists.[10] This particular organization of the canon suggests that, in the view of certain saṃgha members, the true word of the Buddha was represented not merely by translations from foreign languages but also by works of knowledgeable Buddhists in Chinese exegetical tradition.

In addition, during the Eastern Jin period, Shi Dao'an, a famous exegete of Buddhist literature who served as head of the saṃgha in Xiangyang (Hubei), applied certain principles of historical textual criticism to Chinese Buddhist scriptures.[11] Dao'an was well aware that in Buddhist communities outside of China, the authenticity of the Buddha-word was verified through a continuous oral tradition wherein young monks repeated after senior monks the texts that the latter had memorized during their own initiation. Such a method of verification, however, could not be employed by the Chinese saṃgha for two main reasons. First, Chinese Buddhists apparently had problems learning the many different languages involved in the transmission of Buddhist texts; and second, in order to compete with Confucianism, the new doctrine was under pressure to develop a written canon which could compare to the Confucian Classics.[12]

This led to Dao'an's decision to rely on principles of textual criticism already developed in Confucian historiography and use them to gauge the authenticity of Chinese Buddhist texts. In practical terms, according to Dao'an, only those scriptures which were made by known translators approved by the saṃgha could represent the "true words" of the Buddha and thereby constitute a reliable canon.[13] He was vehemently committed to excluding texts of unknown origin from the Buddhist canon. This was meant to guard against forgeries produced in various areas of Central Asia (primarily, the Gansu corridor and Liangzhou). The flow of forgeries to Chinese territories undoubtedly demonstrated the growing popularity of Buddhist scriptures among the Eastern Jin aristocracy, who engaged in imitating and redacting the texts already translated and approved by the saṃgha. Another type of Buddhist scripture Daoan warned about included the abbreviated and redacted texts. These were not considered authentic transmissions of the Buddha's word unless they had been made by trusted monks such as An Shigao 安世高 and Kang Senghui 康僧會.[14] As we will see later, Dao'an's approach to the Buddhist scriptural canon had far-reaching consequences in terms of further development of ideas about the Buddhist scriptures' authenticity among Chinese followers.

At the very end of the Jin period, in 419, yet another significant catalog was published by the saṃgha—the *Zhongjing lu* 眾經錄 (Catalog of Scriptures).[15] The compilation of this work began by order of Shi Huiyuan 釋慧遠 (334–416).[16] After Huiyuan separated from Dao'an and settled at Mount Lu in southern China, he realized that his community was suffering from a shortage of scriptures, the bulk of which remained in Dao'an's possession. Huiyuan dispatched an expedition in search of scriptures, and the expedition returned with both the original texts and the Chinese translations. Huiyuan ordered the translations be made from the originals, and later he ordered that one of his disciples, Shi Daoliu 釋道流 (fl. early fifth century) begin writing a catalog. Daoliu died without finishing his work, but another of Huiyuan's students, Zhu Daozu 竺道祖 (fl. early fifth century), finished it in 419, three years after Huiyuan's death.[17]

The catalog published by two of Huiyuan's disciples was the largest in history of Chinese Buddhism to that point. It comprised four *juan*, whereas all the previous catalogs, including Dao'an's, were only one *juan* long. That divided translations according to the dynasties during which they had been done, distinguishing the translations of the Wei, Wu, Western Jin, and Eastern Jin dynasties. This catalog also attempted to separate authentic scriptures from those believed to be false, although the criteria of authenticity in this case did not include knowledge of the translator, as in Dao'an's catalog. This is evident from the fact that the section of Huiyuan's catalog that contained the inauthentic scriptures was called "False Scriptures from Hexi."[18] *Hexi*, literally "west of the river," indicates areas within the Gansu corridor known for forging Buddhist texts. This means that Huiyuan and his disciples followed Dao'an in assuming that texts produced in areas known for forgery must be signaled in the catalogs in order to warn followers that their origins might be questionable. Yet the principle that only those texts that were translated by known and reliable members of the saṃgha constituted the reliable transmission of Buddha's word in China did not play a crucial role.

Information about Daozu's catalog, the full text of which, unfortunately, has not been preserved, allows us to infer the following points about the saṃgha's view of the canon. First, it may be suggested that by the early fifth century there existed a relatively established notion of the contents of the Chinese Tripiṭaka. For as the story of the *Zhongjing lu* indicates, Huiyuan and his community were left with an incomplete collection of the Tripiṭaka, prompting Huiyuan to send his students in search of the specific missing texts.

Another point concerns taxonomic divisions selected by Huiyuan and/or his disciples for the catalog of scriptures, namely, the decision to divide texts based on the Chinese dynasties in which they were produced. Huiyuan had participated in the debate about monks' obedience to state authorities (as discussed earlier) and taken a decisive position defending the monks' right to remain standing in the presence of state officials. He is also known for writing a lengthy treatise on the exemption of monks from the requirements of civil etiquette on the grounds of their religious beliefs. In the last section of this text, he praised Buddhist monks for their unique contribution to the well-being of all sentient beings because monks can offer the path of salvation from death and suffering, which no government can provide.[19] Yet, despite his view of the Buddhist clergy as a special category of people endowed with sacred powers that are separate from, and even exceeding, the emperor's, he had nevertheless instructed his disciples to organize the Buddhist canon according to the ruling dynasties under whose rule its various texts had been produced.[20]

THE EMPEROR GETS INVOLVED IN THE PROTECTION OF THE BUDDHIST CANON

During the Jin dynasty and the early part of the Nanbeichao period, the saṃgha sought adequate methods to define and protect the authenticity of the Buddha-word. The first noticeable attempt by imperial power to assume the role of guardian and controller of the Buddhist canon was made by Liang Wudi (502–557).

Liang Wudi is well-known as the ideal protector of the Dharma and the first cakravartin in Chinese history. [21] He is also known for exempting monasteries from paying taxes, banning Daoist practices at court and replacing them with Buddhist ones, and promoting Buddhists to the highest positions in his government. Wudi's distinctly pro-Buddhist policies also included prohibiting meat and wine in the ancestral sacrifices, forbidding the use of animals for medicinal purposes, and making regular retreats to Buddhist monasteries.[22]

Liang Wudi's patronage set in place a tradition in which the emperor acted as the ultimate authority guarding the authenticity of Buddhist doctrines and scriptures: this model corresponded to the imperial supervision of Confucian Classics during the Han dynasty. At the same time, his intrusion into the affairs of the saṃgha prompted Buddhists to assert their own ways of establishing criteria of authenticity and canonicity for the Buddhist scriptures.

This conflict between the emperor and the saṃgha, as far as the question of scriptural canonicity is concerned, can be illustrated through the stories of three Buddhist catalogs published during the Southern Liang dynasty (502–557). One is the *Chu sanzang jiji* 出三藏記集 (Collection of Records about the Production of the Tripiṭaka) written in 515/518 by Shi Sengyou 釋僧祐, then head of the saṃgha. The other two were written by court historians—the *Hualin fodian zhongjing mulu* 華林佛殿眾經目錄 (Catalog of Scriptures from the Buddha Palace in the Jetavana Park) in 518 by Shi Sengshao 釋僧 紹 (fl. first half of the 6th century), and the *Liangshi zhongjing mulu* 梁世眾經目錄 (Catalog of Scriptures of the Liang Dynasty) in 520 (or 521?) by Shi Baochang 釋寶唱 (466–?).

Sengyou's work contained a representation of the canon that reflected the positions of the saṃgha's leadership at that time,[23] while Sengshao and Baochang expressed views close to Liang Wudi's. Indeed the emperor directly ordered first, Sengshao, and then Baochang to write an official dynastic bibliography of Buddhist texts *after* Sengyou's account of the Buddhist canon had been completed and presented to the emperor.

Sengshao's attempts to please the emperor were unsuccessful despite his trying to write a better description of the Buddhist cannon than Sengyou's. Sengshao excluded the voluminous historical records for which Sengyou's catalog was famous, and instead of describing *all* translations ever made in Chinese history, he concentrated on texts kept in the emperor's private collection known as the "Buddha Palace in the Jetavana Park." This was the reason for giving his work the title *Hualin fodian zhongjing mulu* (Catalog of Scriptures from the Buddha Palace in the Jetavana Park).[24]

Seeing that Sengshao was unable to carry out his orders, Emperor Wu ordered Baochang[25] to write a dynastic catalog of Buddhist scriptures, and he did this successfully.[26] Baochang obviously delighted the emperor because his catalog was recognized as an official work of the dynasty under an imperially-granted title—*Liangshi zhongjing mulu* (Catalog of Scriptures of the Liang Dynasty)—and Wudi further rewarded Baochang by putting him in charge of the entire collection of Buddhist texts in his palace library. While serving in this position, Baochang produced three complete copies of the canon based on the catalog he had produced.[27] At the same time, Sengyou's catalog, while celebrated and preserved by the saṃgha, received no similar favors from the emperor.

In order to understand the differences between the imperially-chosen and saṃgha-chosen approaches to the Buddhist canon, let us first look at Baochang's taxonomic classifications:

Liangshi zhongjing mulu:

> Mahāyāna scriptures by known translators in many juan 大乘有譯人多卷經
>
> Mahāyāna anonymous scriptures in many juan 大乘無譯人多卷經
>
> Mahāyāna scriptures by known translators in one juan 大乘有譯人一卷經
>
> Mahāyāna anonymous scriptures in one juan 大乘無譯人一卷經
>
> Hīnayāna[28] scriptures by known translators in many juan 小乘有譯人多卷

Hīnayāna anonymous scriptures in many juan 小乘無譯人多卷

Hīnayāna scriptures by known translators in one juan 小乘有譯人一卷

Hīnayāna anonymous scriptures in one juan 小乘無譯人一卷

Earlier translations [i.e. redactions] of scriptures 先異譯經

Dhyāna scriptures 禪經

Vinaya scriptures 戒律

Suspicious scriptures 疑經

Commentaries 注經

Abhidharma 數論

Notes on the meaning [of Buddhist terms] 義記

Names of different [Buddhas and bodhisattvas] arranged in accordance with the occasions [when it is appropriate to call upon them]; 隨事別名

Names of [Buddhas and bodhisattvas] which can be used together and are arranged in accordance with the occasions [when it is appropriate to call upon them] 隨事共名

Avadāna scriptures 譬喻

Epithets of the Buddha 佛名

Dhāraṇī 神咒

As one can see, Baochang separated scriptures of the Mahāyāna traditions from those of the Hīnayāna. He also recognized categories of texts found in the Indic and Central Asian traditions, dividing scriptures according to their derivation from the sūtra-piṭaka, vinaya-piṭaka, or abhidharma-piṭaka. He separated anonymous translations, which might include forgeries, from texts made by known, reliable members of the saṃgha, and indicated whether translations were brief, that is, spanning only one *juan*, or lengthy, occupying several *juan*. This distinction was doctrinally important because the Chinese believed, albeit not always correctly, that the longer translations were closer to the complete original texts and treated shorter texts as abridged versions or incomplete translations. In addition to the above taxonomic categories, Baochang paid attention to what we may call the higher and lower traditions of using Buddhist scriptures. He did not merely account for translations that were mainly used by the clergy and the educated elite, but also featured different characters and pronunciations of the names of the Buddhas and bodhisattvas and explained on which occasions these names might be called upon to receive supernatural assistance—traditions widely associated with folk worship, although undoubtedly used by members of the elite as well.[29] He also listed texts of dhāraṇī (formulaic texts whose chanting was known to produce powerful magic) and epithets of the Buddha similarly known to result in good merit and better reincarnation in the next life.

Finally, Baochang was the first in his time to separate the avadāna literature from other types of translated scriptures. Avadāna, in Sanskrit —"piyu" 譬喻 in the early Chinese translations—refers to a type of narrative that is still the subject of academic discussion.[30] But what can be definitely argued is that Baochang began separating scriptures within the sūtra-piṭaka according to the value of their contents and literary form, unlike Dao'an and Sengyou, both of whom classified translated texts mainly on the basis of their historical textual characteristics and not so much on the basis of their contents.

For comparison, let us examine the taxonomic categories used in Sengyou's catalog.

Chu sanzang jiji:

- A newly compiled list of scriptures 新集撰出經[31]
- A newly compiled list of different translations of scriptures 新集異出經[32]
- A newly compiled list of the ancient redactions of scriptures from the venerable An's [catalog] 新集安公古異經
- A newly compiled list of the anonymous translations of scriptures from the venerable An's [catalog] 新集安公失譯經
- A newly compiled list of different translations of the [same] scriptures made in Liangzhou from the venerable An's [catalog] 新集安公涼土異經
- A newly compiled list of different translations of the [same] scriptures made in Guanzhong from the venerable An's [catalog] 新集安公關中異經
- A newly compiled list with explanations of the Vinaya [texts] which are divided according to the five schools [of Buddhism] 新集律分為五部記錄
- A newly compiled list with explanations of the Vinaya [texts] which are divided according to the eighteen schools [of Buddhism] 新集律分為十八部記錄
- A newly compiled list with explanations of the Vinaya [texts] which are divided according to the four schools [of Buddhism all of which] have spread to China[33] 新集律來漢地四部記錄
- A newly compiled addition to the list of the anonymous translations of scriptures 新集續撰失譯雜經
- A newly compiled list of the digest translations of scriptures 新集抄經
- A newly compiled list of suspicious scriptures from the venerable An's [catalog] 新集安公疑經
- A newly compiled list of the suspicious scriptures and false compilations 新集疑經偽撰雜

- A newly compiled list of scriptural commentaries and various other [historical] records from the venerable An's [catalog] 新集安公注經及雜經志

Sengyou's main concern, as one can see from this taxonomic classification, was to prove that he had followed the earlier famous head of the saṃgha—Dao'an—in all of the latter's ways of describing Buddhist scriptures and separating the authentic words of the Buddha from forgeries.[34] We see that six whole divisions of Sengyou's catalog were taken directly from the work by Dao'an, namely, divisions three through six; and divisions twelve and fourteen too appear to have been copied from Dao'an's catalog. A large portion of the first division, likewise, came from Dao'an's catalog; in addition, two more divisions (ten and thirteen) are nothing more than extensions that Sengyou added to the lists previously compiled by Dao'an. By carefully reading through these six divisions, one can see the continuation of Dao'an's critical approach to Chinese translations, which asserted that only those scriptures that were made by known and saṃgha-approved translators represented the "true words" of the Buddha and constituted the reliable canon.

Sengyou's catalog lacks some essential features that are observed in the catalog by Baochang: Sengyou failed to distinguish between Mahāyāna and Hīnayāna doctrines and did not properly distinguish among scriptures that derived from three different collections—sūtra-piṭaka, vinaya-piṭaka, and abhidharma-piṭaka. These shortcomings were noted by scholars of the Sui and Tang dynasties, who were respectful but critical of of Sengyou's work because of these deficient qualities.

Another difference between Baochang's and Sengyou's approaches to the Chinese Buddhist canon is that the former paid attention to Buddhist worship practiced in the capital by collecting and describing small texts such as the dhāraṇī that called on various Buddhas' and bodhisattvas' names and provided instructions on how to use them for a worshipper's religious needs. Sengyou's work appears to be more scholarly and free of such liturgic aims despite their being highly favored by the court and the emperor.

Sengyou was also not afraid to attack the popular writings—which happened to be among the emperor's favorites—attributed to a certain nun whose textual transmission he did not consider authentic. Shi Sengfa 釋 僧法, according to a story retold by Sengyou, experienced enlightenment after which she began chanting scriptures in Sanskrit. These scriptures were written down and translated into Chinese. Nevertheless, Sengyou proclaimed these to be false even though other scholars had agreed on their doctrinal consistency.[35] Sengyou's doctrinal crusade was also waged against the work of Miaoguang 妙光, who stood trial for forging scriptures whose contents Sengyou considered to be heretical. Sengyou served as senior judge during that trial, and by its verdict Miaoguang was expelled from the monastery and his books were burned. Sengyou wrote at the very end of his catalog that a few titles of the latter's writings were still popular, and this is why he had to warn followers about them. [36]

These methods of Sengyou's approach to the Buddhist canon did not sit well with the imperial powers, leading Liang Wudi to order a new, dynasty-sponsored, account of the Tripiṭaka as soon as Sengyou's work was completed and presented to the court. As we already know, Baochang successfully completed the dynastic catalog of the Buddhist canon of the Southern Liang and was rewarded by the emperor, who promoted him and personally accepted three copies of the canon based on Baochang's catalog.

Yet the saṃgha's ultimate choice was not made in Baochang's favor, but in favor of Sengyou's vision of the canon. Sengyou's catalog has been used as the ideal model by most Chinese Buddhist catalogers, whereas knowledge about Baochang's catalog has nearly disappeared, with the catalog itself being lost by the middle of the seventh century.

That Baochang's positions, overall, did not fit well with those of the saṃgha becomes more obvious when one reads the "Introduction" to the *Gao seng zhuan* 高僧傳 (Lives of Eminent Monks) by Huijiao 慧皎 in which Baochang is criticized anonymously.[37] As a favorite historian at the court, Baochang wrote not only a scriptural catalog but also the life accounts of monks. He was known in particular for a work entitled the *Ming seng zhuan* 名僧傳 (Lives of Famous Monks). Huijiao, the author of the later collection of monks' biographies purposely titled *Lives of the Eminent Monks* (Gao seng zhuan), rebuked Baochang for promoting the idea of a "famous monk," calling it inconsistent with Buddhism and proper monk behavior, and suggested that such views derive from being too close to the court.[38]

In writing the monks' biographies, Baochang invented a classification based on the monks' religious merits which he connected to what might be called monastic professional occupations, such as translator, exegete, artist, performer of magic, and others. Baochang's classification was borrowed by Huijiao and altered, and scholars continue to speculate about whether Baochang's original work is superior to Huijiao's.[39] Nevertheless, in this case, just as with Baochang's scriptural catalog, the saṃgha favored Huijiao and his views by recognizing his biographical account as a standard of perfection and discontinuing the process of copying Baochang's biographical work.

SCRIPTURAL AUTHORITY UNDER THE NORTHERN WEI AND QI DYNASTIES

Only two comprehensive catalogs of Buddhist scriptures were issued during the rule of the northern dynasties, one by Northern Wei (386–534) and another by Northern Qi (550–557). Both were ordered by emperors, with the saṃgha reluctantly following their orders. Because the state exercised strict control over Buddhist affairs in the north, the saṃgha often appeared politically helpless both in times of persecution and in times of active imperial patronage.[40] Not surprisingly, Buddhist scholars under the northern dynasties did not initiate any internal movements aimed to measure the truthfulness of the Buddhist scriptural canon that would remind us of those initiated by Dao'an, Huiyuan, and Sengyou in the south.[41] The level of scholarship required for compiling an efficient bibliographic description of Buddhist texts in the north was lacking, and this is evident by the prolonged struggle of the Northern Wei and Qi dynasties attempting to complete a dynastic catalog that would somehow match that issued for Emperor Wu of the Southern Liang dynasty.

The title *Weishi zhongjing mulu* 魏世眾經目錄 (Catalog of Scriptures of the Wei Dynasty) was modeled after the title of the Southern Liang official catalog, *Liangshi zhongjing mulu*. Its compilation was ordered during the Yongping era (508–512), but it was not finished until the Tianping era of the Western Wei (534–538), taking a quarter of a century for its completion. Not even an order from the head of state was capable of forming an instant group of scholars sufficiently learned in both Buddhist and Confucian scriptural traditions, the requisite combination of skills, to produce a reliable Buddhist bibliography. It is significant that a lay Buddhist, Li Kuo 李廓 (fl. mid-sixth century), and not a member of the clergy, was finally chosen to lead the project.[42]

Li Kuo most likely fulfilled the wishes of the Wei dynastic rulers when he finally finished the catalog because public condemnation of scriptures that taught the so-called nonauthentic doctrines was far greater there than in the south. Notably, Li Kuo did not include a section for the scriptures considered to be merely suspicious but not condemned as false yet. However, he did dedicate three divisions of his bibliographic work to describing texts which had to be excluded from the canon and destroyed because they had been condemned by the government. In the eighth division, he listed false sūtras; in the ninth, he listed false śāstras; and in the tenth division, he provided a list of texts which he explained were "absolutely non-scriptures but which have been erroneously called scriptures by fools" (全非經, 愚人稱經). The most obvious reason for such an impressive collection of condemned texts is the Wei rulers' tight ideological control over the contents of the canon aimed to ensure that no form of antigovernment propaganda was preached by it.

Another notable feature of the *Weishi zhongjing mulu* that probably
reflects state domination over the saṃgha's own priorities and concerns
is the complete lack of Mahāyāna vinaya-piṭaka texts. Only the contents
of the Hīnayāna vinaya-piṭaka were listed in this catalog. The Hīnayāna
vinaya was known to be practiced in foreign countries where the saṃgha
enjoyed relative freedom from the state and was able to follow its own
internal rules of regulation and punishment. China was associated with
practicing Mahāyāna Buddhism, and therefore, the fact that the Mahāyāna
vinaya was altogether absent from the Wei dynasty's catalog appears
significant, most likely suggesting that the Chinese saṃgha under the
northern dynasties was no longer represented by its own monastic rules
and regulations.[43]

Compared to the southern catalogs, the *Weishi zhongjing mulu* did
not include any views on the historical evolution of the Buddhist canon
and did not supply information about the earliest Chinese translations.
It strictly focused on translations made during the northern dynasties;
moreover, it included only those scriptures that were physically accessible
in monasteries and at the court, that is, the texts that were approved
for use and duplication by the chief of the saṃgha who represented the
imperial government.

The *Qishi zhongjing mulu* 齊世眾經目錄 (Catalog of Scriptures of the
Northern Qi Dynasty) was commissioned by the Emperor Wenxuan (r.
550–559) and took more than two decades to be completed. This Northern
Qi catalog no longer recognized the importance of distinguishing scriptures in terms of them being Mahāyāna versus Hīnayāna teachings,
while serious attention was paid to "heterogeneous" teachings favored
by the court.

All in all, the northern catalogs described far fewer scriptures than
the southern catalogs. The *Weishi zhongjing mulu* counted only 427 texts
and the *Qishi zhongjing mulu* counted only 787 texts; by comparison
the *Liangshi zhongjing mulu* counted 1,433 texts and the catalog by
Sengyou, 2,162.

THE SAṂGHA AND EMPEROR DURING THE SUI DYNASTY

Who is in Charge of Eliminating "False" Scriptures?

The Buddhist policies of the Emperor Wen, founder of the Sui dynasty (581–618), are widely known.[44] Very much like the Emperor Wu of the Southern Liang, he went into history as the cakravartin, protector of the Dharma, expanding Buddhist influence into many new and significant areas of Chinese society. Like Liang Wudi, the Sui Wendi depended on the ideal of the cakravartin as a way to legitimize his political power. As a young official of the non-Chinese Northern Zhou dynasty (557–581), Wendi had seized the throne from his sovereign and then successfully united both northern and southern lands under his command. Creating an ideological justification for this new political order was an urgent task. Since Confucian doctrine vehemently opposed the dismissal of any lord who was not implicated in extreme cruelty against his people, Buddhism remained the only doctrine that could serve as a reservoir of ideas pertaining to why and how political power needed to be transferred. The Northern Zhou dynasty (557–581) had actively persecuted Buddhism; thus Wendi's decision was to rely on Buddhist scriptures that praised any king who would step in to protect the Dharma from its imminent destruction.

Not surprisingly, Wendi actively participated in the guardianship of the Buddha's word against perceived perversion and forgeries. One aspect of this activity involved ordering two major catalogs of the Buddhist canon —the *Da Sui zhongjing mulu* 大隋眾經目錄 (Catalog of Scriptures of the Great Sui Dynasty), presented to the throne in 594 by the monk Shi Fajing 釋法經, and the *Sui Renshou nian neidian lu* 隋仁壽年內典錄 (Catalog of the Inner Canon of the Renshou Era of the Sui Dynasty), presented by the monk Shi Yancong 釋彥悰 in 602. The latter catalog was specifically ordered by Wendi to counter views expressed by a lay Buddhist historian, Fei Changfang 費長房, who had written a famous history of Buddhism in China, the *Lidai Sanbao ji* 歷代三寶記 (Records of the Three Treasures throughout the Successive Dynasties) and published it around 597.[45]

The Sui dynasty's first Buddhist scriptural catalog, the *Da Sui zhongjing mulu*, expressed a distinct softening of the government position toward the scriptures proclaimed as inauthentic and routinely destroyed by the rulers of the northern dynasties. Specifically, Fajing eliminated a large division that had a title that severely condemned certain scriptures in the Northern Wei catalog. This simple taxonomic reorganization took the emphasis away from the so-called false scriptures, presenting the canon of the Sui dynasty as being more genuine than that of the northern dynasties. Additionally, many of the texts branded as "false" in the northern catalogs were classified in the Sui dynasty's catalog as being merely suspicious, but not false. For instance, Fajing often appended a note saying that the doctrinal status of a certain text required further investigation.[46]

Of importance is also the fact that Fajing restored a section containing the Mahāyāna vinaya-piṭaka which had been taken out by Li Kuo. This confirms that, under Wendi, the saṃgha's prestige was partially restored in terms of its historical traditions and practices of monastic living.

At the same time, what might be called a "scriptural inquisition" was conducted by the Sui government. According to early Tang-dynasty Buddhist sources, the apocalyptic literature about the coming of the Buddha Maitreya followed by the destruction of the world was burned at Wendi's order. Specifically, it is reported that three hundred scrolls of "false and extravagant" scriptures were confiscated from private collections and publicly destroyed.[47] We observe a peculiar parallel between the Sui and the Southern Liang dynasties here. During the Liang dynasty, which was ruled by a cakravartin just as was the Sui dynasty, it was the head of the saṃgha, Sengyou, who condemned certain texts and ordered them to be destroyed. But under the Sui, the same function was performed by the head of the state.

It must be argued that, under the Sui dynasty, guarding the purity of the Buddhist doctrine became a large-scale dynastic enterprise which some Buddhists viewed as a mostly positive development. The *Lidai*

Sanbao ji illustrated this new position very well. This text, which is both a history of Buddhism in China and a scriptural catalog, was finished in 597 by Fei Changfang 費長房 (fl. mid to late sixth century). Changfang was a former monk who lost his clerical position and monastic status because of persecution in the Northern Zhou dynasty. His privileges were partially restored during the Sui dynasty, and he felt tremendous gratitude toward Wendi, although the latter, for reasons quite unknown to historians, never fully restored his monastic status, merely granting him only certain religious privileges.[48] In a state of extreme loyalty to this monarch, Changfang produced the first history of Buddhism in China that closely blended events pertaining to the spread of Buddhism in this county with its ancient history.

One example illustrating Changfang's reshaping of traditional Chinese history through a Buddhist lens is his retelling of the legend of Houji, founder of the Zhou dynasty (1046–221 BCE). Changfang informed readers that Houji's mother had seen a giant figure in her dream and subsequently became pregnant.[49] The apparent "Buddhicization" of Chinese history happened on two different levels as a result of making changes to the traditional record. First, seeing a giant human figure in a dream points to the story of the Buddha's birth because, according to a well-known Buddhist legend, his mother saw a giant elephant in a dream and then became pregnant with the Buddha. On another level, Changfang's version clearly alludes to the dream of Emperor Ming of the Latter Han dynasty (58–75 CE), who saw a "great figure" in his dream and then sent a military expedition in search of the Buddha's images and scriptures.[50]

Changfang proceeds to change the whole of Chinese history in a similar way in order to prove that Buddhism has been integral to it from the very beginning.[51] In this sense, the *Lidai Sanbao ji* can be rightly compared to the Eusebius' early Christian *History of the Church*[52] or to the *Dīpavaṃsa*[53] in Sri Lanka's, among other texts in which national history has been reinterpreted through the lens of the religious ideals of one new religion to which the whole nation had been already converted.

In a practical sense, Changfang turned the periodic sequence of Chinese dynasties (which he called "lidai" 歷代) into a fundamental principle of classification according to which the entire Buddhist canon was to be organized and verified in terms of its doctrinal truthfulness. He presented the Buddhist canon in such a way that a given text's association with the particular Chinese dynasty that had sponsored its production legitimized that text as a part of the canon. In so doing, he deviated significantly from the principles developed within the saṃgha. Its distinguished leaders, such as Dao'an and Sengyou, sought to verify each text's doctrinal authenticity by associating it with known and reliable translators who worked in China and belonged to the Chinese monastic community; Fajing, the author of the first scriptural catalog of the Sui dynasty, followed this principle, as well. But in the *Lidai Sanbao ji*, only some scriptures were legitimized through the association with respective translators and reliable members of China's monastic community, while others were legitimized through the association with the emperor and the dynasty.[54]

Because Changfang presented the dynastic approval of the Buddhist canon in China as being equal in its truthfulness to the words of Buddha, he was able to assign a higher taxonomic status to indigenous Chinese literature which previously was listed at the very end of scriptural catalogs, and only after all translated texts had been already mentioned. He elevated the status of Chinese commentaries and historical records by listing them alongside translated texts in the same dynastic category; this was based on the fact that these had not been rejected by the dynastic rulers, and therefore, the saṃgha had no reason to give them a lower position in the canon than texts believed to be translations from foreign languages.

As a result of using dynastic approval as proof of doctrinal authenticity, Changfang restored canonical status to several dozen texts which had been pronounced as suspicious and false by other Buddhist bibliographers, including his immediate predecessor, Fajing. This was a radical departure from the rules of textual criticism developed in the saṃgha circles since the time of Dao'an. In fact, the *Lidai Sanbao ji* is the only scriptural catalog in the history of Chinese Buddhism which does not have categories of "suspicious" and "false" scriptures.

Although virtually every known Buddhist author during the period castigated Changfang's work for its lack of scrupulous textual criticism, it took an imperial decree to correct the situation. In 602, Shi Yancong (fl. 557–610) presented a new catalog of the Sui dynasty—the *Sui Renshou neidian lu*—with the specific purpose of altering some of the positions taken by Changfang, especially those concerning inauthentic texts and Chinese indigenous literature. In Yancong's catalog, unlike Changfang's, there is a special division (division number five) that is entirely dedicated to suspicious and false scriptures; however, Yancong's catalog included only a few more works in this category than Fajing's catalog did (209 texts in Yancong's catalog versus 197 in Fajing's), while a good number of works considered to be suspicious and false by the previous catalogers, but restored to a good status by Changfang, had retained the good status in Yancong's catalog.

Unlike Changfang, Yancong did not present material pertaining to dynastic chronicles and listed very few legendary Buddhist events that happened in response to the spread of Dharma. This served as an ideological platform for excluding from the canon all writings (e.g., treatises, commentaries, chronicles) by Chinese Buddhist authors that had been made a prominent part of the canon by Changfang. This move could be a reflection of Wendi's position on such literature. Yancong also made a noticeable change in the way he referred to the name of the canon itself, as expressed in the title of his work—*Catalog of the Inner Canon of the Sui Dynasty (Sui Renshou neidian lu)*. The term "inner canon" became popular in the following Tang dynasty, but this was new for the Sui period. It expressed the idea that the Buddhist canon was protected in the inner quarters of the imperial palace where Wendi's impressive collection of scriptures was being amassed.[55] In this regard, the title of this Sui-dynasty catalog is reminiscent of the Southern Liang dynasty's *Hualin fodian zhongjing mulu* (Catalog of Scriptures from the Buddha Palace in the Jetavana Park) because, in both cases, reference was made to a canon that was both physically and ideologically guarded by the emperor. The saṃgha was sidelined.

NOTES

1. Dao'an, a pivotal figure in early Chinese Buddhism, is credited with the establishment of the vinaya disciplinarian rules for Chinese converts. See Yifa, *The Origins of Buddhist Monastic Codes in China* (Honolulu: University of Hawai'i Press, 2002), 8–13. The best treatment of Daoan's biography is in Arthur Link, "Biography of Tao-an," *T'oung Pao* 46 (1958): 1–48. See also Erik Zürcher, *The Buddhist Conquest of China* (Leiden: Brill, 1959 and 2007), 184–204; and Fang Guangchang, *Dao'an pingzhuan* (Beijing: Kunlun chubanshe, 2004).

2. The debate over monks' privileges allowing them to remain standing in the presence of state officials, including the emperor himself, was first discussed in English by Leon Hurvitz in "Render Unto Caesar in Early Chinese Buddhism: Huiyuan's Treatise on the Exemption of the Buddhist Clergy from the Requirements of Civil Etiquette," *Sino-Indian Studies* 5 (1957): 2–36. Chinese materials pertaining to this first phase of prohibiting monks' independence from political power are collected in a famous anthology of apologetic literature, *Hong ming ji* 弘明集 (Collection [of Notes about] Propagating [the Way] and Illuminating [its Doctrines]) which was recently translated by H. H. Ziegler for the BDK English Tripitaka Translation Series. The decree of 340 was followed by another in 403, with more decrees and debates coming in the following centuries. For a detailed study of these debates in English, see Erik Reinders, *Buddhist and Christian Responses to the Kowtow Problem in China* (New York: Bloomsbury, 2015), chapters 2 and 3; and *Ritual Topography: Bowing and Refusing to Bow in China* (forthcoming).

3. According to Ian Harris, traditional political interdependence existed between the saṃgha and the state in Thailand, where each ruler sought legitimization from the saṃgha. At the same time, the saṃgha was perfectly capable of challenging the state when the latter seemed significantly out of line with the saṃgha's traditional values. See Ian Harris, ed., *Buddhism, Power, and Political Order* (London: Routledge, 2007), 3–4. For a study of the Hindu-Buddhist based philosophy justifying the saṃgha's high political status, see Stanley Jeyaraja Tambiah, *World Conqueror and World Renouncer: A Study of Buddhism and Polity in Thailand* (Cambridge, UK: Cambridge University Press, 1996), part I, and especially pp. 54 and 96.

4. One case in point involves a political struggle between the saṃgha and King Taksin (r. 1767–1782). Taksin sought to impose state regulations which would supersede traditional monastic rules. In protest, high clerics fled the capital, declared the king insane, and started a political campaign that ultimately brought about his abdication. Cf. Yoneo Ishii, "Church and State in Thailand," *Asian Survey* 8 (1968): 864–871.

5. For specific examples of such punishments, see Tanya Storch, "The Past Explains the Present: State Control over Religious Communities in Medieval China," *The Medieval History Journal* 3 (2000): 311–336 . Beginning with the Tang dynasty, monastic disciplinarian codes began resembling imperial laws designed by the state for the regulation of Buddhist communities. Cf. Yifa, *Origins*.

6. *Lidai sanbao ji* (T 2034), 127, b26. It appears that Shixing put together a list of Chinese translations available at the time with the purpose of comparing those to Buddhist scriptures available outside of China, namely, in a Buddhist kingdom of Khotan, for which he left in 260 never to return to China. For more on his trip, see Xavier Tremblay, "The Spread of Buddhism In Serindia: Buddhism Among Iranians, Tocharians, and Turks Before the 13th Century," in Ann Heirman and Stephan Bumbacher, eds., *The Spread of Buddhism* (Leiden: Brill, 2007), 100. For his biography in Chinese, see T 2145, p. 97a–b. Shixing's catalog is analyzed by Tan Shibao in *Han-Tang foshi tanzhen* (Guangzhou: Zhongshan daxue chubanshe, 1991), 94–104.

7. Zhu Fahu is also known under his Sanskrit name as Dharmarakṣa. For details of his biography and translation activities, see Daniel Boucher, "Gāndhārī and the Early Chinese Buddhist Translations Reconsidered: The Case of the Saddharmapuṇḍarīkasūtra," *Journal of the American Oriental Society* 118 (1998): 471–506; and "Dharmaraksa and the Transmission of Buddhism to China," *Asia Major*, Third Series, 19, no. 1–2 (2006): 13-37. For the reference to Fahu's catalog, see T 2034, p. 127, c5. This bibliographic account is also known as the *Nie Daozhen lu* because, in all probability, Nie Daozhen was its actual author. Daozhen lived in Chang'an during the Western Jin (265–317); he was the son of Nie Chengyuan, one of Zhu Fahu's most famous disciples, who had helped him with his translations. On this, see Tan Shibao, *Han-Tang foshi tanzhen*, 104–110. References to the *Nie Daozhen lu* cross-listed with the *Zhu Fahu lu* can be found in T 2034, pp. 63a–64b.

8. For a discussion of its date, see p. 20 of Huang Biji黃碧姬. "Fei Chang-fang *Lidai Sanbao ji* yanjiu," 費長房《歷代三寶紀》研究 *Gudian wenxian yanjiu jikan* 20 (2009): 1–167.

9. This concept was first suggested during the First International Conference, "Spreading Buddha's Words in China" (University of Arizona, March 2011); it was further developed in Zacchetti's "Notions and Visions of the Canon in Early Chinese Buddhism," in Jiang Wu and Lucille Chia, eds., *Spreading Buddha's Word in East Asia: The Formation and Transformation of the Chinese Buddhist Canon* (New York: Columbia University Press, 2015), 87.

10. References to this catalog are in T 2034, p. 74, c7-9. In T 2145, p. 49a-b, and p. 58b-c, we find examples of Mindu's writings related to his bibliographic activities.

11. See reference to his catalog in T 2034, p. 76, b13, where the full title of his catalog, granted to it by the later catalogers, is reproduced. Before that, his catalog was referred to as *Anlu* (An's Catalog). Dao'an's life coincided with the brutal political situation following the collapse of the Han dynasty in 220. Before reaching the age of fifty-three, he migrated through many parts of northern China, building up several Buddhist centers, all of which were forced to disperse due to calamities of the time. In about 365, he settled in Xiangyang where he led a distinguished community of more than three hundred members for roughly fifteen years, until the city was destroyed in 379 and he was forced to move to Chang'an. He died there just six years later still serving as the main leader of the Buddhist community. According to Chen Yinke in *Jinming guan cong gao chuban* (Beijing: Sanlian shudian, 2001), 181–187, Dao'an "invented" Buddhist textual scholarship. According to T. Storch in *The History of Chinese Buddhist Bibliography* (Amherst: Cambria Press, 2014), 31–36, he applied traditional methods that already existed in Chinese book catalogs.

12. On this emulation see Roger Coreless, "The Meaning of Ching (Sutra?) in Buddhist Chinese," *Journal of Chinese Philosophy* 3.1 (1975): 67-72; and Storch, *The History of Chinese Buddhist Bibliography*, 3-11.

13. On the reconstruction of Dao'an's catalog, see Ui Hakuju, *Shaku Dōan Kenkyū* (Tokyo: Iwanamai shoten, 1959) and Fang Guangchang, *Dao'an pingzhuan*. For a successful use of this catalog in reconstructing the earliest reliable authored translations, see Jan Nattier, *A Guide to the Earliest Chinese Buddhist Translations* (Tokyo: International Research Institute for Advanced Buddhology, 2008).

14. For more on Dao'an's criteria of authenticity for the Chinese Buddhist canon, see Zacchetti, "Notions and Visions of the Canon," 89–90; Kyoko Tokuno, "The Evaluation of Indigenous Scriptures in Chinese Buddhist Scriptural Catalogues," in Robert Buswell, Jr., ed., *Chinese Buddhist Apocrypha* (Honolulu: University of Hawai'i Press, 1990): 33–35; and Storch, "Fei Changfang's *Records of the Three Treasures throughout the Successive Dynasties* (Lidai Sanbao ji) and Its Role in the Formation of the Chinese Buddhist Canon," in Wu and Jiang, eds., *Spreading Buddha's Word*, 113–114.

15. This catalog marks the beginning of a period during which Chinese Buddhists referred to the canon as the "zhongjing' 眾經, or "multitude of [Buddhist] Classics." For the study of different terms applied to the Chinese Tripiṭaka, see Jiang Wu, "The Chinese Buddhist Canon Through the Ages," in Wu and Jiang, eds., *Spreading Buddha's Word*, 18–19; and Guangchang Fang, "Defining the Chinese Buddhist Canon: Its Origin, Periodization, and Future," *Journal of Chinese Buddhist Studies* 28 (2015): 1–34. It appears that this catalog was the first (or one of the first) to promote this title for the canon. All the previous catalogs were named after the person who authored the catalog—that is, *Zhu Shixing lu, Zhu Fahu lu, Nie Daozhen lu*, and so forth. Because the term "zhongjing" became widely accepted in the later era, the titles of some earlier catalogs, such as the one by Dao'an, were changed to incorporate this new way of referring to the Buddhist scriptural canon.

16. Huiyuan was well-versed in the Confucian Classics. He was converted to Buddhism by Dao'an and remained his faithful disciple even after he separated from Dao'an due to political calamities of the time; and third, for Huiyuan (very much like for Dao'an), scriptural correctness represented more than a purely scholastic principle, inasmuch as it bore on one's chances for reincarnation in a better place. On Hui-yuan's personal religious views, see Walter Liebenthal, "Shih Hui-yuan's Buddhism as Set Forth in His Writings," *Journal of the American Oriental Society* 70 (1950): 243–259. However, see also Charles B. Jones, "Was Lushan Huiyuan a Pure Land Buddhist? Evidence from His Correspondence with Kumāra-jīva About *Nianfo* Practice," *Chung-Hwa Buddhist Journal* 21 (2008): 175–191. A most substantial study of all materials pertaining to Huiyuan's life and religious activities is in Kimura Eiichi, ed., *Eon Kenkyū*, 2 vols. (Tokyo: Sobunsha, 1960–1962).

17. T 2034, p. 74, a2-6.

338 TEXTS AND TRANSFORMATIONS

18. See T 2034, p. 74, a2-6; and p. 127, c4, for general information about this
    text; for the samples of references to its contents, see 2034, p. 63, a6-8.
19. T 2102, p. 31a-32b
20. The exact reason for such a decision will, probably, remain unknown
    because we lack the actual text of the catalog. One possible explanation
    is that Huiyuan recognized the importance of dynastic sponsorship in
    the production of Buddhist texts even though he insisted that Buddhist
    ritual be observed during the interaction between the saṃgha and secu-
    lar authorities. Another explanation may involve the notion of greater
    reliability of those texts which were produced in Chinese-controlled ter-
    ritories vs. those produced in the areas without Chinese cultural influ-
    ence. This attitude is common to Dao'an's catalog and later catalogs.
21. That is "zhuanlun shengwang" 轉輪聖王, "the wheel-turning emperor."
    The term refers to a universal monarch—in Theravāda Buddhism, the
    ideal of a monarch who rules in accordance with the Dharma. Moreover,
    the cakravartin resembles the traditional Chinese sage-ruler (聖王).
22. Literature about Emperor Wu's Buddhist policies is abundant. The most
    complete account of the above listed actions pertaining to establish-
    ing Buddhism as state religion is Mori Mikisaburō Ryō-no Butei (Kyoto:
    Heigakuji shoten, 1956). See also Andreas Janousch, "The Emperor
    as Bodhisattva: The Bodhisattva Ordination and Ritual Assemblies of
    Emperor Wu of the Liang Dynasty" in Joseph McDermott, ed., State and
    Court Ritual in China (Cambridge, Eng.: Cambridge University Press,
    1999), 112–149; Jinhua Chen, "Pañcavārṣika Assemblies in Liang Wudi's
    Buddhist Palace Chapel," Harvard Journal of Asiatic Studies 66 (2006): 43–
    103; and Tom De Rauw, "Beyond Buddhist Apology: The Political Use
    of Buddhism by Emperor Wu of the Liang Dynasty (r. 502–549)," PhD
    dissertation, Ghent University, 2008.
23. Cf. Arthur Link, "Shih Seng-yu and His Writings," Journal of the Amer-
    ican Oriental Society 80.1 (1960): 17–43.
24. For a discussion of this library and Sengshao's catalog, see Jinhua Chen,
    "Buddhist Establishments within Liang Wudi's Imperial Park," in Jinhua
    Chen and Lori Meeks, eds., Development and Practice of Humanitarian
    Buddhism: Interdisciplinary Perspectives (Hualien, Taiwan: Tzu Chi Uni-
    versity Press, 2007), 18–22. Chen also points out the difficulty in identi-
    fying the exact monk responsible for writing this catalog, because two
    monks with the same name existed at that time (18).

25. Baochang's life is detailed in Tom De Rauw, "Baochang: Sixth Century Biographer of Buddhist Monks...and Nuns?" *Journal of the American Oriental Society* 125 (2005): 203–218.

26. Information about the completion of this catalog by the imperial order is recorded in both Buddhist sources and dynastic chronicles. See *Sui shu* (Beijing: Zhonghua shuju, 1977): 35.1098.

27. T 2060, p. 426, c21-25.

28. In this table and further in my paper, I translate 小乘 as Hīnayāna. However, many American Buddhologists believe that the word "Hīnayāna" is best avoided due to its pejorative implications during early Buddhist history outside of China. See Jan Nattier, *A Few Good Men: The Bodhisattva Path According to the Inquiry of Ugra* (Honolulu: University of Hawai'i Press, 2005), 172–173.

29. De Rauw brings in evidence that it was Baochang's specific knowledge of various powerful prayers to the Buddhas and bodhisattvas that earned him political favors with Wudi. See De Rauw, "Baochang: Sixth Century Biographer," 206.

30. I follow, more or less, the definition given in Robert E. Buswell, Jr. and Donald Lopez, Jr., eds., *The Princeton Dictionary of Buddhism* (Princeton: Princeton University Press, 2014), 81, assuming that, in a nutshell, it refers to the stories which typically illustrate the results of karma and explain how past events have led to present circumstances.

31. In modern editions, including the Taishō, two words have been added to this title, so that it would read: "A newly compiled list of scriptures, vinaya [texts] and treatises" 新集撰出經律論. This was done to correct Sengyou's approach to Chinese Buddhist texts, all of which he called *jing*—"scriptures," or "[Buddhist] Classics," regardless of their proper Buddhist genre. For the original title of this division of Sengyou's catalog, see Yao Mingda 姚名達, *Zhongguo muluxue shi* 中國目錄學史 (Changsha: Shangwu, 1937), 244.

32. In the Taishō edition, p. 5c, where a general list of subdivisions of Sengyou's catalog is presented, two characters 條解 have been added to the title. At p. 13c, where the actual division is presented, the title appears without these two characters.

33. In the Taishō edition, p. 5c, we do not find these separate lists of various types of the vinaya texts. There, at p. 5, only four school-vinaya is mentioned—新集表序四部律. The titles translated in my paper are presented at p. 15b. In Sengyou's catalog, vinaya texts are classified and annotated according to the above-mentioned three divisions: the five

schools of vinaya, eighteen schools of vinaya, and four schools of vinaya whose texts were translated in China.

34. Arthur Link translated the introductory section of the *Chu sanzang jiji*, in which Sengyou had explained taxonomic principles apparent in his approach to Chinese Buddhist scriptures. See Arthur Link, "The Earliest Chinese Account of the Compilation of the Tripitaka," *Journal of the American Oriental Society* 81 (1961): 87–103, and 281–99.

35. The passage is in T 2145, p. 40; it starts in b5 and runs for the following section. In his text, Sengyou refers to her as Nizi (500-?), daughter of a Confucian doctor, who later became a nun under the name Sengfa. For more about Sengfa and her influence on Buddhist and Daoist scriptural traditions, see Robert Campany, "Notes on the Devotional Uses and Symbolic Functions of Sutra Texts as Depicted in Early Chinese Buddhist Miracle Tales and Hagiographies," *Journal of the International Association of Buddhist Studies* 14 (1991), 44-46. See also Chen, "Buddhist Establishments," 24, and Shufen Liu, "The Return of the State: On the Significance of Buddhist Epigraphy and Its Geographic Distribution" in John Lagerwey, ed., *Early Chinese Religion, Part Two: The Period of Division (220-589 AD)* (Leiden: Brill, 2009), 337–39.

36. T 2145, p. 40, b24-c12.

37. Arthur Wright, "Biography and Hagiography: Hui-Chiao's *Lives of Eminent Monks*," in Robert M. Somers, ed., *Studies in Chinese Buddhism* (New Haven: Yale University Press, 1990), 95–98. For more on Huijiao's work and the later Buddhist biographical tradition, see John Kieschnick, *The Eminent Monk* (Honolulu: University of Hawai'i Press, 1997), 4–15.

38. The history of the *Ming seng zhuan* and reasons for Huijiao's negative reception of this text (to the point of refusing to include Baochang's biography into the *Gao seng zhuan*) are discussed in de Rauw, "Baochang," 212-225.

39. There is an ongoing discussion about who was the more capable historian – Baochang or Huijiao. Makita Tairyō and Arthur Wright considered Huijiao's work superior to that of Baochang. However, Koichi Shinohara undoubtedly believes that Huijiao cleverly used Baochang's work without expressing proper gratitude and calls Huijiao's preface "a rather tendentious document that covers up its author's overwhelming indebtedness to Baochang": Shinohara, "Biographies of Eminent Monks in a Comparative Perspective: The Function of the Holy in Medieval Chinese Buddhism," *Chung-Hwa Buddhist Journal* 7 (1994): 484.

40. On the rulers of northern dynasties and Buddhism, , see Kenneth Ch'en, *Buddhism in China* (Princeton: Princeton University Press, 1964), 145–213; Arthur Wright, *Buddhism in Chinese History* (Stanford: Stanford University Press, 1959), 54–56; Whalen Lai, "Society and the Sacred in the Secular City: Temple Legends of the Lo-yang Ch'ieh-lan-chi," in Albert Dien, ed., *State and Society in Early Medieval China* (Stanford: Stanford University Press, 1990): 229–268; and Yi T'ung Wang, tr., *A Record of Buddhist Monasteries in Lo-yang* (Princeton: Princeton University Press, 1984).

41. It is important to make this observation against the background of flourishing Buddhist art and gigantic stone carvings of Buddhist texts, all of which was carried out under imperial orders, but not initiated from within the saṃgha itself. See Katherine Tsiang, "Monumentalization of Buddhist Texts in the Northern Qi Dynasty," *Artibus Asiae* 56 (1996): 233–261. For catalogs of private collections going back to the northern dynasties, see He Mei 何梅, *Lidai hanwen Dazangjing mulu xinkao* 歷代漢文大藏經目錄新考 (Beijing: Shehui kexue wenxian chubanshe, 2014).

42. T 2034, p. 87, b19-21.

43. See the table representing the complete contents of the Wei catalog in Storch, *The History of Chinese Buddhist Bibliography*, 103.

44. See, for instance, Yamazaki Hiroshi, *Zui-no kōso buntei no bukkyō chikokusaku* (Tokyo: Bukkyo hosei keizai kenkyujo, 1971); Arthur Wright, "The Formation of Sui Ideology, 581–604," in John Fairbank, ed., *Chinese Thought and Institutions* (Chicago: University of Chicago Press, 1957), 71–104; and Jinhua Chen, "Śarīra and Scepter: Empress Wu's Political Use of Buddhist Relics," *International Association of Buddhist Studies* 25/1-2 (2002): 33–150, with special attention to section VI, "Ties by Blood and Dharma: A Comparative Study of Emperor Wen and Empress Wu's Political Use of Buddhism."

45. This text's unique ideological principles and taxonomic classification of Buddhist texts will be discussed later in this chapter. For recent studies of the *Lidai sanbao ji*, see Max Deeg, "Zwischen Spannung und Harmonie: Das Problem von Chronologie und Synchronologie in der frühen chinesischen buddhistischen Historiographie," in Peter Schalk, ed., *Geschichten und Geschichte: Historiographie und Hagiographie in der asiatischen Religionsgeschichte* (Uppsala: Acta Universitatis Upsaliensis, 2010): 96–139; and Biji Huang, "Fei Changfang *Lidai sanbao ji* yanjiu. It must be noted that Tan Shibao, *Han-Tang foshi tanzhen*, is highly critical of Changfang's catalog, with the unfortunate result that the valid

information it conveys is disregarded alongside the undeniable forgeries it also contains.

46. See details in Kyoko Tokuno, "The Evaluation of the Indigenous Scriptures."

47. T 2149, p. 333c. See also Erik Zürcher, "Prince Moonlight: Eschatology and Messianism in Early Medieval Chinese Buddhism," *T'oung Pao* second series 68 (1982), 15.

48. One reasonable explanation might be that, while no longer officially a monk, Changfang engaged in activities inconsistent with monastic behavior, such as consumption of wine and sexual intercourse. However, this remains simply a hypothesis because no record explains why he was not ordained as a monk again after the Sui dynasty had restored Buddhism in China. See the discussion of Changfang's clerical status in Biji Huang, "Fei Changfang *Lidai sanbao ji* yanjiu."

49. T 2034, p. 23, a6.

50. Examples of how different versions of this story were used by Chinese Buddhist bibliographers are in T 2145, p. 5, c17-22; and T 2034, p 49, a2-9. A comparison of all known versions may be found in Tang Yongtong, "The Editions of the *Ssu-shih-erh chang-ching*," *Harvard Journal of Asian Studies* 1 (1936), 146-155. On the importance of this text and its background see Robert Sharf, "The Scripture in Forty-Two Sections," in Donald Lopez Jr. , ed., *Religions of China in Practice* (Princeton: Princeton University Press, 1996), 360–371.

51. For detailed analysis of this particular aspect of Changfang's catalog, see Storch, "Fei Changfang's *Records of the Three Treasures*.", and Deeg, "Zwischen Spannung und Harmonie."

52. Eusebius (d. ca. 339), a bishop of Caesarea in Palestine and scholar of the biblical canon, authored the first full-length historical narrative that was written entirely from a Christian point of view (the title of his work is alternatively translated as *Ecclesiastical History*). His account was kept up to date by later Christian scholars, the "continuators," who used his model for a comparative timeline of pagan and Old Testament history. See Robert Grant, *Eusebius as Church Historian* (Oxford: Oxford University Press, 1980).

53. Dīpavaṃsa, or *Chronicle of the Island*, is the earliest surviving Pāli record of Sri Lankan history. Its present form dates from the 4th century C.E. Like the *Lidai Sanbao ji*, it explains the history of Sri Lanka through a Buddhist lens, presenting the entire time prior to the arrival of Buddhism as being demonic and uncivilized. It also presents legendary sto-

ries about the Buddha's visits to the island, delivery of the Buddha's relics by Aśoka's missionaries, and so on. The most reliable critical edition and English translation is still Hermann Oldenberg, *The Dīpavaṃsa: An Ancient Buddhist Historical Record* (London: Williams and Norgate, 1879).

54. Antonino Forte commented on this trend in *A Jewel in Indra's Net: A Letter Sent by Fazang in China to Uisang in Korea* (Kyoto: Scuola italiana di studi sull'Asia orientale, 2000), 57–58; Jinhua Chen also noted this change in the dates provided in the Tang dynasty's catalogs. See "Some Aspects of the Buddhist Translation Procedure in Early Medieval China," *Journal Asiatique* 293 (2005), 648.

55. The word "inner" also stands to represent Buddhist teachings. The title of this catalog, therefore, can be also translated as *Catalog of the Inner [viz. , Buddhist] Canon of the Sui Dynasty*.

CHAPTER 13

YIJING AND THE
BUDDHIST COSMOPOLIS
OF THE SEVENTH CENTURY

Tansen Sen

Buddhist images, ideas, and teachings started reaching Han China (206 BCE–220 CE) in the first or the second century of the Common Era. By this time Buddhism had already gone through manifold changes, doctrinal reinterpretations, and contentious divisions. The texts, practices, and material representations of the teachings of the Buddha differed significantly across most of India.[1] The diverse sites, conduits, and carriers transmitting Buddhism from India to Han and post-Han China resulted in the spread of distinct Buddhist schools and practices, which became more divergent with the incorporation of Chinese beliefs and imaginaries, and interpretations by local sectarian factions. During the subsequent four or five centuries, diverse forms of Buddhist doctrines, texts, and art forms also emerged in Central Asia, Southeast Asia, Korea, and Japan. Despite this diversity, the Buddhist "world" or "cosmopolis" was united through the recognition of the sacred sites in India associated with the life of the Buddha as the central realm of Buddhism. It was here that Buddhists from faraway lands came on pilgrimages and in search for the "true" teachings of Buddhism.

Within this context of the spread of Buddhism and its diversity, the seventh century marked a watershed. The period witnessed brisk movements of pilgrims, missionaries, translators, and artisans; and at the same time, it was discernable for the emergence of multiple centers of Buddhist learning and pilgrimage across most of the continent. The latter development eventually led to the doctrinal fragmentation of the Buddhist cosmopolis, with China-Japan-Korea, Sri Lanka-Southeast Asia, and Tibet-India forming the three main circuits of Buddhist exchanges and interactions in the second millennium CE.[2] Both these aspects can be discerned in the writings of the Tang monk Yijing 義淨 (635–713) who traveled to India between 671 and 695. Yijing also stayed in Palembang on the island of Sumatra for several years and was, therefore, familiar with the Buddhist practices in three different regions of the Buddhist cosmopolis.

The focus of this essay is on two works composed by Yijing in Palembang on his return journey to Tang China (618–907): *Nanhai jigui neifa zhuan* 南海寄歸內法傳 (A Record of the Inner Law Sent Home from the Southern Seas) and *Da Tang Xiyu qiufa gaoseng zhuan* 大唐西域求法高僧傳 (Biographies of Eminent Monks who went to the Western Regions in Search of the Law).[3] Using these two records, the essay examines three facets of Buddhist interactions in Asia, particularly Tang China-India connections, during the seventh century. It first outlines the circulation of people, objects, and knowledge within the Buddhist cosmopolis. Second, it explores the role of the Nālandā Mahāvihara as the center of Buddhist learning. Third, it analyzes some of the issues pertaining to the subsequent fragmentation of the Buddhist cosmopolis, concentrating specifically on the recognition among the Buddhist clergy about the existing diversity of practices and the creation, at the same time, of new sites of learning and pilgrimage outside India.

YIJING AND HIS JOURNEY TO INDIA

The seventh century saw the formation of several unified polities within the Buddhist cosmopolis. This included the Tang Dynasty in China, the empire of Harṣa in what is present-day northern India, the Tibetan empire, the Silla polity in Korea, and the Śrīvijayan thalassocracy in Southeast Asia. Buddhist doctrines and institutions flourished within all these polities, often supported by the respective rulers and elites. The state support and the political stability across most of Asia facilitated the movement of Buddhist monks over long distances; they also accelerated the circulation of Buddhist ritual objects, and contributed to the integration of the Buddhist cosmopolis through the intertwined networks of missionaries and pilgrims, commercial activity, and intraregional diplomacy. During this period, rulers of foreign polities sent emissaries to make offerings at Buddhist sites in the Gangetic region of India, and the Nālandā Mahāvihara became an active center for missionary work and a place of learning for local and foreign monks. Thus, for most part of the seventh century, the Gangetic region remained the center of the Buddhist cosmopolis.

The Chinese monk Xuanzang 玄奘 (c. 600–665) visited India during the first half of the seventh century. The narrative of his journey, which Xuanzang completed shortly after he returned to Tang China in 645, amplified the interest in the sacred sites and learning institutions in India. The *Da Tang Xiyu ji* 大唐西域記 (Records of the Western Regions [visited during] the Great Tang [Dynasty]) was widely read and circulated throughout most of East Asia. Perhaps as a result of the popularity of this narrative, the number of Chinese monks as well as those from the Korean peninsula traveling to the Buddhist holy land for pilgrimage, to acquire Buddhist texts, or to study at the Nālandā Mahāvihara increased significantly. Yijing was one such person, who, similar to the other East Asian Buddhist visitors to India, was familiar with the travelogue of Xuanzang as well as the earlier fifth-century travel record of the region by Faxian 法顯 (337?–422?) known as *Foguo ji* 佛國記 (Records of the Buddhist Polities).[4] In fact, similar to Faxian, Yijing was also interested in the practice of monastic rules (*Vinaya*) in India and made strong arguments for their implementation in China. However, as Ji Xianlin has pointed out, while Faxian was interested in procuring texts that were lacking in China, Yijing had a more advanced agenda of verifying the practice of monastic rules, collecting the Vinaya texts, and translating them.[5]

Yijing was born as Zhang Wenming 張文明 in present-day Jinan, the capital of Shandong Province. He entered a nearby monastery at the age of seven and was ordained at the age of twenty-one. It was almost fifteen years later that he traveled to Chang'an, the capital of the Tang Dynasty, and met with other monks who were planning to visit India. The following year, he proceeded to Yangzhou in the southeast, and from there proceeded to the port town of Guangzhou with the intention of making the journey to India by the maritime route along with a few other Chinese monks. Eventually, however, only one other monk, someone named Shanxing 善行, embarked on the trip to India with Yijing. Their journey was funded by an official in the Lingnan region named Feng Xiaoquan 馮孝詮.[6]

Yijing and Shanxing sailed on a Persian (*Bosi* 波斯) ship. After twenty days they reached Śrīvijaya (Shilifoshi [尸利] 佛逝／室利佛逝), most likely the port of Palembang on Sumatra. Yijing seems to have stayed in Palembang for several months and to have become acquainted with the ruler of the region. It was this ruler who supported Yijing's trip across the Bay of Bengal by finding him accommodation on a "royal ship" (*wang bo* 王舶). Yijing halted in Kedah (Moluoyu末羅瑜; i.e., Malayu) for two months before reaching Tāmralipti (Tanmoliti 耽摩立底) on the Bengal coast in early 673. His companion Shanxing had fallen ill in Palembang and returned to Tang China.⁷ In Tāmralipti, Yijing met a disciple of Xuanzang named Dachengdeng 大乘燈 and decided to study Sanskrit with him before traveling elsewhere in India. A year later, along with Dachengdeng, Yijing joined a group of merchants and continued his journey to "Middle India" (Zhong Tianzhu 中天竺).⁸

Yijing first visited some of the main Buddhist sacred sites in Middle India, which included the Gṛdhrakūṭa Mountain and the Mahābodhi Temple, and then stayed in Nālandā for about ten years. In 685, he took a ship from Tāmralipti to Kedah, where he remained for a year. Yijing then returned to Palembang and lived there for almost six years, traveling to Guangzhou at least once during this prolonged stay. In addition to compiling *Nanhai jigui neifa zhuan* and *Da Tang Xiyu qiufa gaoseng zhuan*, Yijing also translated a few Buddhist texts in Palembang. In 691, he sent with a Chinese monk named Dajin 大津 his two compilations and some of the translations to Chang'an, where Empress Wu Zetian 武則天 (r. 690–705) had recently established her own dynasty and was using Buddhism to legitimize her rule.⁹

Yijing departed from Palembang sometime in 693 and eventually reached Luoyang in 695 and received a grand welcome, with some reports stating that Empress Wu personally greeted him at the city gate.¹⁰ In Luoyang, Yijing worked with foreign monks such as Shicha'nantuo 實 叉難陀 (Śikṣānanda, 652–710) from Khotan and Putiliuzhi 菩提流支 (Bodhiruci, d. 727?) from South India to legitimize Empress Wu's rule. The latter two monks were specifically involved in the manipulation of Buddhist texts to promote Empress Wu as the rightful ruler of China.¹¹ Later, when Yijing started his own translation project, Empress Wu wrote a preface to one of the Buddhist texts.

Yijing continued to be closely associated with the court after the re-establishment of the Tang Dynasty in 705 by Emperor Zhongzong 中宗 (r. 684, 705–710). Similar to Wu Zetian, Emperor Zhongzong wrote preface to one of the translations completed by Yijing and sponsored the monk's other projects. He also provided a special place within the Dajianfu

Temple 大荐福寺 (i.e., the Small Goose Pagoda 小雁塔) in Chang'an for Yijing and his translation team. Additionally, the emperor occasionally invited Yijing to reside in his palace and translate Buddhist texts there. In 713 when Yijing died at the age of 79, the reigning Emperor Xuanzong 玄宗 (r. 712–756) dispatched court official to express condolences, offer gifts, and bestow the posthumous title of Hongluqing 鴻臚卿 (Chief Minister of the Court of State Ceremonial) on the Tang monk. Yijing had translated over fifty Buddhist texts and authored five other works. He also composed a lexicon of Sanskrit words entitled *Fanyu qianzi wen* 梵語千子文 (A Thousand Sanskrit Words).[12] Forty years after the death of Yijing, Emperor Suzong 肅宗 (r. 756–762) constructed a temple called Jinguangming si 金光明寺 in Luoyang to mark Yijing's contributions to the propagation of Buddhism in Tang China.[13]

YIJING AND THE CONNECTIONS ACROSS THE BUDDHIST COSMOPOLIS

Yijing's *Nanhai jigui neifa zhuan* and *Da Tang Xiyu qiufa gaoseng zhuan*, his commentaries in some of the texts he translated, and the circulations of his works to other parts of East Asia provide important evidence on the vibrant exchanges that linked the Buddhist cosmopolis of the seventh century. Yijing's maritime voyage between Tang China and India is one example of the connectivities across the various regions of this Buddhist cosmopolis. When examined together with Xuanzang's *Da Tang Xiyu ji*, which focuses on the networks through the overland routes, it becomes evident that a large part of Asia was integrated through the movement of Buddhist monks who hitchhiked on mercantile ships and caravans. At the same time, support from elites and ruling classes was crucial for sustaining these long-distance movements and connections. The Buddhist cosmopolis of the seventh century, therefore, was one that was integrated through collaborations between itinerant monks, mercantile networks, and the state sponsorship of Buddhist activities.

Yijing's record of his maritime travels is critical not only for charting the networks that connected the maritime space of the Buddhist cosmopolis, but also for understanding the role of Śrīvijaya in fostering Buddhist connections during the second half of the seventh century. Two centuries earlier Faxian had narrated his maritime travel across the Bay of Bengal and the South China Sea and found no evidence of Buddhist practices at the Southeast Asian coast he disembarked. Faxian also described the perilous nature of maritime travel and the contestation among missionaries belonging to different religious traditions.[14] Chinese sources have notices of several other Buddhist monks from different regions of India who took the sea route to China before Yijing's trip. These sources mention that the Buddhist missionaries and pilgrims often sailed on Bosi, Kunlun (Southeast Asia), or Sri Lankan ships.[15] Yijing, as noted earlier, took a Bosi ship from the Tang coast to Palembang. Subsequently, he sailed on a royal ship belonging to the ruler of Śrīvijaya that passed through the Straits of Malacca to Tāmralipti in Bengal. In one of his translations entitled *Genben shuo yiqie youbu baiyi jiemo* 根本說一切有部百一羯磨 (*Mūlasarvāstivādaekaśatakarman*),[16] Yijing describes the route he took on his return journey from Tāmralipti. Sailing from Tāmralipti in the southeast direction for two months, Yijing reached Kedah, which, according to him, was ruled by the Śrīvijayan polity. It took him another month to arrive at the island of Sumatra from Kedah. The sailing time from Sumatra to Guangzhou was about a month. Yijing also details the specific seasons during which the ships set sail from one location to the other and describes the vibrant, albeit still perilous, maritime linkages between Guangzhou and Palembang, and between Palembang and Tāmralipti.

Yijing spent several months (in some cases years) at each of the three locations on his itinerary. While he learned Sanskrit at Tāmralipti for about a year, he was in Palembang for six years engaged in writing and translation, and he lived in Kedah for almost a year during his return trip.

Figure 30. Yijing's Itinerary.

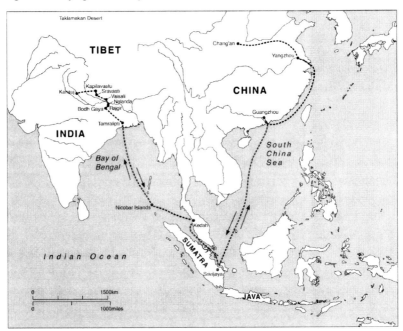

It is not clear what he did in Kedah during his stay. These three locations on Yijing's itinerary were all key sites for Buddhist practices and
transmissions: the importance of Tāmralipti as a learning center was
already noted by Faxian in the fifth century; the so-called Buddhagupta
inscription found in Kedah and dated to the fifth century is recognized
as the earliest evidence of Buddhism in maritime Southeast Asia; and the
founding of Śrīvijayan thalassocracy centered at Palembang in the mid-
seventh century contributed to the flourishing of Buddhism in the islands
of Sumatra and Java. Additionally, Guangzhou, which is also mentioned
on Yijing's itinerary, was already a major destination for Buddhist monks
from India in the third century.[17] It is evident from his itinerary that
by the second half of the seventh-century maritime Southeast Asia had
become intimately enmeshed into the network of Buddhist interactions.

Palembang in particular had already attained the reputation of a hub for Buddhist activity, for which reason Yijing recommends that Chinese monks wishing to travel to India should study there for a year or two.[18]

The maritime route described by Yijing was also used by Korean monks traveling to India. In his *Da Tang Xiyu qiufa gaoseng zhuan,* Yijing mentions two unnamed Korean monks who first went to the Tang capital Chang'an and then took the maritime route through Palembang to India.[19] Monks from Jiaozhou 交州 (present-day northern Vietnam), according to him, traveled through this maritime route as well, although one of these Jiaozhou monks sailed from Palembang to Sri Lanka and from there to West India (*Xi Tianzhu* 西天竺).[20] Additionally, Yijing points out that the monk Dachengdeng had, as a child accompanied his parents, to Dvaravati polity (Duheluobodi 社和羅鉢底 in present-day Thailand) before returning to Tang China with a court diplomat and subsequently becoming a disciple of Xuanzang. Clearly, a number of sailing options existed for the Buddhist monks when traveling between coastal China and Southeast Asia, and between Southeast Asia and South Asian sites since the Bay of Bengal region was connected to the ports located in the South China Sea through various mercantile and shipping networks.

Yijing also speaks of monks who took the overland routes through Central Asia, Tibet, or Burma to reach the sacred sites and learning centers in the Gangetic region during the seventh century. The monk Xuanzhao 玄照, for example, passed through Lanzhou (in present-day Gansu Province), the Hexi Corridor (also in present-day Gansu Province), trekked across the Hindukush and Pamir ranges, reached Tukhāra and subsequently entered Tibet. From Tibet he traveled to Jālandhara (in the present-day Punjab State of India) and eventually reached Bodh Gayā and Nālandā. On his return journey Xuanzhao passed through Nepal and Tibet before reaching Luoyang.[21] The Korean monk Hyŏnt'ae 玄太 also used the route through Tibet and Nepal.[22] Similar to the maritime route, the passageway through Tibet had become a popular conduit for monks traveling between India and China during the second half of the seventh century. Monks from China and elsewhere also traveled to the Gangetic region through Sichuan and eastern regions of India and through Kashmir and Afghanistan. However, the Gangetic region was not the only destination for some of these monks. Several Chinese monks, such as the one from Jiaozhou mentioned earlier, went to Sri Lanka to venerate the Tooth Relic housed there; others went to sites in West India, and some stayed in Kashmir or Nepal.

Another important facet of Yijing's records relates to the intimate connections between the itinerant monks and the courts in Tang China, Kashmir, and the polities in Southeast Asia. Especially in the case of Tang China, some monks who appear in Yijing's accounts were recruited by the court to undertake tasks on behalf of the emperor. Xuanzhao was recalled from India by the Tang emperor Gaozong 高宗 (r. 649–683) and then tasked to bring the longevity physician named Lujiayiduo 盧迦溢多 (Lokāditya?) to China.[23] Princess Wencheng 文成 in Tibet, who was given in marriage to the Tibetan ruler Khri Songtsän Gampo (r. 629–649) by the Tang court, provided support to the monk during his travel.[24] A Sogdian monk called Sengjiabamo 僧伽跋摩 (Saṃghabhara?) was similarly ordered by the Tang emperor to accompany an embassy to India.[25] Additionally, some of the Chinese monks are reported to have traveled with Tang diplomats touring polities in India. At least on two occasions the monks returned to Tang China together with these diplomats through the maritime route. Although these two episodes are mentioned in passing in Yijing's work, they are the earliest records of Chinese diplomats traveling between China and India through the maritime route.[26]

It is clear from Yijing's accounts that the circulation of objects also facilitated the integration of the Buddhist cosmopolis. The same Xuanzhao who was recruited by the Tang emperor received an additional request to procure medicinal herbs from the polity in West India called Luocha 羅荼 (Lāṭa?). The Sogdian Sengjiabamo is reported to have made copies of the images of the Buddha and Avalokiteśvara when he was in India and taken them back to Tang China.[27] Buddhist texts were the most common objects carried from India to China. Yijing himself conveyed Buddhist texts containing 500,000 ślokas, some of which he had already translated into Chinese when at Nālandā. Xuanzang's disciple Dachengdeng, according to Yijing, brought Buddhist images and texts in the other direction, from China to South Asia, presumably to donate to local monastic institutions. In the same manner, Yijing notes the need for paper and ink from China[28] to use in his translation projects when he was residing in Śrīvijaya. Moreover, Yijing describes a futile attempt made by a Chinese monk to steal the Tooth Relic from Sri Lanka.[29] Thus, objects associated with Buddhist activities circulated in many different directions and in multiple forms and ways.

Similarly, several aspects of the circulation of knowledge can be discerned from the writings of Yijing. The routes traversed by monks outlined above, for instance, are evidence of knowledge about the modes of transportation, the halting places, the learning centers, the sacred sites, the geographical contours, and the perils of sea travel shared among monks living in different parts of Asia. Yijing's reports also suggest that the opportunity to learn languages, especially Sanskrit, existed at several places across the Buddhist cosmopolis. This included monasteries in India, Sumatra, and Tang China. Yijing's *Nanhai jigui neifa zhuan* is especially noteworthy for the detailed descriptions of customs and practices in Indian monasteries. Since he was primarily interested in the monastic rules, Yijing provides a meticulous record of how monks in India lived in monastic setting and often compared these to the clergy in China. This comparison of Chinese and Indian monastic customs based on eyewitness accounts, discussed later in this essay, served to inform the Buddhist clergy elsewhere of the daily routine in Indian monastic institutions. It was perhaps for this reason that Yijing's *Nanhai jigui neifa zhuan* circulated widely in East Asia, including among Japanese monks, who did not visit the Buddhist holy land before the seventeenth century.[30] Similarly, the Vinaya texts translated by Yijing were carried to places such as Dunhuang and Central Asia, where they were copied or excerpted

for further dissemination.[31] Indeed, one of Yijing's main contributions
to fostering the connections within the Buddhist cosmopolis may have
been the transmission of knowledge about monastic rules and practices
through his works.

Nālandā as the Center of the Buddhist Cosmopolis

Yijing studied at Nālandā Mahāvihara for almost a decade between
675 and 685. The description of the institution that he provides is
detailed and wide-ranging. It includes depictions of the architecture,
notices on the daily lives of monks, and an account of the areas located
in the vicinity of the monastic institution. Yijing also reports on the
presence of foreign monks from Tang China, Korea, and other regions
of the Buddhist cosmopolis at the monastery. A detailed section on the
Mahāvihara appears in the *Da Tang Xiyu qiufa gaoseng zhuan*[32] where
Yijing notes that the monastery was founded by the "ancient king"
Shilishuojieluodiedi 室利鑠羯羅昳底 (Śrīsakrāditya, i.e., the Gupta King
Kumāragupta, r. c. 415–455) for the north Indian *bhikṣu* Heluoshepan
曷羅社槃 (Granthavatsa?). The later Gupta kings, according to Yijing,
continued to sponsor the expansion of the monastery and eventually
made it into the most spectacular and imposing monument in the region.

The full name of the monastery was Shilinalantuomohebiheluo 室
利那爛陀莫訶毗訶羅 (Śrīnālandāmahāvihāra), rendered into Chinese
by Yijing as the "Place where the Auspicious Dragon Lived." "Śrī," he
explains, was an appellation used by kings and high officials and meant
"auspicious" or "honorable." The term "Nālandā," according to Yijing,
originated from the word "Najialantuo" 那伽爛陀 (Nāgalanda), the name
of a dragon who lived in the vicinity of the monastery. "Biheluo" (*vihara*)
Yijing points out, meant "dwelling place" and argues that it would be
incorrect to translate the word merely as "temple." Yijing also provides
the layout of the monastic institution, describing the residences for
the monks, the multistoried buildings, the various temples, as well as
the *caitya*s and other monuments within the monastery complex. The

stupas, decorated with gold and precious stones, housed sacred relics. Yijing gives an estimate of 3,500 monks living in the monastery, which possessed 201 villages donated by several generations of rulers for the upkeep of the monks.

Writing about the organizational structure and lives of monks at the monastery, Yijing notes that the oldest person, irrespective of his "virtues," was appointed the director. There were also a "head of the temple" (*sizhu* 寺主), a person in charge of calculating and announcing time, someone who oversaw the affairs of the monks, another who inspected the dwelling quarters, somebody assigned to organize the meals, and a few who looked after the finances of the monastery. Writing about the director of duties (Karmadāna) and his task of keeping time, Yijing explains, "At the end of the first watch, the director of duties strikes a drum in a loft of the monastery to announce the time for the monks. Such is the way of using the clepsydra in Nālandā Monastery. At dusk and dawn, a drum is beaten for one stretch at the gate. These miscellaneous affairs are performed by servants or porters. From sunset to dawn, the ordinary monks are not obliged to sound the bell, nor is it the duty of servants; the director of duties has to do it himself."[33]

There were eight courtyards with three hundred rooms in the monastery.[34] Specific rules were followed when assigning these rooms to monks residing at the monastery. Yijing writes that, "all the rooms are distributed in order of seniority to the last person."[35] The monks were required to follow the rules of the Nālandā monastery and those found breaking them were expelled. Also expelled were monks who used money without prior consent. After describing the strict rules at the monastery, Yijing emphasizes that the "uninterrupted prosperity of the monastery is due to nothing else but the observance of the Vinaya rules by the monks."[36]

Yijing reports about a "Zhina" 支那寺 (or "Cina") Temple that existed in the vicinity of Nālandā. Built in the late third century by the King Shilijiduo 室利笈多 (Śrīgupta) for the Chinese monks visiting the region, the temple was in ruins during Yijing's visit. At one point during the early Tang period, Yijing says, there may have been around twenty Chinese monks living at the temple. The king of East India 東天竺, to whom the land at that time belonged, was quoted by Yijing as offering repairs to the temple if any monks from Tang China visited the region again. The king also promised to endow several villages for its maintenance.[37]

The most impressive aspect of Yijing's record of the Nālandā Monastery is the biographies of monks from different regions of the Buddhist cosmopolis who traveled expressly to study there. The monk Xuanzhao from the present-day Shaanxi Province lived in Nālandā for three years studying *Mādhaymikaśāstra* and *Śataśātra* under the monk Jinaprabha, and *Yogācāryabhūmiśāstra* with the master Ratnasiṃharatna. The monk Daoxi 道希 from Shandong Province studied Mahayana texts.[38] Many foreign monks were unable to return to their homelands and died at Nālandā. A monk named Āryavarman 阿離耶跋摩 from Silla in Korea, for example, died near the Dragon Spring at the age of seventy.[39] Another Korean monk called Hyeŏp 慧業 seems to have also passed away in the vicinity of Nālandā.[40] For monks in East Asia, the writings of Yijing confirmed many of the descriptions given by Xuanzang and sustained the popularity of Nālandā among the local followers of Buddhism.

THE DIVERSITY AND SEGMENTATION OF THE BUDDHIST COSMOPOLIS

Already from the early phase of the spread of the doctrine it was apparent that diversity rather than universalism would define the world of Buddhism. In China, the rendition of Sanskrit texts into the Chinese language and the commentaries written upon them laid the foundation of this diversity. Additionally, the incorporation of Chinese beliefs and the production of apocryphal texts made the practice of Buddhism in China distinct from other places. The same trajectory took place in Korea and Japan, in Tibet, and in Sri Lanka. This diversity created multiple Buddhisms across the Buddhist cosmopolis, each place having its unique sets of texts, images, and rituals. As mentioned earlier, the pilgrimage sites and learning centers in the Gangetic region unified this diverse Buddhist cosmopolis. Even this aspect of Buddhism started changing in the seventh century when pilgrimage sites and learning centers began emerging in China and elsewhere. Mount Wutai, for instance, promoted by the Chinese clergy as the abode of the bodhisattva Mañjuśrī, was eventually recognized as such by foreign monks, including those from India.[41] Yijing was one of the first writers to point out the recognition of the Chinese mountain as a pilgrimage site by the Indian clergy.

From an early phase of the transmission of Buddhism, members of the Chinese clergy were aware of the diversity of Buddhist schools and practices, especially the existence of divisions between Theravada and Mahayana. Faxian and Xuanzang when they traveled to India made it a point to categorize the Buddhist monastic institutions they encountered into Theravada / Hinayana or Mahayana. Yijing continued this practice, but he was more interested in pointing out the diverse monastic rules employed by the Buddhists living in different places. He reports:

> In all of the five parts of India, as well as the various islands of the South Seas, people speak of the four nikāyas, but the number of followers of the nikāyas varies at different places. In Maghadha all four nikāyas are in practice, but the Sarvāstivāda-nikāya is the one most flourshing. In Lāṭa and Sindhu--names of countries in West India--three of the nikāyas have few followers, but the Sāṃmitīya has a large number of adherents. In the north all monks follow the Sarvāstivāda-nikāya, though one may sometimes meet with followers of the Mahāsāṃghika-nikāya. In the south all monks follow the Sthavira-nikāya, while the other nikāyas have few followers. In the countries at the eastern frontier, all four nikāyas are practiced in various ways.

> In the Island of the Lion, all monks belong to the Sthavira-nikāya, while the Mahāsāṃghika-nikāya is repulsed. In the South Seas there are more than ten countries where only the Mūlasarvās-tivāda-nikāya is predominant, though one may occasionally find

some followers of the Sāṃmitīya-nikāya. Recently a few adherents of the other two nikāyas have also been found here.

In all these countries [of Southeast Asia] the people follow Buddhism, but mostly of the Hinayana School, except in Malayu where there are a few Mahayana believers.

....

In this country (i.e., Champa) the majority of the monks belong to the Sāṃmitīya-nikāya, with only a few adherents of the Sarvāstivāda-nikāya.

....

In East China, however, the main principles of Buddhism practiced are those of the Dharmagupta School, while in Central China the Mahāsāṃghika-nikāya was also followed at various places in old times. South of the Yangzi River and outside the [local] mountain range, the Sarvāstivāda-nikāya fourished in former times.[42]

On the categorization of Buddhist practices into "Hinayana" and "Mahayana," Yijing notes:

In the regions of North India and the South Seas, what is prevalent is purely Hinayana, while in the Divine Land of China, the monks the great teachings in their minds. At other places both Mahayana and the Hinayana are practiced in a mixed way. Through an examination of their practices, we see no differences in their disciplinary rules and restrictions. Both of them classify the Vinaya rules into five sections and practice the four noble truths. Those who worship bodhisattvas and read Mahayana scriptures are named Mahayanists, and those who do not do so are called Hinayanists.[43]

Specifically, with regard to China, Yijing recommends that the Confucian values of loyalty toward the rulers and filial practices related to parents must continue within the framework of Buddhist Vinaya rules. "But," he points out, "errors and mistakes have crept in during the course of transmission, so that disciplinary rules have become discrepant. Long-standing irregular forms of conduct may become regular practices which are contrary to moral principles."[44] Yijing's *Nanhai jigui neifa zhuan* was composed with the aim to highlight these irregularities by illustrating the correct implementation of the Vinaya rules in India and eventually to "expunge" the various offenses committed by the Chinese clergy in their practice of Buddhism. Therefore, he carefully outlines differences in the practice of Buddhism in India and China. Sometimes he recommends that the Chinese clergy change their ways; at other times, however, he explains that the disparities were due to cultural differences and suggests that the practices could continue. Yijing admits that he did not know much about the practice of Vinaya in India when he was in China. "I should say with a sigh," he laments at the beginning of his book, "that when I was in the Divine Land of China, I thought of myself as knowing the Vinaya well, and little imagined that after coming here to India, I should have found myself ignorant of the subject. Had I not come to the west, how could I have seen such correct rules and regulations?"[45]

Writing about culinary practices and eating habits, for example, Yijing remarks that when having meals monks in India sat on chairs with their feet on the ground. In China, however, he notes that initially the monks sat squatting on their heels when eating. Later, they started sitting cross-legged at meal times. Yijing argued that since the Buddha sat with his feet on the ground, the correct way for the Chinese clergy was to also adopt this practice. "Disciples of the Buddha," he advocated, "should follow the example of the Buddha. Even if it is hard for them to keep the rules, they must not deride them."[46]

Similarly, criticizing the practice of self-immolation among the Buddhists in China, Yijing writes, "the guilt of committing suicide is next only to a breach of the first section [of the four grievous faults] of the disciplinary rules. When I examined the Vinaya-piṭaka, I never saw any passage allowing one to commit suicide." [47]

When discussing the use of spoons and chopsticks, Yijing acknowledges the fact that there were no chopsticks in India, "nor," he points out, "are they mentioned in the Vinaya texts of the four schools of Buddhist monks."[48] Since chopsticks are "neither allowed nor disallowed," he further explains, "if nobody derides or talks about the use of chopsticks, they may well be utilized in China." Similarly, in the case of cleansing one's body or robes before offering salutations, Yijing makes an exception for the Chinese monks: since they live "in a cold country, it is rather difficult for them to behave in accordance with the teachings, even though they wish to do so."[49]

These distinctions and variations increased after the seventh century with the emergence of local pilgrimage sites and learning centers, as well as the strengthening of indigenous teachings, practices, and art forms. Mount Wutai was one of the key places outside India that augmented China's status as a central Buddhist realm. Already in the seventh century, monks from India had started frequenting Mount Wutai to pay homage to Mañjuśrī. A Sri Lankan named Śākyamitra may have been one of the first such monks.[50] Yijing confirms the fact that monks in India recognized the Chinese mountain as a sacred site. "In India," he reports, "it is said in praise [of the Chinese people] that as Mañjuśrī is now living in Bing-zhou [in China], the people there are blessed by his presence, and thus they should be admired and praised."[51] The promotion of the Maitreya cult by Empress Wu Zetian during the last quarter of the seventh century, the popularity of indigenous Buddhist schools in China, and the decline of several monastic towns in India also contributed to the recognition of China as a central Buddhist realm.[52] Although monks from China continued to make pilgrimage to the holy sites in India, engagement with Indian Buddhism and the yearning to learn from Indian ideas and practices gradually faded between the eighth and tenth centuries. Yijing's record of his travels and monastic practices in India turned out to be the last such composition by a Chinese monk.

CONCLUSION

The seventh century was clearly the most vibrant period for Buddhist interactions across most of Asia. The doctrine, in various forms and practices, received the support of political regimes in India (such as by Harṣa), Southeast Asia (especially by the rulers of the Śrīvijayan polity), and East Asia (including by Wu Zetian in China). The doctrine was also accepted by newly formed states such as Tibet and had penetrated Japan. The expansion of commercial activity facilitated the movement of Buddhist pilgrims, preachers, ritual objects, as well as paintings and statues. These movements, in turn, intensified the circulation of knowledge and ideas across the Buddhist cosmopolis. The learning centers in Nālandā, Palembang, Dunhuang, and Chang'an underpinned these transmissions and circulations of Buddhist monks, objects, and ideas, as did the traditional pilgrimage sites in the Gangetic region and the emerging ones in East and Southeast Asia. The Buddhist cosmopolis was, therefore, a highly interconnected sphere within Asia with multidirectional movements, transmissions, and learning. At the same time, this Buddhist cosmopolis was extremely diverse with the mixing of distinct languages, practices, and art forms.

The writings of Yijing discussed above are important sources for understanding some of these dynamics of the seventh-century Buddhist cosmopolis. They confirm the existence of several overland and maritime routes that connected the Korean peninsula to India. His writings also demonstrate the diversity of people and polities involved in fostering intra-Asian connections. Yijing also records the widespread translation activity of Buddhist texts undertaken at places such as Nālandā, Palembang, and Chang'an. Additionally, it becomes clear from his writings that the practice of Buddhism, including the use of monastic rules, differed from place to place. Some of these differences were due to the specific Vinaya tradition the monastic institutions preferred to follow; and at other times distinct cultural and ecological factors played an important role in the creation of unique rituals and practices.

Moreover, Yijing's writings indicate that he wanted the Chinese clergy to model their practice of Buddhism on the traditions he witnessed in India. In fact, he frequently criticized Chinese deviations from these practices and blamed the errors that took place in the course of transmission of the doctrine from India to China. Despite his efforts, however, the post-seventh century phase marked further deviation from the practices and teachings formulated in India. In fact, neither the efforts of Yijing nor that of Xuanzang before him to promote the practices and teachings prevalent in India in Tang China were successful. The establishment of new Buddhist schools in China, the emergence of highly localized traditions, and the fear of a coming demise of Buddhism in India all contributed to the perpetuation of the divergences, resulting eventually in the formation of a segmented Buddhist world in the tenth to eleventh centuries and a decline in the Buddhist connections between India and China. The seventh century, therefore, also marked the beginnings of this untangling of the Buddhist cosmopolis.

NOTES

1. "India" in this essay refers to the area that now comprises of the Republic of India, Pakistan, and Bangladesh.

2. On this post-seventh century fragmentation of the Buddhist cosmopolis, see Tansen Sen, *Buddhism, Diplomacy, and Trade: The Realignment of Sino-Indian Relations, 600–1400* (Honolulu: University of Hawai'i Press, 2003).

3. Wang Bangwei ([1988] 2009; 1995) has undertaken a detailed study of Yijing's writings, including annotating *Nanhai jigui neifa zhuan* (T. [54] 2125) and *Da Tang Xiyu qiufa gaoseng zhuan* (T. [51] 2066). There are also Western-language translations of these two works; see Édouard Chavannes, *Mémoire composé à l'époque de la grande dynastie T'ang sur les religieux éminents qui allèrent chercher la loi dans les pays d'occident par I-Tsing* (Paris: Ernest Leroux, 1894); Latika Lahiri, tr., *Chinese Monks in India: Biography of Eminent Monks Who Went to the Western World in Search of the Law During the T'ang Dynasty* (Delhi: Motilal Banarsidass, 1986); Li Rongxi, tr., *Buddhist Monastic Traditions of Southern Asia: A Record of the Inner Law Sent Home from the South Seas* (Berkeley: Numata Center for Buddhist Translation and Research, 2000); J. Takakusu, *A Record of the Buddhist Religion as Practiced in India and the Malay Archipelago (AD 671–695)* (Delhi: Munshiram Manoharlal Publishers Pvt. Ltd, [1896] 1982).

4. For an overview of the travels of Faxian, Xuanzang, and Yijing to India, see Tansen Sen, "The Travel Records of Chinese Pilgrims Faxian, Xuanzang, and Yijing: Sources for Cross-Cultural Encounters between Ancient China and Ancient India," *Education About Asia* 11.3 (2006): 24–33.

5. Ji Xianlin, *Zhong-Yin wenhua jiaoliu shi* 中印文化交流史 [History of China-India cultural exchanges] (Beijing: Xinhua chubanshe, 1991), 83.

6. *Da Tang Xiyu qiufa gaoseng zhuan*, T. 2066: 7c15–17; Wang Bangwei, *Nanhai jigui neifa zhuan jiaozhu* 南海寄歸內法傳校注 [Annotation of a record of the inner law sent home from the Southern Seas] (Beijing: Zhonghua shuju, 1995), 2–6. Yijing's biography appears in Zanning's 贊寧 (919–1001) *Song gaoseng zhuan* 宋高僧傳 (T. [50] 2061: 710b–711b).

7. Yijing's maritime journey from Lingnan to Tāmralipti and his return from Tāmralipti to Palembang is described in *Da Tang Xiyu qiufa gaoseng*

zhuan, T. 2066: 7c15–8b14. The return journey is detailed in *Genben shuo yiqie youbu baiyi jiemo*, T. 1453 as well (see below).

8. Ibid., and T. 2066:4b18–4c10; Wang, *Nanhai jigui neifa zhuan jiaozhu*, 6–9.

9. On the use of Buddhism for political purposes by Empress Wu, see Antonino Forte, *Political Propaganda and Ideology in China at the End of the Seventh Century: Inquiry into the Nature, Authors and Function of the Tunhuang Document S. 6502 Followed by an Annotated Translation* (Napoli: Istituto Universitario Orientale, 1976).

10. This is similar to the reception Xuanzang reportedly received when he returned from India. In both cases the reports of rulers welcoming the Buddhist monks at the city gates were most likely hagiographical.

11. Forte, *Political Propaganda and Ideology in China.*

12. For a detailed examination of this work, see Prabodh Chandra Bagchi, *Deux lexiques Sanskrit-Chinois: Fan Yu Tsa Ming de Li Yen et Fan Yu Ts'ien Tseu Wen de Yi-Tsing, Tome 1–2* (Paris: Librairie Orientaliste Paul Geuthner, 1929).

13. Yijing's interactions with Wu Zetian and other Tang rulers appear in his biography included in the *Song gaoseng zhuan*, T. 2061: 710b–711b.

14. Tansen Sen, "Buddhism and the Maritime Crossings," in *China and Beyond in the Mediaeval Period: Cultural Crossings and Inter-Regional Connections*, edited by Dorothy Wong and Gustav Heldt (Amherst and Delhi: Cambria Press and Manohar Publishers, 2014), 39–62.

15. On the Buddhist interactions between India and China through the maritime routes, see Sen, "Buddhism and the Maritime Crossings."

16. *Genben shuo yiqie youbu baiyi jiemo*, T. 1453: 477c.

17. Sen, "Buddhism and the Maritime Crossings."

18. *Genben shuo yiqie youbu baiyi jiemo*, T.1453: 477c26–28.

19. *Da Tang Xiyu qiufa gaoseng zhuan*, T. 2066: 2c10.

20. Ibid., T. 2066: 4a22–4b6.

21. Ibid., T. 2066: 1b26–2a22.

22. Ibid., T.2066: 2c2.

23. On the presence of Indian longevity physicians in Tang China, see Sen, *Buddhism, Diplomacy, and Trade*, 44–51.

24. *Da Tang Xiyu qiufa gaoseng zhuan*, T.2066: 1b26–2a22.

25. Ibid., T.2066: 4c15.

26. On China's engagement with the Indian Ocean world in the first millennium CE, see Tansen Sen, "Early China and the Indian Ocean Networks,"

in *The Sea in History: The Ancient World*, edited by Philip de Souza and Pascal Arnaud (Suffolk: Boydell & Brewer, 2017), 536–547.

27. *Da Tang Xiyu qiufa gaoseng zhuan*, T.2066: 4c11–12.
28. Ibid., T. 2066: 4b20-21.
29. Ibid., T. 2066: 3c2–c18. See also Tansen Sen, *India, China, and the World: A Connected History* (Lanham: Rowman & Littlefield, 2017), 151.
30. Fabio Rambelli, "The Idea of India (*Tenjiku*) in Pre-Modern Japan: Issues of Signification and Representation in the Buddhist Translation of Cultures," in *Buddhism Across Asia: Networks of Material, Intellectual and Cultural Exchange*, edited by Tansen Sen (Singapore: Institute of Southeast Asian Studies, 2014), 259–290.
31. Chen Ming, "Vinaya Works Translated by Yijing and Their Circulation: Manuscripts Excavated at Dunhuang and Central Asia," *Studies in Chinese Religion* 1.3 (2015): 229–268.
32. *Da Tang Xiyu qiufa gaoseng zhuan*, T.2066: 5a–6c. See also Wang Bangwei, *Da Tang Xiyu qiufa gaoseng zhuan jiaozhu* 大唐西域求法高僧傳校注 [Annotation of the biographies of eminent monks who went to the western regions in search of the law] (Beijing: Zhonghua shuju, [1988] 2009), 112–116.
33. Li, *Buddhist Monastic Traditions of Southern Asia*, 132.
34. Ibid., 139–140.
35. Ibid., 83.
36. Ibid., 63.
37. *Da Tang Xiyu qiufa gaoseng zhuan*, T. 2066: 5a15–16.
38. Ibid., T.2066: 2a28–2b14.
39. Ibid., T.2066: 2b19–25.
40. Ibid., T.2066: 2b26-2c1.
41. Sen, *Buddhism, Diplomacy, and Trade*.
42. *Nanhai jigui neifa zhuan*, T.2125: 205b–206c; translated in Li, *Buddhist Monastic Traditions of Southern Asia*, 11–13.
43. Li, *Buddhist Monastic Traditions of Southern Asia*, 14.
44. Ibid., 17.
45. Ibid., 63.
46. Ibid., 23.
47. Ibid., 164–165.
48. Ibid., 86.
49. Ibid., 87.
50. Sen, *Buddhism, Diplomacy, and Trade*, 79–80.
51. Li, *Buddhist Monastic Traditions of Southern Asia*, 146.

52. Sen, *Buddhism, Diplomacy, and Trade*, chapter 2.

CHAPTER 14

COUNTDOWN TO 1051

SOME PRELIMINARY THOUGHTS
ON THE PERIODIZATION
OF THE BUDDHIST ESCHATON IN HEIAN AND LIAO

Mimi Yiengpruksawan

The principle of Dharma's end has been studied and debated for generations. There are numerous writings about its place in Buddhist discourse.
Of particular note is the body of scholarship that has emerged in recent
years on the impact of belief in the Buddhist eschaton on Japanese cultural
production in the premodern era.[1] This material has elucidated much but
not the curious history of the temporal scheme itself as it emerged in
the eleventh and twelfth centuries, which gave this end time a starting
date in 1052,[2] and which, perhaps astoundingly, was held in common
by Japanese and Kitan prognosticators of the Heian (794–1185) and Liao
(907–1125) periods respectively. Indeed, a case can be made that the
construction of the Phoenix Hall at Byōdōin in Kyoto Prefecture and the
restoration of the North Pagoda at Chaoyang in Liaoning Province were
conceived with precisely that date in mind. This chapter takes up the
implications of what might seem at first glance rather obtuse questions

of the sort only a calendar enthusiast might wish to explore. Why such a specific date, for example, and does it presuppose the existence of an absolute linear chronology and calendrical system held in common by a handful of Buddhist regimes? In addressing such questions, broader observations become possible which point to the existence in north Asia of a cultural bloc within the broader Mahāyāna cosmopolis.

Coming to terms with temporal consciousness is surely a *Sisyphusarbeit* under any circumstances and even more so with respect to the distant past. As David W. Pankenier has cautioned, the modern "presentist perspective" may defeat attempts at understanding the nature of time and temporality in cultures with differing world views.[3] But Heian writers have bequeathed many hints from inside their social world which indicate a temporal map sensitive to the fleeting, random nature of things but equally possessed of a clear sense of things past and things to come in linear order. The celebrated writer Murasaki Shikibu 紫式部 (ca. 973–ca. 1014), author of *Tale of Genji*, speaks of the times in which she situates her protagonists as *konse* 今世 or *ima no yo* 今の世, "the present world," to be distinguished from *mukashi* 昔, "the past," and *kotai* 古代, "antiquity."[4] While it is true that Murasaki sets the story nearly a century earlier, likely in the reign of Daigo 醍醐天皇 (r. 897–930), her contemporaries, among them the senior statesman Fujiwara no Sanesuke 藤原実資 (957–1046), use the same language to speak of their own "present world."[5]

Many will note that distinguishing the present from the past is an obvious temporal scheme utilized across cultures, and so it is. However, in Murasaki's context it is a nomenclature freighted with the anticipation of decline. Indeed the "present world," juxtaposed against "antiquity," is seen as a darkening age, a kind of *tenebris*, wherein the Dharma has finally begun its devolution as prophesied in more than a millennium of Buddhist commentary.[6] The tone is epitomized by Murasaki when she rues that Genji was destined to be born in the latter days in "this troubled realm of the rising sun." Her frequent use of the phrases *sue no yo* 末の世 "degenerate age" and *yo no sue* 世の末 "latter days" deepens the qualities of loss and resignation at the heart of the story she tells.[7] Even the courtier Fujiwara no Yukinari 藤原行成 (972–1028), a man disinclined to accept the inevitability of a degenerate age, nonetheless tells in his diary of hearing people say that now is the period of the end of the Dharma.[8] This is the language of *eschatos*—of last things and farthest points along an axis of decline.

Yukinari and Sanesuke are equally conscious of living in the last days of the Dharma—a condition they typically refer to as *matsudai* 末代 (Ch. *modai*) "end age", *masse* 末世 (Ch. *moshi*) "end world," and *Buppō metsujin* 佛法滅尽 (Ch. *Fofa miejin*) "annihilation of the Dharma." Yukinari provides an apt example of how courtiers deployed such language to rationalize the circumstances in which they found themselves. He learns that a royal directive has been bungled and consults with the Minister of the Left, Fujiwara no Michinaga 藤原道長 (966–1028), who ascribes the error to stupidity brought on by *matsudai*.[9] Sanesuke is prone to invoking *matsudai* and *masse* to explain a range of phenomena including civil and monastic disturbances, breaches in court protocol, astronomical anomalies, and fires. He reserves terms like "annihilation of the Dharma" for violence perpetrated by monks.[10] Even the Saigū or High Priestess of the Ise Shrine, embroiled in a confrontation with the monarchy in 1031, goes so far as to cite *matsudai* as a contributing factor. The priestess also issues a grim oracle in which she proclaims that the midpoint of the Destiny of the One Hundred Kings has been reached under the new monarch Go Ichijō 後一条天皇 (r. 1016–1036) in 1016.[11]

Fujiwara no Sukefusa 藤原資房 (1007–1057)—Sanesuke's grandson and one of the most informative (if petulant) of Heian diarists on matters of political decorum—belonged to the same generation as the priestess and shared her gloomy outlook. He is so prolific in his invocation of *matsudai* in the 1030s and 1040s that he seems to take eschatological crisis as a personal affront. In 1038, for example, as a confrontation erupts among Tendai (Ch. Tiantai) factions with respect to the appointment of the Tendai Zasu (Tendai Prelate), he speaks with sorrow of the destruction of the Dharma in its latter days.[12] When the main sanctuary at Toyouke Shrine in the Ise complex suddenly collapses in September 1040, Sukefusa sees it as a sign that the world is winding down. Even the reigning monarch Go Suzaku 後朱雀天皇 (r. 1036–1045) becomes convinced that, as a ruler in *matsudai*, he has been abandoned by the gods.[13]

In other words for Murasaki and her contemporaries, the dark ages lay ahead and not behind. The contrast in thinking with Francesco Petrarch's is striking, for whom the future promised a return to light after a long darkness. There was also the existential threat of what amounts to a scheduled rupture in time. Akazome Emon 赤染衛門 (956–1041) makes note of it in *Eiga monogatari* 栄華物語 (Tale of Flowering Fortunes), her partially fictionalized account of the life and times of Michinaga completed around 1030. She writes that, by the third year of Kannin (1019), the end of the Semblance Dharma had come, even in India, where the places once frequented by Buddha and his disciples have become vacant, without any remaining traces of their activities.[14] This remarkable statement suggests, first, that Akazome is cognizant of her times as marking a period of transition from one epoch to another. Second, by using the technical term Semblance Dharma, or Zōhō 像法 (Ch. Xiangfa), Akazome demonstrates her familiarity with the tripartite scheme utilized by Mahāyāna commentators to sequence the decline of the Dharma, namely, True Dharma, or Shōbō 正法 (Ch. Zhengfa); Semblance Dharma; and End or Latter Dharma, or Mappō 末法 (Ch. Mofa).

It comes as a real surprise, then, that the term *Mappō* as such is so rarely encountered in the Heian archive. Murasaki does not use it, nor do Yukinari, Sanesuke, or Michinaga. For the most part, and perhaps surprisingly so given later developments, the same appears to be true for their associates in the monastic community. The Tendai monk Genshin 源信 (942–1017), a contemporary of Murasaki and likely part of her circle, does indeed rely on the idea of the Latter Dharma but is parsimonious with the term "Mappō" proper as evidenced in his *Ōjō yōshū* 往生要集 (Essentials of Salvation) of 985.[15] Shingō 真興 (935 – 1004), a prominent

Hossō scholar at the court of Ichijō 一条天皇 (r. 986–1011), briefly discusses the term Mappō in his commentary on a seventh-century Sanlun (J. Sanron) text, but he, too, does not dwell on it.[16] Nor does the influential Tendai ritualist Kōgyō 皇慶 (977–1049), although he is known to have been a proponent of tantric activity to protect against the ill effects of the Latter Dharma.[17] It is only in the commentaries and proselytizing of the Pure Land clerics Hōnen 法然 (1133–1212) and Shinran 親鸞 (1173–1263), and especially that of the Lotus Sutra proponent Nichiren 日蓮 (1222–1282), that Mappō takes center stage as a word, concept, and spiritual condition. In other words, the term Mappō does not become ubiquitous in Japanese religious and social discourse until after the last decades of the twelfth century.[18]

On the rare occasion that the term Mappō does appear in a Heian record prior to the late eleventh century, it is to mark a specific date. In the fall of 1052, or the seventh year of Eishō, Sukefusa hears that the venerable temple Hasedera has been lost to fire. He writes in his diary that this has occurred in "the first year of Mappō" 末法最年 *Mappō no sainen.* Several weeks later he notes that the temple's statues were rescued even though this is a rare event during Mappō (when presumably such statues would have been destroyed).[19] Interestingly the authors of *Fusō ryakki* 扶桑略記 (Abbreviated Annals of Japan), writing a century or so later, also recognize the seventh year of Eishō—1052—as marking the time when Mappō was entered.[20] More than 400 years later the authors of *Nihon teikō nendai ki* 日本帝皇年代記 (Chronicle of the Monarchs of Japan), a recently discovered chronicle in the Iriki'in family archive, noted the same date for Japan's entry into Mappō.[21] Akazome's comment about reaching the end of the Semblance Dharma is consistent with this temporal map. Moreover, it underlines one of the most important observations to be made about her world: many of its denizens believed they were living at the end of one Buddhist epoch and the beginning of another. Assuredly this is the impression given by the scholar Ōe no Mochitoki 大江以言 (955–1010) when he writes in 1008, to memorialize the recently deceased monk Kaku'un 覚運 (953–1007), that here on the cusp of Mappō there are few sages.[22]

How did commentators of the following generation handle information that the Latter Dharma—that is, Mappō—had begun in 1052, as the authors of *Fusō ryakki* stated? Certainly diarists such as the courtiers Fujiwara no Moromichi 藤原師通 (1062–1099), Fujiwara no Tadazane 藤原忠実 (1078–1162), and Fujiwara no Munetada 藤原宗忠 (1062–1141) made regular use of general terms like *matsudai* and *masse*.[23] But they, too, were parsimonious in their usage of the word Mappō. On one of the few occasions that Munetada did use it, in 1093, it was to explain the ferocity of monastic protests.[24] Interestingly both Munetada and his close associate Moromichi, like Sukefusa in the case of the Hasedera statues, registered relief that, "even as the years speed ahead into Mappō," the Dharma continues to deliver miracles.[25] An observation made by Moromichi, on a summer's night in 1096 after a cooling rain, is pertinent here. We are supposed to have entered *matsudai*, he notes. But the sun and moon are still shining, the hundred-king destiny has yet to be fulfilled, and a gentle rain falls tonight.[26]

As Michele Marra insightfully noted, talk of end times notwithstanding, Munetada, in particular, was not necessarily convinced that it had actually arrived.[27] But the important point here is that Sukefusa in 1052, Munetada in 1095, and Moromichi in 1096 were writing from the other side of a temporal divide marked by the year 1052, when, as Sukefusa states, the world had entered Mappō. Thus the Buddhist historian Jien 慈円 (1155–1225) is entirely justified in using the phrase "latter days" (*yo no sue*) for the time period covering the regency of Fujiwara no Yorimichi 藤原頼通 (1017–1068) through the monarchy and cloistered rule of Toba 鳥羽天皇 (r. 1107–1123).[28] Such calendrical precision has implications. On the one hand it makes clear a rational basis for the concern about end times voiced by Heian writers especially in the early decades of the eleventh century. On the other it begs a question: where did it come from?

END TIMES

Obviously the concept of end time as an integral component of Mahāyāna Buddhism was known in the Japanese archipelago long before Sukefusa's observations in 1052. Indeed, there is longstanding opinion that a calendar date 500 years earlier—552—was recognized as marking the transition to the Latter Dharma as understood by Japanese clerics. However, this view for the most part derives from a source of the thirteenth century, *Kōtaiki* 皇代記 (Chronicle of the Reigns), which figured in the writings of later commentators concerned with the timing of the Buddhist eschaton.[29] There is certainly some evidence in support of a mid-sixth century dating. For example the monk Kyōkai 景戒 (757?–after 822), in *Nihon ryōiki* 日本霊異記 (Account of Supernatural and Strange Tales of Japan) in 787, says that 236 years have passed since entry into the Latter Dharma.[30] But the commentaries of Sanron and Tendai scholars at the turn of the ninth century, just a few decades after Kyōkai's claim, suggest that the matter was not settled, as Marra and Mark L. Blum have shown.[31] The Sanron monk Anchō 安澄 (763–814), for example, discusses various chronologies for the eschaton in his *Chūron soki* 中論疏記 (Commentary on the Middle Treatise) but does not go so far as to identify his own times as falling within Mappō.[32] His famous contemporary Saichō, in *Shugo kokkai shō* 守護国界章 (Defense of the Country) in 818, states that "the Latter Dharma (Mappō) is very near."[33]

It has been claimed that Saichō, founder of the Tendai order in Japan, understood the Latter Dharma to have already begun in his lifetime. This view is based primarily on *Mappō tōmyō ki* 末法灯明記 (Lamp of the Latter Dharma), a work ascribed to Saichō focusing on the challenges of monastic life in the period of the Latter Dharma. Wakamizu Suguru made a strong case that this text is likely a twelfth-century forgery, and indeed its first known mention is in the teachings of Hōnen.[34] Saichō's heirs, among them Annen 安然 (841–915?), did indeed concern themselves with end times but here, too, there is no evidence that the Latter Dharma was understood to have already begun. Indeed, Annen uses the term *matsudai* to refer to the temporal frame in which he is writing.[35] However it is clear that, as expressed by Saichō, the Latter Dharma was closing in. By 984, when Fujiwara no Tamenori 源為憲 (d. 1011) completed *Sanbōe* 三宝絵 (The Three Jewels), it appeared to be imminent. "We may now be in the Period of the Imitated Teaching," he wrote. "But surely only a few years of this interim period remain to us."[36]

Such forecasts suggest that, by the turn of the eleventh century, a final countdown was underway for the Latter Dharma's advent as understood by Japanese commentators. Certainly, the conditions were ripe for millenarian thinking. After decades of relative epidemiological stability, with only sporadic visitations of smallpox, Kyoto was engulfed by at least ten catastrophic outbreaks of smallpox, measles, influenza, and possibly plague between 995 and 1030. This was more than twice the number of outbreaks recorded for the preceding fifty years, and the human cost was high.[37] For example Yukinari, who contracted measles in the summer of 998 and nearly died, wrote of the contagiousness of the disease and its power to seize even the strongest of men.[38] The outbreak had come right after smallpox in 994–995, when, according to Akazome's *Eiga monogatari*, "great numbers of people sickened and died...and their corpses littered the streets."[39] It was followed by influenza in 1000–1001, which left behind a city full of corpses (including that of Murasaki's husband of just three years) and an eschatological turn of mind.[40] The appearance of SN 1006 on Kyoto's southern horizon in May of 1006—the largest supernova in history—only contributed to the growing sense of doom.[41]

This period also saw intensification of commercial and cultural exchange throughout transmarine East Asia by way of the mercantile activities of Chinese sea traders hailing primarily from Mingzhou. Building on decades of monastic contact with Buddhist centers of learning on the continent, Japanese monks boarded Chinese ships for the crossing, and then made their ways to Bian, or Kaifeng—capital of the Northern Song dynasty—as well as to Wutaishan, Tiantaishan, and the many monasteries of Taizhou, Mingzhou, and Suzhou. Kaifeng boasted a great center of learning, Taiping Xingguosi, where Song Taizong 宋太宗 (r. 976–997) had sponsored the opening of a translation center in 980 as part of an ongoing effort to update and expand the Chinese Buddhist Canon. This effort saw first fruit with the publication of the Kaibao edition of the Canon in 983, for which 130,000 woodblocks had been carved in Chengdu and brought to a facility next to the translation center for printing and distribution.[42]

There were many dhāraṇī texts among the translations and recensions produced at the center in an ongoing effort to supplement what had already been published (or released for circulation in manuscript form). Of these quite a few touched on the efficacy of specified rituals and spells in combating the tribulations of Dharma's end. Although the word "Mofa" (i.e., Mappō) is deployed sparingly in these works, multiple references to end times—*moshi, modai*—suggest it was certainly on the minds of translators and their advisors. For example, the recension of the *Jñānolkā-dhāraṇī* (Dhāraṇī of the Buddha of the Lamp of Knowledge), by Dānapāla (Ch. Shihu 施護, fl. late tenth century), makes reference to the end world or *moshi* whereas the Tang-period version does not.[43] The decision to render into Chinese a major part of the *Mañjuśrīmūlakalpa* (Primary Ritual Ordinance of Mañjuśrī) equally suggests an emergent preoccupation with end times. Its translator, Devaśāntika (Ch. Tianxizai 天息災, fl. 980–1000), generates a consistently apocalyptic tone in the multiple mentions of proper ritual procedures to combat the conditions of the Latter Dharma—Mofa—through vocalization of spells presented in the text.[44] Indeed the preface to Song Taizong's decree in 988, ordering the translation of Buddhist texts, cites Tianxizai to note that the Semblance Dharma is like a shadow of the true teachings, which are everlasting.[45]

Exposure to works like the *Mañjuśrīmūlakalpa* may explain the growing interest among Northern Song clerics in the sequencing of the Latter Dharma. For example, *Shishi yaolan* 釋氏要覽 (Essential Readings for Buddhists), a Buddhist dictionary compiled in 1019 by the monk Daocheng

道誠 (fl. early eleventh century), has an entry on the True Dharma which covers timetables for the True, Semblance, and Latter Dharma respectively.[46] Perhaps more pertinent is *Weimojing lüeshou chuiyu ji* 維摩經略疏垂裕記 (Notes on the Brief Commentary on the Vimalakīrti-nirdeśa-sūtra; 1015) by the Tiantai (Shanwai) scholar Zhiyuan 智圓 (976–1022). In the timeworn scholastic habits of his community, Zhiyuan here comments on a commentary by the Tiantai patriarch Zhanran 湛然 (711–782), which in turn is a distillation of a commentary by Tiantai founder Zhiyi 智顗 (538–597) on the *Vimalakīrti-nirdeśa-sūtra* (Sutra of Instruction on Vimalakīrti; Ch. *Weimojing*). Although each of the commentaries mentions end times, only Zhiyuan discusses the three stages of Dharma's decline.[47]

In the Kitan case such sequencing took on what might be called a real-time coefficient by involving a deadline, or so the inscriptions at Chaoyang seem to suggest. Recent scholarship has shown that the Liao capital at Yanjing (near modern Beijing) was a major Buddhist center with its own sutra translation apparatus where newly acquired texts were rendered into Chinese. It is clear that the Liao regime, especially under Liao Shengzong 遼聖宗 (r. 982–1031) and Liao Xingzong 遼興宗 (r. 1031–1055), supported a wide-ranging campaign to promote and disseminate the Dharma in the Kitan territories. A xylographic edition of the Canon was published in two formats, large font and small font, which were circulated in scroll and booklet form respectively.[48] Scholars estimate the imprint of the main part of the Liao edition to have been completed by 1030. At present the edition is known only in fragmentary form, but Chikusa Masaaki has shown that it was for the most part collated with the Kaibao edition.[49] Thus it is likely that the Kitans held in common with their Chinese neighbors a Buddhist community preparing for Dharma's end.[50]

The pragmatism of the Kitan court in this endeavor is exemplified by the stone edition of the Chinese Buddhist Canon at Yunjusi on Fangshan near Beijing (Yan).[51] Carving began in the early seventh century when the monk Jingwan 静琬 (fl. seventh century) pledged to have the Buddhist scriptures carved in stone in order to preserve the Dharma in the time of Mofa. It had faltered by the end of the eighth century but was revived in 964–965 under Liao jurisdiction. Extant stone tablets were reorganized, and subsequent carving went forward based on the Liao edition of the Canon. It was a massive project, eventually yielding thousands of tablets, whose impetus clearly lay in Jingwan's pledge. Indeed, his vow to preserve the Buddhist scriptures is echoed in the inscription by a Liao official and his monastic advisor on a stele commemorating the restoration of Yunjusi in 965. They seek, through the durability of stone, to safeguard Buddha's teachings in the many worlds and ages that lie ahead. In 1005 the stele was recut and another inscription added, which states that through the medium of stone the teachings will be preserved until the coming of Maitreya—that is, the Future Buddha who appears after the eschaton.[52]

Preserving the Buddhist teachings in stone is a logical step to take in preparing for a future inhospitable to the Dharma. Another is to do so with an explicit chronology in mind. An inscription on a tablet carved at Yunjusi in 1058 helps elucidate the importance of such a temporal map. It explains that carving of sutras in preparation for the extinction of the Dharma had slowed by 1027 but was revived after Xingzong came to the throne and in 1038 subsidized the project.[53] Interestingly this subsidy coincided with the restoration of the North Pagoda at Chaoyang in a region under the administrative jurisdiction of Xingzong's eastern capital Dongjing.[54] Originally a timber structure, the Chaoyang North Pagoda was built on the site of the palace of the second Northern Yan (407–436) king shortly after his territory was engulfed by Wei Taiwu 魏太武 (r. 424–452) of Northern Wei (386–535). In 1044, officials overseeing the district of Bazhou (Chaoyang) under Xingzong's government restored the pagoda. Numerous objects were deposited as relics in the cella at the top of the pagoda and in its underground crypt. What links Yunjusi and the North Pagoda is a target date which both were apparently conceived to meet—and which lines up neatly with contemporary Heian prognostications across the sea.

Two inscriptions at the Chaoyang North Pagoda specify that target date with precision. One is carved on the exterior of a stone relic box commemorating emplacement of ritual objects in the cella; the other on a stone dhāraṇī pillar sealed inside the crypt. The relic box is inscribed 大契丹重熙十二年四月八日午時再葬 像法更有八年入末法, "deposited at noon of the 8th day of the 4th moon of the 12th year of the Chongxi reign (May 19, 1043) of the Great Kitan state, with eight years remaining of Xiangfa (Semblance Dharma) followed by entry into Mofa (Latter Dharma)." The words on the pillar read 大契丹重熙十三年歲次甲申四月壬辰朔八日己亥午時再葬, 訖像法更有七年入末法, "deposited at noon on day ren/chen (8) of the 4th moon of the 13th year of the Chongxi reign (May 7, 1044) of the Great Kitan state, with seven years remaining of Xiangfa followed by entry into Mofa." When converted to the Julian calendar the respective countdowns yield a date of February 22, 1051, for the transition to begin. In other words, not only did Kitan prognosticators have in hand a means to making such a calculation; they were also forecasters.[55]

The concordance with the Heian dating, as expressed by Sukefusa with respect to the burning of Hasedera in 1052, is striking and invites scrutiny. Several factors must be taken into consideration here due to the somewhat unexpected nature of this finding. Given the physical distance separating Kyoto from the Liao capitals at Beijing and Dongjing, and the lack of primary evidence for direct contact, it is worth asking how such a shared computation came about. The question raises other problems which have befuddled monks and academics alike: what year did Buddha enter Parinirvāṇa, how many years have elapsed since then, and when will the Buddhist eschaton get underway? Not surprisingly there is a capacious modern literature on this set of issues, to which the present work is deeply indebted.[56] In addition a corollary question arises which, perhaps due to its intractability, has not seen comment. To wit, who maintains the absolute chronology of the Dharma, and how, when year counts are simultaneously regnal (cyclical) and linear depending on local needs in the social control of time. A brief examination of these matters narrowed to the East Asian frame yields insights into the broader significance of the countdown to 1052 in Heian and Liao.

TIME SCALES AND PARINIRVĀṆA DATES

When Tamenori completed *Sanbōe*, and said that only a short time remained of the Semblance Dharma, he also provided a time scale for the Buddha's death relative to his temporal coordinates—that is, "in the winter of the second year of Eikan," or 984.[57] According to that scale Buddha had died 1,933 years *bp*—before present—which, when counted backward from 984, gives 949 BCE as the year when Buddha died. In other words, any countdown implied knowledge of a before-present scale associated with a linear (teleological) chronology. And indeed Buddhist commentators had a variety of scales for calculating time elapsed since the death of Buddha. The Sui-period monk Fei Changfang 費長房 (fl. 562–598), in his catalogue of Buddhist texts *Lidai sanbao ji* 歷代三寶紀 (Records of the Three Treasures throughout the Successive Dynasties), mentions several *bp* scales counting back from 597, the year he completed his catalogue. He gives each scale relative to the reign dates of the kings of Zhou (ca. 1046–256 BCE). From Fei's *bp* scales it is possible to derive a wide range of death dates for Buddha as theorized in 597: 1005 BCE, 810 BCE, 648 BCE, 598 BCE, 549 BCE, and 485 BCE.[58] Fei had his own opinion—608 BCE—based on a time scale relative to the *Chunqiu* 春秋 (The Spring and Autumn Annals).[59]

Centuries later Annen, writing in *Kyōjijō* 教時諍 (Different Views on the Teachings and Time, 876), referenced Fei but utilized yet another *bp* scale, with a commencement date in the fifty-second year of King Mu of Zhou 周穆王, which computes to 953 BCE as the year that Buddha entered Parinirvāṇa—which is close Tamenori's dating of 949 BCE.[60] Kyōkai may well have applied a similar scale when, in *Nihon ryōiki*, he counted back 1,722 years from 787 to arrive at 935 BCE.[61] The origin of this time scale assuming a mid-tenth-century BCE date for Buddha's demise is not known, but much has been speculated. The Sanlun master and "outstanding Buddhist apologist" Falin 法琳 (572–623), writing in *Poxielun* 破邪論 (Treatise on Refuting Error) in 622, provides an important hint. During a debate between the Buddhists and Daoists at the Tuoba court under Xiaoming 魏孝明 (r. 516–528) in the first year of Zhengguang (520), he reports, the Buddhist team gained an advantage by claiming that Buddha was born in the twenty-fourth year of the reign of King Zhao of Zhou 周昭王 and died in the fifty-second year of the reign of King Mu of Zhou. On being challenged the Buddhists cited as sources a biography of King Mu along with the now-lost *Zhoushu yiji* 周書異記 (Strange Accounts of the Book of Zhou) and *Han faben neizhuan* 漢法本內傳 (Inner Tradition on the Foundation of the Dharma under the Han). Falin used the information to calculate that—as of 622–1,577 years had elapsed since Buddha entered Parinirvāṇa. In other words, Buddha died in 955 BCE.[62]

This story is the starting point for what was to become the most widely utilized Buddhist chronology in the Sinophone world after the sixth century CE, with Buddha's death set in the fifty-second year of King Mu at approximately midpoint in the tenth century BCE. Fei, in his discussion of various *bp* scales, credits the King Mu dating to Fashang 法上 (495–580), a prominent monk associated with the Northern Qi (550–577) court, who transmitted it to a monk from the kingdom of Goguryeo 高句麗 (traditional dates 37 BCE – 668 CE).[63] According to Lewis Lancaster, the King Mu dating, by way of the disciples of Xuanzang 玄奘 (602–664), even made its way to Dunhuang.[64] It remained in place for centuries, for the most part displacing an older tradition—subscribed to by Fei in his preference for 608 BCE—according to which Buddha was born in the tenth year of King Zhuang of Zhou 周莊王.[65] Sometimes the fifty-third year of King Mu was cited in records as the death date, but for the most part the fifty-second year was favored by commentators.[66]

Thus Annen, in referencing the fifty-second year of King Mu in his dating of the Buddha's death to 955 BCE, was squarely in the continental mainstream. Indeed, the King Mu chronology appears to have been well established among Japanese commentators by the eighth century, if not earlier. For example, the Hossō monk Zenju 善珠 (727–797), working back from the year that Han Mingdi 漢明帝 (r. 58–75) dreamed of a golden man, and citing the fifty-second year of King Mu, provides a *bp* scale which yields 953 BCE for Buddha's death date.[67] Anchō utilized the fifty-third year dating and presumably subscribed to the same scale give or take a few years. Annen's teacher Enchin 圓珍 (814–891) likely did the same with his King Mu dating in his *Jukkeshū* 授決集 (Collection of Instructions; received from the Abbot of Yuezhou Kaiyuansi, 884).[68]

It is evident that, by dating Buddha's demise to 949 BCE, Tamenori stood on precedent going back to Fashang. He was also in step with the views of a few Northern Song commentators contemporary with him. For example, the Chan scholar Daoyuan 道原 (fl. early eleventh century), in his *Jingde chuandeng lu* 景德傳燈錄 (Record of the Transmission of the Lamp Compiled in the Jingde Era; 1004), gives a biography of Buddha including his death and the distribution of his relics in the fifty-second year of King Mu. Daoyuan also provides a *bp* count which yields the date 950 BCE.[69] However, in contrast to the general acceptance of the King Mu dating among Heian writers, their Northern Song counterparts did not always agree on the death date for Buddha.

For example, Zanning 贊寧 (920–1001), a distinguished Vinaya master attached to the court of Song Taizong, provides an overview of various dating schemes for the death of Buddha in his *Da Song seng shi lüe* 大宋僧史略 (Topical Compendium of the Buddhist Clergy Compiled in the Great Song Dynasty) of 999. He notes that there is much disagreement but seems to favor the King Mu chronology.[70] His contemporary, Zhiyuan, for instance, follows Fei Changfang in favoring a birth date in the reign of King Zhuang and death date in that of King Kuang of Zhou 周匡王. In his commentary on the *Vimalakīrti sutra* and its commentaries, he calculates that Buddha died 1,661 years *bp*—that is, in 646 BCE.[71] In other words a consensus view did not appear to exist among Northern Song commentators with respect to the chronology of Buddha.

The Liao case, on the other hand, suggests not only a consensus among Kitan prognosticators with respect to the chronology of Buddha but a firm death date along with an apparently unique system of backward counting —akin to the "T-Minus" scale of a rocket launch—to the year 1051 for the beginning of the eschaton. As noted, Heian commentators were also familiar with this dating system. However, it appears not to have been utilized by Northern Song forecasters.[72] That the countdown was a logical extension of the King Mu chronology seems clear enough. Some useful insights are gained when so empirical an approach to measuring the arrow of time—calendrical and mathematical—is considered in juxtaposition with eschatological time as theorized by contemporary Buddhist thinkers.

SEQUENCING THE ESCHATON

Modern scholarship has set the reign dates for King Mu at 956–918 BCE according to the Xia-Shang-Zhou Chronology Project—too short a span to accommodate fifty-two years on the throne. However, the traditional dates—1001–946 BCE—remain relevant to discussion of Buddha's death date relative to sequencing of the eschaton.[73] The latter has been a topic of concern in the Buddhist world at least since the second century CE, and various staging timetables have been proposed. For Heian writers assessing the level of decline in their time, as for their contemporaries across the sea, there were two timetables in circulation, both tripartite in nature. One timetable set the duration of the True Dharma as extending 500 years beyond the death of Buddha; the Semblance Dharma as extending 1,000 years beyond the end of the True Dharma; and the Latter Dharma as extending 10,000 years beyond the end of the Semblance Dharma. The other had the True Dharma at 1,000 years beyond the death of Buddha but otherwise remained the same. Obviously the 500-year disparity made a difference in the calculations.

By the time that Akazome made reference to the scheme in 1019, the lengthiest option for the True Dharma was current. For example, Shingō states in his commentary on a Yogācāra treatise that the True Dharma lasts 1,000 years. His Chinese contemporaries Zhiyuan and Daocheng also subscribe to this model.[74] A substantial tradition of analysis and commentary on the duration of the Dharma lay behind such thinking across a number of Buddhist schools. For example, the Sanlun master Jizang 吉藏 (549–623) provided an overview of the problem in his *Fahua xuan lun* 法華玄論 (Commentary on the Lotus Sutra) and leaned toward the longer option, as did his younger contemporaries Falin and Daoxuan.[75] Of course the shorter option of 500 years was much older, having been theorized in the *Candragarbha sūtra* and promoted by the Tiantai patriarch Huisi 慧思 (515–577).[76] But it was not a prevailing opinion even in the time of Huisi. The same can be said for the Japanese case. It is clear from comments by Anchō, Kūkai, and Annen that, like their Chinese counterparts, they favored the longer option. Anchō in *Chūron soki* gives an analysis of the various timetables and their sources, as noted, even making reference to a legendary stele inscription at Jetavana-vihāra in support of the 1,000-year span.[77]

As noted it has been asserted that 552 marked the first year of the Latter Dharma from the perspective of Japanese writers in the Nara and Heian periods. However, the evidence for this is weak. While it is true that Shōtoku Taishi explained the 500-year span in his commentary on the *Śrīmālādevīsiṃhanāda-sūtra*, written ca. 609–611, it is not clear from his wording that this was a commitment to the year 552 as marking the Latter Dharma.[78] Kyōkai did indeed favor the 500-year option and saw the year 565 as the start date for the Latter Dharma—or so it seems. But some scholars have questioned the authenticity of the section of *Nihon ryōiki* whence this evidence derives.[79] The same is true for *Mappō tōmyō ki*, a work associated with Saichō but probably written in the twelfth century. Its writer subscribes to the 500-year span and claims that the Latter Dharma is underway.[80] But this is not the typical view of someone thinking about the Buddhist eschaton at the turn of the eleventh century. Rather it belongs to a later period and the likes of works like *Kōtaiki*. In other words, it is a back formation not entirely relevant to the Heian context.

With respect to that Heian context—the world of Tamenori and Murasaki—a paradigm was in place which made inevitable the conclusion that the Buddhist eschaton was imminent. Borrowing from Michel Foucault, this might be described as an epistemic condition, in the sense that contemporary Buddhist science, relative to time and the duration of the Dharma, allowed no other possibility. Certainly, the axiomatic logic was unassailable. Buddha had died in the fifty-second year of King Mu, or 949 BCE, as Tamenori's *bp* scale confirmed; the experts agreed that the True Dharma had survived for a period of a thousand years and then been replaced by the Semblance Dharma for another period of a thousand years, which was about to end in 1051. Thus, the Latter Dharma would begin in earnest in 1052 just a few decades hence. When Murasaki has Genji observe that the arts in his day have grown superficial, in a memorable scene from the *Tale of Genji* as he prepares his daughter's trousseau, he blames it on the end time and the shallowness which arises as the Dharma attenuates. Murasaki may be engaging in hyperbole, but the observation has a certain truth to it given the calculations.[81]

TIPPING POINT 1052

The precision of counting down to 1051, and assigning epochal significance to it, suggests the existence of a coherent system for predicting the onset of the Buddhist onset. So far there is evidence that, by the end of the eleventh century, this system was held in common by Kitan and Japanese prognosticators. That it may have been known to their counterparts in Korea is suggested by an entry in *Goryeosa* 高麗史 (History of Goryeo; 1451) which records how King Munjong 文宗 (r. 1046–1083) in the third month of the sixth year of his reign—1052—ordered five different kinds of calendar in order to better predict the future. As Yannick Bruneton has shown, the Goryeo court was famous for its diviners, astrologists, and calendar makers. That Munjong mustered these resources early in 1052 hints at sensitivity to the year itself as marking a watershed.[82] Such sensitivity appears not to have been shared by Northern Song commentators. It is certainly true that Daoyuan assigned Buddha a death date of 950 BCE, in keeping with a tradition going back to Fashang, but his contemporaries Zanning and Zhiyuan did not. In short Northern Song experts differed among themselves and did not seem to attach particular significance to the year 1052.

The articulation of such a countdown is momentous for two reasons. First, it constituted a feat of calendrical coordination. Second, and more importantly, it set an inexorable start date for the Buddhist eschaton in the very near future. The Latter Dharma loomed over the world like *Melancholia*'s moon. It sparked action to protect what remained of the Dharma and to provide solace in the waning of its energies. The restoration project at Chaoyang North Pagoda is one example, with its inscriptions counting down to 1051, and the relics and texts deposited inside it. As Youn-mi Kim has shown, these relics and texts suggest that the upper cella was intended to function as a "miniature ritual altar related to the famous Buddhist incantation known as the *Uṣṇīṣavijayā dhāraṇī* (Superlative Spell of the Buddha's Crown)," which would generate the protective powers of the spell in perpetuity.[83] By 1052 there were five Chinese versions of the dhāraṇī's ritual text in circulation, one of which—a translation from the Sanskrit by the Indian monk Divākara ca. 676–688—explained its efficacy during the Semblance and Latter Dharma.[84] The dhāraṇī pillar in the pagoda's underground crypt also makes reference to the *Uṣṇīṣavijayā dhāraṇī* but includes other spells on its four sections, some of them in Siddhaṃ script. Nine dhāraṇī texts occupy the pillar's surface, three of which offer protection in the period of the Latter Dharma.[85]

Another example of a Buddhist project likely undertaken with the Latter Dharma in mind is the Phoenix Hall at Byōdōin. Few have remarked just how thoroughly its iconographical program was driven by strategies to offset the effects of the Latter Dharma, but the evidence is there.[86] The hall was sponsored by Fujiwara no Yorimichi who, as the son of Michinaga, had grown up in the years that Murasaki was writing *Tale of Genji* and was well exposed to Sanesuke's constant invocation of *matsudai* to explain the times in which they lived.[87] Yorimichi designed the Phoenix Hall to enshrine a large gilt-wood statue of an esoteric form of Amitābha whose dhāraṇīs—two of them inscribed in Siddhaṃ script on the surface of a small wooden disk placed inside the statue—provide protections against the effects of the Latter Dharma.

Construction of the Phoenix Hall was more or less contemporary with that of the Chaoyang North Pagoda. It began in 1052 when Yorimichi converted his villa on the west bank of the Uji River into a Buddhist temple. The Phoenix Hall was built that year and consecrated in the spring of 1053. It was given the form of traditional representations of Amitābha's palace in Sukhāvatī, a paradise outside of time and beyond the reach of the Latter Dharma. The hall's location not far from the boisterous rapids of the river, which it faced, seems to have been related to the longstanding association of that river and its environs with sadness and loss, as mentioned multiple times in *Tale of Genji*.[88] Such sentiments would have been well suited to a time when the Dharma was understood to be transitioning to full-scale devolution. Chants and incantations directed at Amitābha certainly offered solace, by granting an encounter with Amitābha, to be sure, but also by their very periodicity. This is exemplified in the circle of dhāraṇīs on the disk inside the statue, figured no doubt on the turning of a wheel, but also calling to mind the Dharmacakra (Wheel of the Dharma) whose internal combustion as it turns disseminates the Buddha's teachings. Like the ritual altar producing a self-generating *Uṣṇīṣavijayā dhāraṇī* inside the incantatory space of the Chaoyang North Pagoda's cella, the Phoenix Hall offered a setting in which the Dharma might, at least for a moment, be held in place against the stream of time.

CALENDARS

With these considerations in mind, and specifically with respect to the countdown to 1051, it is hard to imagine that the Heian and Liao parallels are accidental. On the assumption, then, that Kitan and Japanese prognosticators held in common both the countdown and a community to which it mattered, two broader implications are worth exploring. The first has to do with measurement of linear time. As noted, various *bp* scales were utilized by commentators seeking to situate the birth and death dates of Buddha relative to their own time. All such scales are based on an absolute dating system—linear dating—which runs parallel to finite regnal dates (e.g. 949 BCE vs. King Mu 52). Herbert Franke once noted that, in contrast to the Judeo-Christian and Islamic traditions, "in China no supranational absolute chronology has evolved" and thus the "real dates" of Buddha cannot be derived from Chinese sources.[89]

Although this is certainly true, it does not preclude the development of an absolute chronology for Buddha specific to the Sinophone world and utilized by its Buddhist scholars and forecasters. First, all prognosticators— be they based at the Northern Song, Liao, Goryeo, or Heian courts— utilized lunisolar calendars which were intimately related. Whether it was the *Yingtian li* 應天曆 (Corresponding Heavens) and its derivatives in Northern Song; the *Daming li* 大明曆 (Great Enlightenment) in Liao; or the *Xuanming li* 宣明曆 (J. *Senmyō reki*, Manifest Enlightenment) in Goryeo and Heian, each reckoned time through the "stems and branches" binomial sexagenary cycle for year and day counts repeating itself through natural time. The calendar maker determined a hypothetical first day of a "year zero" or epoch. It began at midnight on the new moon of the eleventh month in the solar period Dongzhi 冬至 (at winter solstice), with sun, moon, and five planets in position, and the first day as *jia/zi* (1) of the sexagenary cycle. For example, the creators of the *Yingtian li*, under Song Taizu 宋太祖 (r. 960–975) in 964, set their reference (epoch) date at 4,285,558 years prior to 964, when the calendar was adopted. The epoch date for the *Daming li* was 51,939 years prior to 463, when the calendar was promulgated under Song Wudi 武帝 of Liu-Song (r. 420– 422), to be adopted centuries later at the court of Liao Shengzong in 994. For the *Xuanming li*, created for Tang Muzong 唐穆宗 (r. 820–824) in 822, it was an astounding 7,070,138 years prior.[90]

It is clear enough, then, that fully articulated linear chronologies were available to those seeking to calculate years elapsed since the reign of King Mu, for example, but were such calendars accurate? Records of astronomical events suggest that some of them were. For example, NASA's "Five Millennium Canon of Lunar Eclipses" has a total lunar eclipse, No. 07408, occurring on January 30, 1078. The Heian courtier Minamoto no Toshifusa 源俊房 (1035–1121), who was utilizing the *Xuanming li*, saw this eclipse and recorded it in his diary, *Suisaki* 水佐記, on day *geng/shen* (14) of the intercalary twelfth moon of the first year of Shōryaku—that is, on January 30, 1078.[91] And, because calendars provided a more or less accurate linear chronology aligned with astronomical events, they were routinely consulted in order to establish the veracity of historical events mentioned in discussions at court or in contemporary writings. For example, Sanesuke, having encountered in 1012 a citation referring to a portentous event at the court of Tang Taizong 太宗 (r. 627–649) on the seventh day of the fourth moon of the seventeenth year of Zhenguan, or April 20, 643, checked this date against a Chinese calendar which had recently come into his possession, and found it to be wrong.[92]

Sanesuke was a notorious stickler for proper documentation of events, so when he was told in 1014 that the statue of Yakushi (Skt. Bhaiṣajyaguru) at Kōryūji was supposed to have its eyes ritually opened on day *geng/yin* (5) of the fifth month of every *yin* (tiger) year, he decided to investigate. To do so, and working with a monk from Kōryūji, Sanesuke consulted a calendar he referred to as the *Fan li* 梵曆 (J. *Bon reki*), using it to check entries for all eye-opening rituals recorded since the transfer of the Japanese government from the old capital of Nara to the new capital of Heian, which took place in 794.[93] This calendar sees only sporadic mention in a small number of eighth-century horoscopic Buddhist astrology texts such as *Kaiyuan zhanjing* 開元占經 (Kaiyuan Omen Classic) by Gautama Siddhārtha (Qutan Xida, 瞿曇悉達, fl. early 8th century) and a commentary on the *Mahāvairocana-abhisaṃbodhi-tantra* by Yixing 一行 (683–727).[94] Its title—"Sanskrit" or "Brahman" calendar—suggests a Buddhist association.

Sanesuke's use of the *Fan li* to check dates sheds light on yet another chronological system available to Heian prognosticators. Judging from how it is described in *Kaiyuan zhanjing* and Yixing's commentary—as explaining the order of the planetary days of the week—the *Fan li* was an hemerology or "omens" calendar which likely also included ephemerides determining positions of the moon and planets on given days in relation to the twelve zodiacal mansions and twenty-seven (or twenty-eight) lodges. As such it drew on Indian and Persian astrocalendrical science as exemplified by the *Xiuyao jing* 宿曜經 (J. *Sukuyō kyō*, Sutra of Constellations and Luminaries, T.1299) which had been translated by Amoghavajra (Bukong Jingang 不空金剛; 705–744) in 759 and 764, and the *Qiyao rangzai jue* 七曜攘災決 (Methods for Averting Disasters under the Seven Luminaries), translated in 865. These books were part of the armamentarium of Buddhist horoscopy as practiced at the Heian court under the aegis of specialists known as Sukuyō masters 宿曜師 (J. Sukuyōshi). Indeed, Sanesuke had consulted such a horoscope—a Sukuyō *kanmon* 宿曜勘文 or Sukuyō report—to avoid attending an event at the palace in 1014.[95]

Astronomical and astrological prognostications of this sort relied on ephemerides or astronomical tables giving the positions of celestial objects over time. The *Qiyao rangzai jue* contained a data set of this nature going back to the tenth year of the Zhenguan era, or 794. It is likely that the *Fan li* contained some of the same astronomical data, which might explain why Sanesuke was able to use it to check dates as far back as the move to Kyoto in 794.[96] As such the *Fan li* calls to mind (and may be related to) at least two other calendars utilized for horoscopy in Sanesuke's day. One, the *Qiyao li* 七曜曆 (Seven Luminaries), was predominantly mathematical and, as its title suggests, provided calculations pertaining to lunations, eclipses, and the motions of the planets. It was consulted when, as in the case of a lunar eclipse in August 1031, the prediction differed from the actual event—which Sanesuke believed negatively affected his fate.[97]

The other calendar, the *Futian li* 符天曆 (Betokened Heaven), was
a recent arrival, having been brought to Kyoto by the Japanese monk
Nichien 日延 (fl. late tenth century) on his return from a visit to the
kingdom of Wu/Yue 吳越 (904–978) in 957. Nichien had been asked by a
prominent astrologer at the Heian court to obtain a new calendar based
on the most recent continental developments in calendrical science,
which he did through his contacts in the Tiantai monastic community,
at a hefty price.[98] The purchase probably did not disappoint, for this
"atypical canon of unknown origin" had some breathtaking features. Its
epoch or start date—set by the calendar maker Cao Shiwei 曹士蔿 (fl.
eighth century) during the Jianzhong era (780–783) under Tang Dezong
唐德宗 (r. 780–805)—was the relatively recent fifth year of the Xianqing
era, or 660. Moreover, in a departure from longstanding calendrical
practice, the epoch began, not in the solar period Dongzhi at the winter
solstice, but in Yushui 雨水, with the sun in the constellation Pisces at
330-degree longitude, and the sun and moon in conjunction—that is,
at the vernal equinox. According to Nakayama Shigeru's calculation,
which is supported by ephemerides available through NASA/JPL, this
was Julian day 1962169, or Sunday, February 16, 660.[99]

These features of the *Futian li*—that it began in Pisces at the vernal
equinox on a Sunday—imply a linear chronology of considerable age,
scale, and tenacity. Setting aside the focus on the vernal equinox in Pisces
as the start point of the tropical (solar) year, which brings to mind the
global system of astrological ages based on the earth's axial precession and
the Age of Pisces specifically, the role of Sunday is pivotal here. It has been
well noted that calendar makers at the Heian court were familiar with the
seven-day or planetary week and marked accordingly the personalized
astrological almanacs, or *guchūreki*, they supplied annually to high-
ranking courtiers. Such almanacs were typically used as templates for
diaries. Holographs of Michinaga's diary show that words deriving from
the Sogdian names of days of the week, rendered in Chinese logograms,
were entered in red ink above month and day counts written in black ink.
For example, on the day Mīr or Myr 蜜 (J. Mitsu, Ch. Mi), the twenty-

first day of the first month of the second year of Kannin, Michinaga made preparations for a banquet. This date converts to Julian day number 2092921.5 or 2092922, in either case Sunday, February 9, 1018.[100]

This is not as extraordinary as it may seem. The *Xiuyao jing* provides instructions for the seven-day week, including the relevant Sogdian words for each of the days, as did the *Qiyao li* familiar to Sanesuke.[101] Most of the astrocalendrical books consulted by Sukuyō masters and other specialists at the Heian court, primarily the Onmyō (Ying Yang) masters 陰陽師 (Onmyōshi) from the Bureau of Divination, contained information about calculating the days of the week. Proper identification of Sundays or "Mīr Days" was crucial. According to a twelfth-century biography of the tantric master Kūkai 空海 (774–835)—credited with promoting the *Xiuyaojing* and other horoscopic Buddhist teachings—the art of calculating Sundays, which he had introduced, was known in the Daidō era (806–810). However, within just a few decades it was being said that, because calendar makers did not know how to calculate Sundays anymore, confusion reigned in assigning dates and astrological values.[102]

A catalog of books in the palace library in the time of Uda 宇多天皇 (r. 887–897), compiled by Fujiwara no Sukeyo 藤原佐世 (847–898), shows that technical knowledge relating to the seven-day week was certainly available by the end of the ninth century, in Chinese works such as *Qiyao xunxing fa* 七曜巡行法 (Procedures on the Rotation of the Seven Planets) and Xijing's *Qiyao xingchen biexing fa* 七曜星辰別行法 (Procedures for Distinguishing the Movements of the Stars according to the Seven Planets; T1309). The *Futian li* was also among the books in the library.[103] Although the *Futian li* no longer exists except in fragmentary form, there is a reasonable likelihood that it contained instructions on the seven-day week given its role in the casting of horoscopes. The *Qiyao li* and *Fan li* in Sanesuke's possession would also have included discussion of the seven days of the week. Thus, it is reasonable to expect that, by the time Michinaga was writing his diary, calendar makers knew how to properly identify Sundays and thus insure the accuracy of their work.

As for Northern Song calendrical practice, Marc Kalinowski has shown that a day count based on the twenty-eight lodges was favored. However, he also notes that this was "a mere duplicate of the seven-day week notation already current in Tang times."[104] The work of the translation center in Kaifeng included a number of texts relating to astrology and the seven planetary days, such as the *Mañjuśrīmūlakalpa* and *Grahamātṛkā dhāraṇī* (Dharani of the Sacred Planet Mothers; T1303).[105] Indeed, as noted by Kam-Wing Fung, the *Yingtian li* likely included a method for calculating the seven days of the week. That the *Yingtian li* was created by an Islamic astronomer together with a Chinese mathematician at the court of Song Taizu—Ma Yize 馬依澤 (921–1005) and Wang Chu'ne 王處訥 (913–982)—lends support to this view.[106] Annotated calendars from tenth-century Dunhuang typically include designation of Sundays and sometimes other days of the week. For example, and exactly as seen in Michinaga's diary, the creator of an almanac (British Library, S.95) for the third year of Xiande (956) entered the logogram "Sunday" (i.e., "Mi") in red ink above the appropriate numerical day counts.[107] In other words, from Dunhuang to Heian, calendar makers held in common a system for extracting dates—and specifically Sundays—in a linear progression likely calculated on the basis of ephemerides provided by the *Qiyao li*, *Fan li*, or even *Yingtian li*.

Utilization of the seven-day week in Liao and Goryeo is difficult to assess given the paucity of primary information relating to their respective calendar systems. The authors of *Liaoshi* do not mention the seven-day week when they provide technical information about the *Daming li* including its calendrical and astronomical tables. However, the *Xingming zongkuo* 星命總括 (Compendia of Astrology and Divination; 984), an astrological manual by the Kitan official Yelü Chun 耶律纯 (fl. tenth century), sheds some light here. Chun notes in the preface that, while ambassador at the Goryeo court, he studied the stars and astrology with a Goryeo national master, including those relating to the seven luminaries or days of the week.[108] It also bears noting that the *Qiyao li* was among the calendars ordered by the Goryeo king in 1052.

All things considered, and bearing in mind the calibration of dating systems and calendrical practices in Northern Song, Liao, Goryeo, and Heian, the existence of a widely held linear chronology, along with techniques for calculating days of the week, surely facilitated the kind of countdown needed to forecast the Latter Dharma. Like a master clock running quietly in the background, a global mechanism was in place according to which—across local calendars—the Latter Dharma could be predicted down to the year, month, and probably even the day. The origins of this mechanism remain an enigma for now. But it is certain that, for a system of this scale to work, there had to be periods of sustained political, cultural, and technological exchange across multiple borders. It is here that the second implication of the countdown to 1051 comes into view.

CONTACT

If Northern Song prognosticators were familiar with this countdown, they appear to have left neither documentary nor epigraphic evidence that such was the case, as noted. Certainly, anyone utilizing the 949 BCE death date—as did Daoyuan—would have deduced the significance of the year 1051 in the staging of the Dharma's efflorescence and decline. However, attention to both date and countdown is yet to be demonstrated. Of course, this may be an accident of limited access to relevant materials. There are ongoing efforts to document Buddhist stone inscriptions in Sichuan and Shandong, for example, and as such material becomes available, a different story may well emerge. The Dunhuang manuscripts similarly hold promise. But for the time being the countdown to 1051 appears to have been the province of prognosticators in Liao, Heian, and possibly Goryeo. In other words it was held in common by several north Asian kingdoms each with its own history of interaction with— and emulation of—the Chinese state especially under the Tang emperors. This introduces the second of the broader implications posed by Heian and Liao concurrence with respect to the Latter Dharma's timing.

An observation made by Erik Zürcher some years ago bears mentioning here. He wrote that the *Zhoushu yiji* and *Han faben neizhuan*—the now-lost texts whence the King Mu dating derives—may have had a "northern origin" because they are first mentioned in connection with the Buddhist-Daoist debate at the Tuoba court in 520.[109] It is also worth noting that Fashang, who rose to high Buddhist office under Wenxuan 齊文宣 (r. 550–559) of the Northern Qi, was instrumental in promoting the King Mu dating, as reported by Fei Changfang in *Lidai sanbao ji*. Fei also reports that Fashang transmitted the King Mu dating to Ŭiyŏn 義淵 (fl. early eighth century), a Korean monk who had been sent by the king of Goguryeo to study with him. Among the king's goals was to learn how many years had passed since Buddha's death.[110]

The pivotal role of the Northern Dynasties in the promotion of Buddhism is another factor to be considered. It was the Buddhist culture of Northern Wei, and to some degree Northern Qi and Northern Zhou, whose influence was strongly felt in the Asuka region as Japan's first Buddhist regime took shape. Transmission—texts, objects, technology—came by way of diplomatic and monastic exchange with the Korean kingdoms of Baekje 百済 (traditional dates 18 BCE–660 CE), Silla 新羅 (traditional dates 57 BCE–935 CE), and Goguryeo, each with its own ties to Northern Dynasties cultures. The advent of the Tang state shifted the geopolitical balance of power out of the north, and its cosmopolitan Buddhist culture, like an incoming tide, engulfed and transformed whatever it encountered. However, the foundations of Buddhism and Buddhist culture, on the Korean peninsula and in the Japanese archipelago, had been laid long before the Tang expansion, with Northern Dynasties building blocks.

In 1990, thousands of Buddhist texts, in fascicle and booklet form, were investigated by a team of researchers led by Ochiai Toshinori at the temple Nanatsudera 七寺 in Nagoya.[111] This "Nanatsudera Canon" had been transcribed at the end of the twelfth century at the request of a local governor and was long believed to be a copy of the Kaibao edition.

However, to the researchers' surprise, among the Nanatsudera texts were those which appear to have been lost by the time that the authoritative Tang-period catalogs *Kaiyuan shijiao lu* 開元釋教錄 (Record of Śākyamuni's Teachings from the Kaiyuan Era; 730) and *Zhenyuan xinding shijiao mulu* 貞元新定釋教目録 (Zhenyuan Revised List of Canonical Buddhist Texts; 800) had been compiled. Since these vulgates served as the templates for the Kaibao and later editions of the Chinese Buddhist Canon (whether handwritten or printed), Ochiai and others came to the conclusion that some Nanatsudera texts had reached Buddhist establishments in Asuka and Nara before 730.

Perhaps the most famous example is the *Foshuo Piluo sanmei jing* 佛説毗羅三昧經 (The Scripture of *Piluo* Samādhi, Spoken by the Buddha). It is listed in both vulgates as spurious and thus excluded from the canon.[112] According to Ochiai this scripture had a very long history as an apocryphon and is even remarked upon as dubious by the monk Dao'an道安 (312–385) of Eastern Jin 東晋 (317–420). However, it is present among the Nanatsudera texts. "Any student of Chinese Buddhism would certainly stare open-mouthed in wonder," writes Ochiai. "As this would mean that in the Nanatsudera Canon, copied between 1175 and 1180, there has been discovered a text composed in China as early as the third or fourth century AD."[113] Another example is the *Foshuo bi'an shenzhou chengjiu jing* (J. Bussetsu Higan jinshu jōju kyō) 佛説彼岸神咒成就經 (Scripture of the Accomplishing of Magical Spells for Reaching the Other Shore, Spoken by Buddha), or *Bi'an Sutra*. It takes up a moment of despair deep in the past, when the Latter Dharma had finally come to the world vacated by Buddha Fragrant Sandalwood—the 76th predecessor of Śākyamuni—and there was great suffering. Śākyamuni uses this lesson from the past to transmit, by way of Mañjuśrī, the spells and even the sutra itself as a means to coping with the Latter Dharma and attaining salvation in a pure land.[114]

Ochiai notes that neither Chinese nor Japanese catalogs mention the *Bi'an Sutra*, which he assesses to be a non-canonical work compiled in

China and transmitted to Japan quite early.[115] Indeed its roots appear
to lie in a corpus of works circulating independently of the canonical
literature since earliest times. What makes this particular apocryphon
noteworthy, of course, is the emphasis on the Latter Dharma. Given the
Liao and Heian concordance in dating the onset of the Latter Dharma,
there is a reasonable expectation that the *Bi'an Sutra* may have been
held in common as well. To date there is no evidence for this sutra in
the Liao epigraphic archive, nor has it been documented among texts
recovered from Liao sites. Perhaps it is better to say that the presence
of the *Bi'an Sutra* in the Nanatsudera Canon allows two preliminary
deductions. First, it is among a number of very old Chinese texts kept
in circulation—their non-canonical status notwithstanding—since the
fourth or fifth centuries, even after these texts had been lost in China.
Second, and as such, it demonstrates an inclination toward preservation
of the deep Buddhist past which lay beneath the Tang overlay.

That the Kitans shared in this formative Buddhist past is obvious but
bears repeating. With their Xianbei pedigree and period of tributary status
under the Northern Wei, the Kitan leadership certainly was in a position
to lay claim to that heritage once a consolidated Liao state emerged
in north China in the early decades of the tenth century. Moreover,
Buddhism likely had come to the Kitan tribes by way of their Tuoba
overlords, who—after a short period of anti-Buddhist persecutions in the
early fifth century—embraced the Buddhist scholars who came to their
courts. Indeed, it was at the court of Xiaoming that the King Mu dating
may have been established. Xiaoming's predecessor Wencheng 魏文成
(r. 452–465) had initiated carving of five Buddhist cave temples out of
the sandstone cliffs at Wuzhoushan 武州山—today known as Yungang
—near his capital at Pingcheng (Datong). In this "definitive affirmation
of Buddhism," Piero Corradini writes, some aspects of Tuoba power
came to be instantiated as the complex grew to encompass more than
two hundred caves.[116]

Over the ensuing centuries, with the north under Tang suzerainty, the rock-cut caves at Yungang were maintained by local patrons but gradually fell into decline. It would be members of the Liao royal family and their affiliates who, as at Fangshan and Chaoyang, would bring Yungang back into favor. Indeed, Sofukawa Hiroshi has noted that the Liao period was the period of restorations at Yungang.[117] This is certainly confirmed by a stele inscription from Yungang discovered by the historian Su Bai in 1962, who found a transcription in fascicle 4,650 of the *Yongle dadian* 永樂大典 (Yongle Encyclopedia) in the library at Peking University. The inscription dates to 1147 and reports that ten Yungang temples (caves) were refurbished under Liao patronage. Even Xingzong's mother, the dowager Fatian 法天 (d. 1058), sponsored renovations there in 1049 (Chongxi 18).[118] Fatian and her relatives by no means limited their Buddhist patronage to restoration projects, it should be said. Fatian herself had sponsored, also in 1049, the Śākyamuni Relic Pagoda 釋迦佛舍利塔 at Qingzhou 慶州 in what is now Inner Mongolia's Balin Left Banner. However, in the impulse to restore caves at Yungang is glimpsed a commitment to preserving, not only the cultural productions of Northern Wei ancestors, but equally the Buddhist foundations of the Liao state.

Of course, the Kitans had also been Tang tributaries. The transformation of the Kitan khaganate into a dynasty under Yelü Abaoji 耶律阿保機 (Liao Taizu 遼太祖; r. 907–926) owed much to the strategic adaptation of Tang models of government and civil society to a late Northern Dynasties political and cultural base. To some degree this is mirrored in Liao material culture, where—as François Louis has shown—Kitan aristocrats relied on Chinese craftsmen to combine Tang designs and techniques with the steppe traditions of the north.[119] In certain areas of Buddhist scholarship, such as the preservation and transmission of texts, the Liao monastic community tended to adhere to early Tang precedents. As noted the Liao edition of the canon was collated with the Kaibao edition, except for one important caveat. Whereas the format for the Kaibao xylographic imprint was 23–50 lines of text per printing block, and fourteen characters per line, the Liao format per block was typically thirty-eight lines and seventeen characters. According to Chikusa and others, the Liao carvers followed an "orthodox" transcription tradition—as seen also at Fangshan—going back to the Tang period and even earlier in northern regions not affected by the instability of regimes to their south.[120]

The picture that emerges, from Heian to Liao, is one framed by a shared Northern Dynasties heritage and the inclination to actively conserve some vestiges of an older identity and history in the wake of the Tang cultural juggernaut. Of course, preserving the past is an integral aspect of human society broadly considered. However, in this specific case it allowed for the continued viability of selected Buddhist traditions which otherwise might have been lost, be they Buddhist sutras, certain rock-cut caves, calendrical systems, or the notion that the first day of the Latter Dharma could be calculated precisely according to an absolute chronology whose epoch was set on the day that Śākyamuni died. Although Tamenori surely was not thinking about a debate at the Northern Wei court when he stated that Buddha died in 949 BCE, and in so doing aligned himself with the King Mu dating and a countdown shared with his Kitan neighbors, its echoes were there.

There is reason enough to think that the alignment of the Liao and Heian countdowns was sheer happenstance—the by-product of a Northern Dynasties heritage held in common under a Tang veneer. Indeed, it is close to impossible to make a case using traditional historical records that those who adhered to those countdowns, in Beijing or Dongjing on the one hand and Kyoto on the other, were ever in direct contact prior to the 1090s.[121] Nonetheless, there is food for thought if material culture is taken into consideration. For example, the Phoenix Hall at Byōdōin shares a number of features with Liao architectural practices, most prominently the removal of weight-bearing pillars from the inner sanctuary, emplacement of a colossal statue in a proportionately small space, lavish utilization of mirrors, and articulation and design of metal fixtures.[122] In the late 1990s, from a purely art historical and formalist perspective, Ogawa Hiromitsu demonstrated the extraordinary correspondence—too close to be random

—between the landscape paintings on the interior walls and doors of the Phoenix Hall and those on the walls of the inner burial chamber of Liao Shengzong's tomb at Qingling 慶陵 in Qingzhou.[123]

Ogawa did not pursue the implications of his analysis, as that was not his goal, but the discovery is noteworthy. It places in perspective what Tsunematsu Mikio 常松幹雄 calls the "riddle tile" found among the many eleventh-century terracotta roof tiles unearthed during excavations in the 1980s in and around the port city of Hakata 博多 in what is now Fukuoka Prefecture.[124] Home to the Dazaifu regional command, and since the eighth century the official port of entry into the kingdom of Japan, Hakata was also the trading town to which Chinese seagoing merchants had been bringing their wares since the 980s. It should come as no surprise that hundreds of Longquan celadon shards have been unearthed in Hakata, along with terracotta roof tiles with designs characteristic of government buildings and Buddhist temples seen in Heian, Goryeo, and Northern Song.

Among the eleventh-century tiles recovered from Hakata is a category of eave-end tile—Tsunematsu's "riddle" tile—which at first glance appears to be sui generis. It bears a distinctive design on its face, reminiscent of a fern frond, with a scalloped lower border. In fact, this type of eave-end tile, as Tsunematsu shows, is characteristic of those excavated from the sites of the sanctuary halls in front of the tombs of Shengzong and Xingzong at Qingling. According to Tsunematsu, the derivation is likely the Buddhist architecture of Goguryeo or its successor state Balhae 渤海 (698–926), and by the eleventh century it was utilized throughout northeast China.[125] Perhaps amazingly "fern-frond" tiles have also been unearthed at the site of Jōmyōji 浄妙寺, in Uji, which was refurbished by Michinaga in 1005 to commemorate his Fujiwara ancestors in their graves nearby. Judging from Michinaga's other cultural productions—including gigantic Buddhist halls reminiscent of the colossal architecture favored by Liao patrons as seen at Fengguosi 奉國寺 in Liaoning Province—there is certainly room for speculation that he may have drawn inspiration from his Kitan contemporaries.[126]

This in turn raises the inevitable question: but how? In 1012, Michinaga reported in his diary that he had received a fascicle of "compositions from Great Liao" 大遼作文 (J. *Dai Ryō sakubun*) sent him by Jakushō, a Japanese monk living in Kaifeng with whom he had close ties. The writings were delivered to the Dazaifu authorities by a Chinese merchant and forwarded to Kyoto. There is no way of knowing what these writings from Great Liao were about, since Michinaga provides no details, but based on his choice of words, they were not official documents.[127] That they were delivered by a Chinese merchant—one Zhou Wenyi 周文裔 (fl. eleventh century), who was well known in Dazaifu and counted Michinaga and Yorimichi among his clients—offers an important perspective on a state of affairs in which Michinaga found himself receiving writings from the Liao kingdom by way of a Chinese merchant on behalf of a Japanese monk living in Kaifeng.

It bears noting here that Michinaga and his peers at the Heian court likely were well aware of that Liao kingdom despite lack of evidence for direct contact. Given the strong diplomatic and trade relations linking Wu/Yue under Qian Yuanguan 錢元瓘 (Wenmu 文穆; r. 932–941) and Qian Chu 錢俶 (Zhongyi 忠懿; r. 947–978) to the Heian government under the regencies of Michinaga's great-grandfather Tadahira 時平 (880–949) and grandfather Morosuke 師輔 (909–960), it is impossible to imagine that no one talked about the Liao powerhouse gaining ground in northeastern China. After all Wu/Yue—as Edmund H. Worthy notes—was "the first of the Chinese states to establish relations with the Kitans" and the Kitans for their part "stood to gain from diplomatic and commercial relations with the wealthy state of Wu/Yue." Relations between Wu/Yue and Heian were equally strong. "No other state during the Tang-Sung transition period," Worthy writes, "developed such extensive relations with Japan."[128] It is reasonable to expect that an envoy to the Heian court from Wu/Yue, such as Cheng Xun 承勳 (fl. early tenth century) on behalf of Qian Yuanguan in 935, would have brought news of the Kitans.[129]

The history of relations between the kingdom of Balhae and that of Japan, in which envoys from Abaoji's government eventually had a role to play, also deserves comment. Located at the northern end of the Korean peninsula, and encompassing what are now Primorye in the Russian Federation and the Chinese provinces of Jilin, Heilongjiang, and Liaoning, Balhae sent thirty-four missions to Japan by way of the so-called Bokkai (Balhae) sea route across the Eastern Sea (Sea of Japan). The route went from what is now Posyet Bay in Vladivostok to Fukura Harbor 福浦港 on the Noto Peninsula 能登半島, in what is now Ishikawa Prefecture, and to Tsuruga Harbor 敦賀港 in what is now Fukui Prefecture, not far from Kyoto. Approximately fourteen missions were sent from Nara and Kyoto to Balhae. Relations were strong for nearly two centuries, with a Balhae envoy even introducing the *Xuanming li*—the "newest Chinese calendar"—to the Heian court in 858.[130] Balhae was annexed by the Kitan state in 926, after which it was known as Dong Qidan 東契丹 (East Kitan), but some of its diplomatic personnel apparently remained in place. For example, Bae Gu 裴璆 (fl. early tenth century), who had represented Balhae at the Heian court in 920, made his way to Kyoto again in 930 as the envoy of the Dong Qidan (Liao) government.[131]

Obviously, the Kyoto visited by Bae in 930 and by Cheng Xun in 935 was not the Kyoto of Michinaga in 1012. Had Michinaga sought information about contact with Dong Qidan or Wu/Yue prior to his time, there were certainly historical documents for him to consult in his own library or in the offices of the secretariat of the Council of State.[132] But two generations would have passed by then, with no official record for any contact with the Kitan government. However, those very records intimate the existence of other avenues of communication. For example, Cheng Xun was a merchant as well as Qian Yuanguan's envoy to the Heian court.[133] As such he belonged to a seagoing community of traders who had been carrying diplomatic missions on their ships for decades, along sea routes crisscrossing the region from Hangzhou and Mingzhou on the coast of what is now Zhejiang Province to Hakata, with ports of call on the islands of Tsushima and, sometimes, Jejudo. In other words, the stage was already set for the exponential increase in cultural exchange throughout this region which would begin at the close of the tenth century.

By the time that Zhou Wenyi brought some Liao writings to Michinaga, in 1012, so extensive was cross-regional traffic in goods and ideas that complete lack of Kitan participation in the system seems unlikely. It might be better to consider the possibility that a few Kitan traders and monks were on the Chinese ships and managed in one way or another to make contact with some of their Japanese neighbors across the sea. Scholars tend to focus on the Dazaifu regional command, and its port city of Hakata, in painting an official portrait of Heian relations—diplomatic and otherwise—with the world abroad. However other harbors were open if not officially so, such as Tsuruga, where Chinese merchants sometimes settled on a temporary basis. According to Murai Shōsuke, looking at Heian government records, there was a peak in such activity in the 990s, and again in the 1120s. He furthermore suggests that, by the late eleventh century, Kitan traders were in evidence along the Echizen coast.[134]

Although Murai makes a case that, for much of the eleventh century, the historical record is silent with respect to any Chinese (not to mention Kitan) presence along the western seaboard of the Japanese archipelago, it bears mentioning that the main harbors associated with the Balhae route—Fukura and Tsuruga—remained active during this period. There was also Tosaminato 十三湊 to the north, on the Tsugaru Peninsula in what is now Aomori Prefecture, facing west toward Posyet Bay and, due to optimal wind and current conditions part of the year, well within reach of Liao territory. Tosaminato receives short shrift in the modern literature. But excavations have shown that it was a major entrepôt in the tenth and eleventh centuries, of a size comparable to that of Dazaifu, and heavily invested in trade in northern goods such as fur, eagles' wings, and minerals (tin, gold) in exchange for textiles and high-fired wares from Goryeo and Northern Song.[135]

Most importantly, Tosaminato was integrated into the overland trunk routes linking metropolitan Kyoto to Mutsu and Dewa provinces—a region called Ōshū which encompassed what are now Aomori, Akita, Yamagata, Iwate, Miyagi, and northern Fukushima prefectures. Heian courtiers had an appetite for goods from this remote region, and when the commanding officer of the Chinjufu (Ōshū) regional command returned to Kyoto bearing gifts for Michinaga in 1014, people jostled to see what he had to offer: quivers, horses, eagles' wings, gold nuggets, silks, cottons, and hemp cloth.[136] Ōshū boasted a booming economy in horses, furs, and gold, to be sure, but it was not suited to silk production. Nor were its inhabitants easily policed by the Heian authorities. Thus, independent trade and even diplomatic contact with the Kitans, by way of Tosaminato and possibly Fukura, cannot be ruled out. Indeed, it is likely that the silks purchased by Michinaga in 1016, through a provisional market offering goods from Mutsu, were imported via Tosaminato likely having passed through Kitan hands.[137]

In sum, it is important to bear in mind that, if there are parallels to be found linking Liao and Heian culture—such as the countdown to 1051— they are likely the manifestation of a shared Northern Dynasties heritage with its own traditions embedded locally but shared globally through ongoing contact and reinforcement. When Taira no Masakado 平将門 (d. 940) revolted in 939 in Hitachi Province on the southern border of Mutsu, to name himself the "new emperor" in contradistinction to the "original emperor" on the throne in Kyoto, he did so in emulation of Abaoji, whose annexation of Balhae set in motion the Liao dynasty. Masakado was dead in battle by 940, but as David T. Bialock notes, his was "an affiliation with a much broader East Asian geopolitical sphere."[138] That sphere was already ancient by the time that Masakado rose to power, with an integrated circuitry of trade facilitating the flow of goods, information, and ideas. It is in this context that the countdown to 1051 comes fully into view as an artifact of history from the periphery taking center stage in the Latter Dharma.

TIME

In 1040 Yorimichi secretly imported a printed version of what he identified to Sukefusa as a Chinese calendar 唐暦. He had requested it the previous year, in the midst of an ongoing and increasingly bitter dispute over prediction of eclipses between the two principal calendar makers at court, namely, Kamo no Michihira 賀茂道平 (fl. eleventh century) and the monk Shōshō 證昭 (fl. eleventh century). There was nothing more mortifying than getting it wrong, and calendar makers vigorously defended their prognostications. Yorimichi must have grown weary of the squabbling and ordered delivery of a Chinese calendar for comparison. As Sukefusa reports, the calendar came from Silla—a common appellation for Goryeo among Chinese, Kitans, and Jurchens—by way of Yorimichi's contacts at the Dazaifu headquarters. Moreover, he was pleased to say, it was an exact match with the calendar prepared by Michihira.[139]

The test came a few days later, with the solar eclipse of February 15, 1040 (NASA "Five Millennium Catalog of Solar Eclipses," No. 07217). Michihira, in concordance with the Chinese calendar imported by Yorimichi, predicted that the eclipse would begin at approximately 12:30 p.m. (Uma Roku Koku, 午六剋), cover eleven fifteenths of the sun, and end at approximately 3:45 p.m. (Saru San Koku, 申三剋). His rival Shōshō predicted the same start time but had the eclipse extend to thirteen fifteenths of the sun—nearly a total eclipse—and end later. As it happened, the eclipse began just before 3:00 p.m. (Saru Koku), covered eleven fifteenths of the sun, and ended at 3:45 p.m. Michihira was praised for his accuracy in predicting both the size of the eclipse relative to the solar disc and the time that it ended. For those already rattled by thoughts of the Latter Dharma, such as Go Suzaku, such accuracy mattered. He enthused that eclipses could be predicted and were not a manifestation of *matsudai*.[140]

On learning that Yorimichi's newly acquired Chinese calendar was a match with that of Michihira, Sukefusa was thrilled. It is a great boon to have a calendar on which everyone can agree, he noted, for otherwise it is difficult to know what is correct when predictions are made. Certainly, this was a matter which caught the attention of those concerned with the management of time in a world perceived as devolving, and herein lies its greater significance. For if ever there was a period of intense scrutiny and reform of calendars, it was the tenth and eleventh centuries at the Northern Song, Liao, and Heian courts. In a little over a century, between 961 and 1075, Northern Song prognosticators utilized six official calendars in succession. Although the first calendar, the *Qintian li* 欽天曆 (Celestial Veneration) had been appropriated from the Later Zhou court in a raid on Kaifeng in 961, the others were produced by the Northern Song calendar makers themselves. Of these the *Yingtian li* (adopted in 964) had the greatest durability with updated sequels issued as the *Qianyuan li* 乾元曆 (The Heavens; 981) and *Yitian li* 儀天曆 (Celestial Ritual; 1001). Although it was not an official calendar, the *Futian li* was also consulted. If the holdings of the Imperial Library are any indication, as listed in *Songshi*, Northern Song rulers had access to an enormous collection of calendars and calendrical treatises.[141]

Liao, Goryeo, and Heian prognosticators utilized only one official calendar each during this same period. As noted the *Daming li*, first introduced at the fifth-century Liu-Song court, was promulgated under Liao Shengzong in 994 and remained the official calendar until the end of the dynasty. The *Xuanming li*, created for Tang Muzong in 822, was adopted as the official Goryeo calendar during the reign of Taejo 太祖 (r. 918–943) and remained so until the fourteenth century.[142] It became the official Heian calendar much earlier, in 862 during the reign of Seiwa 清和天皇 (r. 858–876), and remained in effect much longer as the official calendar of successive Japanese regimes through the seventeenth century. By contrast the *Xuanming li* remained in effect in China for only seventy-one years, until 892, when it was replaced by the more advanced

Chongxuan li 崇玄曆 (Venerating the Profound).[143] The longevity of the *Xuanming li* in Goryeo and Heian is remarkable.

This is especially true because, certainly for Heian prognosticators using the *Xuanming li* computational models and ephemerides, the odds against making consistently accurate predictions were close to insurmountable. As John M. Steele has noted, calculations for the *Xuanming li* were based on observations taken at the imperial observatory at Yangcheng (Gaocheng), in what is now Henan Province. The difference in longitude between Yangcheng and Kyoto guaranteed "a systematic error making all of the predicted times early" which only worsened the longer the calendar was in use.[144] Under these circumstances it makes sense that Sanesuke, already in 1012, was querying a monk just back from Kaifeng about the calendar currently in use in Northern Song.[145] Yorimichi's decision to secretly acquire a Chinese calendar in 1039, along with the disputes between Michihira and Shōshō over prediction of eclipses, similarly suggests problems with the calendrical system in use at the Heian court.

But which Chinese calendar did Yorimichi import? Before proposing an answer, the *Daming li* deserves scrutiny. It was not the first calendar adopted by the Kitans, whose prognosticators had initially utilized the last of the Tang calendars—the *Chongxuan li*—when the calendar makers of the fallen Later Jin 後晉 (936–947) were brought to Zhongjing from Kaifeng in 947. However, the *Daming li* was named the official calendar —the first to be issued by the Kitan state—under Liao Shengzong after it was presented to him in 994 by the governor of Kehan Prefecture in what is now Huailai County, Hebei.[146] Interestingly the *Daming li*, the second of the great calendars produced for the Liu-Song court, had seen use across a number of regimes during the Six Dynasties period but fell out of favor after 589 with the Sui rise to power. As noted it had been designed "by the unrivaled calculator Zu Chongzhi," and its accuracy was later attested when the mathematician Su Song in 1077 compared the Liao calendar—i.e. the *Daming li*—with the Northern Song calendar currently in use—the *Fengyuan li* 奉元曆 (Revering Origins; 1023)—and found the latter to be incorrect.[147] Perhaps there is something to the legend that the Liu-Song kings loved calendars and counting.[148]

Another calendrical test on a wider scale was conducted at the Northern Song court in 1078 as recorded in *Liaoshi*. At that time the Northern Song calendar was compared with the calendars in use at the Liao, Goryeo, and Riben (Heian) courts. The Liao and Japanese calendars—i.e. the *Daming li* and *Xuanming li*—were shown to be aligned in the calculation of solar periods for specific sexagenary years and in the determination of first days of months. The Northern Song calendar showed some consistency with the Liao calendar but appears to have been closer to the Goryeo calendar. Surprisingly there was no match between the calendars utilized by the Goryeo and Heian courts despite both being identified as the *Xuanming li*. Instead the Heian calendar aligned with the Liao calendar.[149] As pointed out by Endō Mitsumasa and Ōtani Mitsuo, this concordance is also seen in the utilization of intercalary months, as in the case of the lunar eclipse recorded by Minamoto no Toshifusa in 1078.[150]

The provenance of Yorimichi's secretly imported calendar becomes relevant here. Although he does identify it as a Chinese calendar, he does not say it is from Great Song (Northern Song)—a term otherwise common in the writings of his time.[151] There is also the secrecy involved —Yorimichi says he ordered it on the sly 密々—as if engaged in an illicit activity, e.g. private trade outside the system regulated by way of the Dazaifu authorities. If silk from Mutsu, why not calendars? Given the concordance of the Heian and Liao calendars by the end of the eleventh century, it is surely within the realm of possibility that by 1040 Yorimichi and Michihira had encountered the *Daming li* and its data. As noted, Michihira bested the monk Shōshō in predicting a solar eclipse.

Shōshō's disadvantage may have been longstanding reliance on the *Xuanming li* among Sukuyō prognosticators, who would also have utilized the *Futian li* and other horoscopic texts to prepare almanacs for courtiers like Sukefusa. It is likely that miscalculations had crept into their observations over time due to conservatism or human error.

Shōshō appears to have been especially stubborn about the accuracy of his prognostications even when shown to be patently wrong, as the stand-off with Michihira indicates. Interestingly Sukefusa—on the basis of an almanac without doubt prepared by Shōshō or one of his disciples—identifies the solar eclipse of February 15, 1040, as falling on a Sunday, which is inaccurate: it occurred on a Friday. In earlier years such identifications had been accurate: Yukinari's almanac correctly identified the twenty-eighth day of the sixth month of the eighth year of Kankō (July 31, 1011) as a Tuesday.[152] The adage appears to have been true. Without proper identification of Sundays, a calendar might fall into chaos. Shōshō was lambasted for his errors.

It is small wonder that, with the Latter Dharma on the near horizon, calendrical accuracy was a priority. What distinguishes the Liao and Heian case is the precision with which their prognosticators met the challenge. On the one hand their calendrical system, based on the *Daming li* to which the Japanese *Xuanming li* apparently had been calibrated, enabled correct predictions. On the other they held in common a cultural heritage whose wellspring was to be found in the Northern Dynasties but also drew on Tang tradition. In a sense this reality is reflected in the staying power of the Liao and Heian calendars, even as the Northern Song regime produced one after another. This is not to say that Liao and Heian were necessarily intertwined in any direct way. Rather, the connection was akin to parallel processing configured through a shared main memory—in this instance a cache of habits, histories, and things consistent with northern cultural traditions. In the early decades of the eleventh century, perhaps triggered by interregional trade, a concurrence of the Liao and Heian worlds took shape by way of calendars and the countdown to 1051.

In the broader sweep of history, a countdown and a calendrical system may seem minor details. But by considering them, a few more pebbles are set in place to build a foundation for understanding the urgency with which the Buddhist eschaton was greeted in the early years of the eleventh century across the Sinophone world. This was a world far more entangled and integrated than scholars have tended to think, especially in the north Asian zone, where a combination of tradition, trade, and geopolitics existed shadowlike on the edges of the Tang political and cultural order until the dynasty fell and its influence receded like the outgoing tide. The turbulent tenth century, in which the Kitan, Korean, and Japanese states took shape in the wake of the Tang imperium, was a time of great challenges. If by the end of that century some people came to believe that the world was ending, it was probably not without reason. At least on the Mahāyāna front all the models were predicting that, like climate change today, its forcing mechanisms were in place and would take effect soon. One can only admire the cool efficiency with which, their calendars and instruments at the ready, atop the bedrock of a northern tradition going back generations, Liao and Heian prognosticators faced the future.

NOTES

1. For example, see Michele Marra, "The Development of Mappō Thought in Japan (I)," *Japanese Journal of Religious Studies* 15: 1 (March 1988), 25–54, and "The Development of Mappō Thought in Japan (II), 15:4 (Dec. 1988), 287–305; Mark L. Blum, *The Origins and Development of Pure Land Buddhism* (Oxford and New York: Oxford University Press, 2002), 77–87; and Hubert Durt, "La Date du Buddha en Corée at au Japon," in Heinz Bechert, ed. *The Dating of the Historical Buddha, Die Datierung des historischen Buddha, Part 1* (Göttingen: Vandenhoeck & Ruprecht, 1991), 458–489.

2. In keeping with longstanding practice in fields necessitating accurate reconciliation of ancient dates, calendars, and astronomical phenomena (e.g., archaeoastronomy) dates prior to 1582, when the Gregorian calendar was adopted and decreed by Pope Gregory XIII, are given according to the Julian calendar and occasionally in Julian day numbers. Conversion of Chinese and Japanese dates is based on Furukawa Ki'ichirō 古川麒一朗 et al. *Nihon rekijitsu sōran Guchūreki hen Kodai zenki* 日本暦日総覧, 具注暦篇, 古代前期 [The Japanese luni-solar calendar for the 6th and 7th centuries] (Tokyo: Hon no Tomosha, 1996), 4 vols.; Furukawa et al. *Nihon rekijitsu sōran Guchūreki hen Kodai chūki* 日本暦日総覧, 具注暦篇, 古代中期 [The Japanese luni-solar calendar for the 8th and 9th centuries] (1996), 4 vols.; Furukawa et al. *Nihon rekijitsu sōran Guchūreki hen Kodai kōki* 日本暦日総覧, 具注暦篇, 古代後期 [The Japanese luni-solar calendar for the 10th and 11th centuries] (1994) 4 vols.; Hong Jinfu 洪金福, ed. *Liao Song Xia Jin Yuan wu chao ri li* 遼宋夏金元五朝日歷 [Sino-Western calendar for the five dynasties Liao-Song-Xia-Jin-Yuan A.D. 900–1400] (Taipei: Zhongyang Yanjiuyuan Lishi Yuyan Yanjiusuo, 2004); Redshift Astronomy Software; and the calendar converter at Fourmilab Switzerland http://www.fourmilab.ch/documents/calendar/.

3. David W. Pankenier, "Temporality and the Fabric of Space-Time in Early Chinese Thought," in Ralph M. Rosen, ed. *Time and Temporality in the Ancient World* (Philadelphia: University of Pennsylvania Museum of Archaeology and Anthropology, 2004), 136.

4. For *konse* see *Genji monogatari* 源氏物語 (henceforth GM), "Suetsumuhana 末摘花," in Abe Akio 阿部秋生, Akiyama Ken 秋山虔, Imai Gen'e 今井源衛, and Suzuki Hideo 鈴木日出男, ed. *Shinpen Nihon koten*

bungaku zenshū 新編日本古典文学全集 [Complete works of Japanese classical literature; revised] (henceforth SNKBZ; Tokyo: Shōgakkan, 2015), vol. 20, p. 293, "Miyuki 行幸," vol. 22, p. 312, and "Wakana I 若菜上," vol. 23, p. 32. For *mukashi* see GM, "Takekawa 竹河," in SNKBZ, vol. 24, p. 109; for *kotai* see GM, "Suetsumuhana," in SNKBZ, vol. 20, p. 293; "Miyuki," vol. 22, pp. 312, 314.

5. For example, see *Shōyūki* 小右記 (Diary of Fujiwara no Sanesuke), Kankō 8/7/11 (Aug. 12, 1011), in *Dai Nihon kokiroku* 大日本古記録 [Records of Japan] (henceforth DNK; Tokyo: Iwanami Shoten, 1952–1991), vol. 10, pt. 2, p. 180, and Chōwa 1 (Kankō 9)/5/24 (June 16, 1012), pt. 3, p. 27.

6. For a recent study touching on darkness and apocalyptic eschatology in Chinese Buddhism and Daoism from the third through eighth centuries see April D. Hughes, "Waiting for Darkness: Judgment, Salvation, and Apocalyptic Eschatology in Medieval China," PhD dissertation, Princeton University, 2014.

7. For "troubled realm" see GM, "Wakamurasaki 若紫," in SNKBZ, vol. 20, p. 224. For "degenerate age" and "latter days" see GM, "Umegae 梅枝, " in SNKBZ, vol. 22, p. 415, "Fuji no Uraba 藤裏葉," in SNKBZ, vol. 22, p. 438, "Wakana II若菜下, " in SNKBZ, vol. 23, p. 198, 199; and "Yadoriki 宿木," in SNKBZ, vol. 24, p. 380.

8. *Gonki* 権記 (Diary of Fujiwara no Yukinari 藤原行成), Chōhō 長保 2/6/20 (Jul. 23, 1000), in *Zōho shiryō taisei* 増補資料大成 [Historical materials, revised edition] (henceforth ZST; Kyoto: Rinsen Shoten, 1965), vol. 4, p. 132a.

9. *Gonki*, Chōhō 2/8/15 (Sept. 15, 1000), in ZST, vol. 4, p. 149a.

10. For civil and monastic unrest see *Shōyūki*, Eiso 1/10/1 (Nov. 2, 989), in DNK, vol. 10, pt. 1, p. 203, Chōtoku 3/4/17 (May 25, 997), vol. 10, pt. 2, p. 32, Kannin 3/4/12 (May 19, 1019), vol. 10, pt. 5, p. 134, Kannin 3/11/22 (Dec. 20, 1019), vol. 10, pt. 5, p. 212, and Jian 3/10/28 (Dec. 13, 1023), vol. 10, pt. 6, p. 224; for breaches in court protocol see Chōhō 1/11/2 (Dec. 12, 999), vol. 10, pt. 2, p. 68; for astronomical anomalies see Chōgen 4/7/24 (Aug. 14, 1031); for fires see Chōgen 4/7/24 (Aug. 14, 1031), vol. 10, pt. 9, p. 11. For "annihilation of the Dharma" see *Shōyūki*, Chōwa 2/4/8 (May 20, 1013), in DNK, Vol. 10, pt. 3, pp. 104–105, and Chōwa 5/3/10 (Apr. 19, 1016), in DNK, vol. 10, pt. 4, p. 165.

11. *Shōyūki*, Chōgen 4/8/4 (Aug. 24, 1031), in DNK, vol. 10, pt. 9, p. 16. The Priestess is Princess Senshi 婦子女王 (1005–1081). The prophecy of One Hundred Kings (Hyakuō no Un 百王運) is encrypted in a steganographic

character-riddle called the Yabataishi野馬台詩, or Poem of Yabatai (Yamato; i.e., Japan), which predicts the demise of Japan's monarchy after 100 generations. Circumstantial evidence points to the origin of the character-riddle sometime in the ninth century, but it is little mentioned until the twelfth century. Sanesuke's is possibly the earliest reference to it in connection with a datable historical event. For a recent study of the prophecy see Komine Kazuaki, *Yabataishi no nazo* 野馬台詩の謎 [The riddle of the poem of Yabatai] (Tokyo: Iwanami Shoten, 2003).

12. *Shunki* 春記 (Diary of Fujiwara no Sukefusa), Chōryaku 2/10/12 (Nov. 11, 1038), in ZST, vol. 7, 5b–6a. Sukefusa's despair over his career as a courtier—he felt that he did not receive the recognition he deserved—contributed to his woebegone outlook and gave him further reason to invoke *matsudai*.

13. *Shunki*, Chōkyū 1/8/11 (Sept. 19, 1040), in ZST, vol. 7, pp. 104b–105b, Chōkyū 1/8/23 (Oct. 1, 1040), vol. 7, p. 112a, and Chōkyū 1/9/9 (Oct. 17, 1040), vol. 7, p. 182b3, 183a5.

14. *Eiga monogatari*, "Utagai うたがひ," in Yamanaka Yutaka 山中裕, Akiyama Ken 秋山虔, and Ikeda Naotaka 池田尚隆, ed. SNKBZ, vol. 32, p. 199.

15. See *Ōjō yōshū*, T2682.84.46c24–27. It is certainly true, as Marra shows in "The Development of Mappō Thought (I)," 40–50, that Genshin utilized the concept of the Buddhist eschaton in order to promote the *nenbutsu* and Pure Land faith more generally, but his use of the term Mappō remains minimal by comparison with his successors writing in the thirteenth and fourteenth centuries.

16. *Yuishikigi shiki* 唯識義私記 (Personal Comments on the Doctrine of Consciousness-Only), T2319.71.349c09–350a16.

17. For example, Kōgyō was an advocate of the Ichiji Kinrin (Ekâkṣara-uṣṇīṣa-cakra) Rite as a protective measure during the period of Mappō; see *Shijūchō ketsu* 四十帖決 (Forty-Notebook Collection), compiled by his disciple Chōen 長宴 (1016–1081) in the late twelfth century; see *Shijūchō ketsu*, T2408.75.877c28, and *Gyōrinshō*, T2409.76.44a27–44b13, 62a11–12.

18. Marra, "The Development of Mappō Thought in Japan (II)," 287–288; Blum, *Origins and Development*, 84–87; Asai Endō, "Nichiren Shōnin's View of Humanity: The Final Dharma Age and the Three Thousand Realms in One Thought-Moment," *Japanese Journal of Religious Studies* 26, No.3-4 (Fall 1999), 239–259.

19. *Shunki*, Eishō 7/8/28 (Sept. 23, 1052), in ZST, vol. 7, 232b–233a, and Eishō 7/9/7 (Oct. 2, 1052), 233a.

20. *Fusō ryakki*, Eishō 7/1/26 (Feb. 29, 1052), in *Shintei zōho kokushi taikei* 新訂増補国史大系 [A library of Japanese history, revised edition] (henceforth SZKT; Tokyo: Yoshikawa Kōbunkan, 2003), vol. 12, 292.

21. See Yamaguchi Takamasa 山口隼正, "*Nihon teikō nendai ki* ni tsuite —Iriki'inke shozō mikan nendai ki no shōkai, Chū" 「日本帝皇年代記」について、入来院家所蔵未刊年代記の紹介 (中) (On the *Nihon teikō nendai ki*—An Introduction to a Previously Unknown Chronicle in the Iriki'in Collection, Part 2), *Nagasaki Daigaku Kyōikugakubu Shakai Kagaku ronsō* 長崎大学教育学部社会科学論叢, no. 65 (June 2004), 3.

22. *Tame Kaku'un Sōzu shijūkūnichi ganmon* 為覚運僧都四十九日願文 [Dedicatory address on the forty-ninth day observation for Bishop Kaku'un], dated Kankō 4/12/10 (Jan. 20, 1008), in *Honchō monzui* 本朝文粋 [Literary essence of our court], fasc. 14, Ganmon 2 願文下 [Dedicatory addresses, 2], in SZKT, vol. 29, p. 352.

23. For Moromichi on *matsudai* see, for example, *Gonijō Moromichi ki* 後二条師通記 [Diary of Fujiwara no Moromichi], Kōwa 1 (Jōtoku 3)/3/15 (Apr. 8, 1099), in DNK, vol. 7, pt. 3, p. 266. For Munetada on *matsudai* and *masse* see, for example, *Chūyūki* 中右記 [Diary of Fujiwara no Munetada], Jōtoku 1 (Eichō 2)/Intercalaris 1/24 (Mar. 10, 1097), in DNK, vol. 21, pt. 3, p. 159, Chōji 1/6/21 (July 14, 1104), pt. 5, p. 171, Chōji 2/8/30 (Oct. 9, 1105), pt. 6, p. 86, and Tennin 1 (Kajō 3)/4/2 (May 14, 1108), pt. 7, p. 262. For Tadazane on *matsudai* and *masse* see for example *Denryaku* 殿暦 [Diary of Fujiwara no Tadazane], in Kōwa 4/8/28 (Oct. 11, 1102), in DNK, vol. 13, pt. 1, p. 148, and Eikyū 4/7/12 (Aug. 21, 1116), pt. 4, p. 249.

24. *Chūyūki*, Kanji 7/8/8 (Sept. 1, 1093), in DNK, vol. 21, pt. 1, p. 224, and Kanji 7/8/29 (Sept. 22, 1093), vol. 21, pt. 1, p. 231.

25. *Gonijō Moromichi ki*, Eichō 1 (Kahō 3)/9/16 (Oct. 4, 1096), in DNK, vol. 7, pt. 3, p. 220; *Chūyūki*, Kahō 2/5/27 (July 1, 1095), in DNK, vol. 21, pt. 2, p. 224, Eichō 1/5/23 (June 16, 1096), Jōtoku 2/5/1 (June 2, 1098), pt. 4, p. 27, and Kajō 1/8/21 (Sept. 20, 1106), pt. 6, p. 202.

26. *Gonijō Moromichi ki*, Eichō 1/6/14 (July 6, 1096), in DNK, vol. 7, pt. 3, p. 200.

27. Marra, "Development of Mappō Thought (I)," 51.

28. *Gūkanshō* 愚管抄 [Some modest views], in Okami Masao 岡見正雄 and Akamatsu Toshihide 赤松俊秀, ed. *Nihon koten bungaku taikei* 日本古典文学大系 [Compendium of Japanese classical literature] (Tokyo: Iwanami Shoten, 1967), vol. 86, 325.

29. *Kōtaiki*, in keeping with *Nihon shoki*, records that Buddhism reached Japan from the Korean kingdom of Baekje 百済 in the thirteenth year of the reign of King Kinmei 欽明 (r. 539–571), or 552, and notes that this was 1,480 years after the death of Buddha; see *Kōtaiki*, in Hanawa Hokinoichi塙保己一, ed. *Gunsho ruijū* 群書類聚 [Classified collection of Japanese texts] (Tokyo: Zoku Gunsho Ruijū Kanseikai, 1992), vol. 3, fasc. 31, p. 170. For a discussion of *Kōtaiki*, which exists in several versions and may originally date to the twelfth century, see Yoshida Kazuhiko 吉田一彦, "*Nihon shoki* bukkyō denrai kiji to mappō shisō, Sono ni" 日本書記仏教伝来記事と末法思想, その二 [The account of the introduction of Buddhism in *Nihon shoki* and the notion of the final Dharma, part 2], *Ningen bunka kenkyū*人間文化研 究 [Studies in humanities and culture], no. 9 (2008), 1–2.

30. *Nihon ryōiki* (*Nihonkoku genpō zen'aku ryōiki* 日本国現報善悪霊異記), "Preface by Kyōkai of Nara," formal title "Nara no Ukyō no Yakushiji no Shamon Kyōkai shirusu" 諾楽の右京の薬師寺の沙門景戒録す [Recorded by Kyōkai of Yakushiji in the right capital of Nara], in Nakada Norio, ed. SNKBZ, vol. 10 (2008), part 3, p. 241.

31. Marra, "Development of Mappō Thought I," 39–40; Blum, *Origins and Development*, 82–83.

32. *Chūron soki*, T2255.65.22c14–15, 51b15–16.

33. *Shugo kokkai shō*, T2362.74.177b28: 末法太有近.

34. *Mappō tōmyō ki*, in Eizan Gakuin 叡山学院, ed. *Dengyō Daishi zenshū* 伝教大師全集 [Collection of works by Dengyō Daishi Saichō] (Sakamoto: Hieizan Tōsho Kankōsho, 1926–1927), 485. Wakamizu Suguru 若水俊, "Mappō tōmyō ki no seiritsu kō" 末法灯明記の成立考 [Thoughts on the emergence of *Mappō tōmyō ki*], *Ibaraki Joshi Tanki Daigaku kiyō* 茨城女子短期大学紀要 [Bulletin of Ibaraki women's college], no. 1 (1972), 19–31. For Hōnen see *Kurodani Shōnin gotōroku*黒谷上人語燈録 [Records of the sayings of the venerable of Kurodani], T2611.83.143c07–27.

35. *Futsū jubosatsukai kōshaku* 普通授菩薩戒廣釋 (Extensive Exploration of the Universal Bodhisattva Precepts Ordination), T2381.74.767a05.

36. Edward Kamens, *The Three Jewels: A Study and Translation of Minamoto Tamenori's Sanbōe* (Ann Arbor: Center for Japanese Studies, University of Michigan, 1988), 92.

37. Smallpox struck Kyoto in 977, with a low die-off, but after that there were no major outbreaks of infectious disease until 995, when a virulent epidemic of smallpox—probably *Variola major*—took many lives. Over

the next thirty-five years it was followed by measles in 998; influenza in 1001; plague in 1015 (buboes were reported); influenza in 1017; smallpox in 1020–1021; measles in 1025; influenza in 1028; mumps in 1029; and influenza in 1030. By comparison, there had been only four major outbreaks of infectious disease in the Kyoto region in the preceding thirty-five years: mumps in 959; likely influenza in 960 and 966; and, as noted, smallpox in 977. For a chronology of epidemics see Hattori Toshirō 服部 敏良, *Heian jidai igaku no kenkyū* 平安時代医学の研究 [Research on medicine in the Heian period] (Tokyo: Kagaku Shoin, 1980), pp. 287–327. For smallpox see *Nihon kiryaku* 日本紀略 [Abbreviated Japanese annals], Shōryaku 5/3/26 (May 9, 994) and 4/24 (June 5, 994), in SZKT, vol. 11, p. 177, and *Sakeiki* 左経記 [Diary of Minamoto no Tsuneyori 経 頼], Kannin 4/3/21 (Apr. 6, 1020), in ZST, vol. 6, p. 91, *Nihon kiryaku,* Jian 1/2/25 (Apr. 9, 1021),p. 255, and *Shōyūki*, Jian 1/2/14 (Mar. 29, 1021, in DNK, vol. 10, pt. 6, p. 13. For measles see *Nihon kiryaku*, Chōtoku 4/7 *hoc mense* (July–Aug, 998), p. 190, and Manju 2/9 *hoc mense* (Sept–Oct, 1025), p. 263. For plague, see *Nihon kiryaku*, Chōwa 4/3/27 (Apr. 18, 1015), p. 234, and *Shōyūki*, Chōwa 4/4/19 (May 9, 1015), pt. 4, p. 10. For mumps see *Nihon kiryaku*, Chōgen 2/10 *hoc mense* and *ultima mense* (Nov–Dec, 1029), pp. 275–276, and *Shōyūki*, Chōgen 2/8/18 (Sept. 28, 1029), pt. 8, p. 153. For other outbreaks of infectious disease see *Nihon kiryaku*, Chōhō 3 *hoc anno* (1001), p. 199, and *Gonki*, Chōhō 3/2/9 (Mar. 6, 1001), in ZST, vol. 4, p. 196b; *Nihon kiryaku*, Kannin 1/6/14 (Jul. 10, 1017), p. 244, and *Shōyūki*, Kannin 1/7/6 (Jul. 31, 1017), pt. 4, p. 205; *Midō Kanpaku ki*, Kannin 1/6/29 (Jul. 25, 1017), in 御堂関白記 [Diary of Fujiwara no Michinaga], in DNK, vol. 1, pt. 3, p. 108; *Nihon kiryaku*, Chōgen 1/5/3 (May 29, 1028), p. 272; and *Shōyūki*, Chōgen 3/6/25 (Jul. 28, 1030), pt. 8, p. 181.

38. *Gonki*, Chōtoku 4/7/2 (Jul. 27, 998), in ZST, vol. 4, p. 37a, Chōtoku 4/7/7 (Aug. 1, 998), p. 39a, Chōtoku 4/7/12 (Aug. 6, 998), p. 40a. The high mortality rate was due to the disease's newness. Except for a possible outbreak recorded in 552 measles was unknown in Japan until 998; see Nakajima Yōichirō, *Byōki Nihonshi* 病気日本史 [History of disease in Japan] (Tokyo: Yūzankaku, 1995), pp. 59–62. There is evidence that measles worldwide was an emergent infectious disease at the time that it arrived in Japan in 998, which may explain its morbidity; see Yuki Furuse, Akira Suzuki, and Hitoshi Oshitani, "Origin of Measles Virus: Divergence from Rinderpest Virus between the 11th and 12th Centuries," *Virology Journal* 7: 52 (2010), 1–4.

39. William H. and Helen Craig McCullough, trans., *Tale of Flowering Fortunes* (Stanford: Stanford University Press, 1980), vol. 1, p. 168; see also *Eiga monogatari*, "Mihatenu yume みはてぬゆめ," in SNKBZ, vol. 31, p. 203.

40. Murasaki had married Fujiwara no Nobutaka 藤原宣孝 (d. 1001) in 998; see Haruo Shirane, "The Aesthetics of Power: Politics in the Tale of Genji," *Harvard Journal of Asiatic Studies* 45, no. 2 (Dec. 1985), 638.

41. *Gonki*, Kankō 3/6/24 (Jul. 21, 1006), in ZST, vol. 5, p. 60a; *Midō Kanpaku ki*, Kankō 3/7/13 (Aug. 9, 1006), in DNK, vol. 1, pt. 1, p. 185.

42. The Kaibao edition or Kaibaozang 開寶藏, after the Kaibao 開寶 Era (968–976), was initiated in 971 by Song Taizu 宋太祖 (r. 960–975); it is also known as the Shu edition, or Shuban 蜀版 (i.e., Sichuan edition). For the Kaibao edition see Jiang Wu, Lucille Chia, and Chen Zhichao, "The Birth of the First Printed Canon: The Kaibao Edition and its Impact," in Jiang Wu and Lucille Chia, ed. *Spreading Buddha's Word in East Asia: The Formation and Transformation of the Chinese Buddhist Canon* (New York: Columbia University Press, 2016), 145–180. For the translation center see Tansen Sen, "The Revival and Failure of Buddhist Translations during the Song Dynasty," *T'oung Pao*, Second Series, vol. 88, Fasc. 1/3 (2002), pp. 27–80.

43. The full title of Dānapāla's recension, T1398, is *Foshuo zhiguang mie yiqie yezhang tuoluoni jing* 佛説智光滅一切業障陀羅尼經 (Skt. *Jñānolkādhāraṇī-sarvadurgatipariśodhanī*, Dhāraṇī of the Gnostic Lamp which destroys all Karmic Hindrances); see T1398.21.915b03–04, b15–17. The Tang-period work, T1397, is *Zhiju tuoluoni jing* 智炬陀羅尼經 (Skt. *Jñānolkā-dhāraṇī*), and it contains no references to end times. Other dhāraṇī texts translated by Dānapāla which mention the end time include T1047, T1370, T1376, and T1408.

44. For the apocalyptic language of the *Mañjuśrīmūlakalpa*, see Glenn Wallis, *Mediating the Power of Buddhas: Ritual in the Mañjuśrīmūlakalpa* (Albany: State University of New York Press, 2002). pp. 106–109, and *Wenshushili genben yigui jing* 文殊師利根本儀軌經 (*Mañjuśrīmūlakalpa*), Chapter 18 (Section 24 in the Sanskrit version), T1191.20.884a02–884c26; Chapter 22 (Section 28), T1191.20.894a21–894c12; and Chapter 28 (Section 34), T1191.20.903c09–0904a05. For the efficacy of spells and incantations during the Latter Dharma, see *Wenshushili genben yigui jing*, T1191.20.884b26-27; see T1191.20.894a25–28 for the efficacy of rituals and mantras generated by Mañjuśrī (Miao Jixiang 妙吉祥, "Wonderful and Auspicious").

45. *Da Song xinyi sanzang shengjiao xu* 大宋新譯三藏聖教序 [Preface to
the new translation of sacred texts under great song], Duangong 1/10
(Nov–Dec 988), in Zeng Zaozhuang 曾棗莊 and Liu Lin 劉琳, ed. *Quan
Song wen* 全宋文 [Complete collection of song prose] (Shanghai and
Hefei: Shanghai Cishu Chubanshe and Anhui Jiaoyu Chubanshe, 2006),
360 vols., vol. 4, fasc. 78, p. 407. Part of the preface can also be found *Fozu
Lidai tongzai* 佛祖歷代通載 [Comprehensive registry of the successive
ages of the Buddhas and the patriarchs) by Nianchang 念常 (1282–1323);
see T2036.49.659a2–b9.
46. *Shishi yaolan*, T2127.54.286a22–b05.
47. *Weimojing lüeshou chuiyu ji* 維摩經略疏垂裕記 [Notes on the brief
commentary on the Vimalakīrti-nirdeśa-sūtra], T1779.38.726c17–21,
737a19ff. For Zhanran's commentary see *Weimojing lüeshou* 維摩經略疏
[Brief commentary on the Vimalakīrti-nirdeśa-sūtra], T1778; for Zhiyi's
commentary see *Weimojing xuanshou* 維摩經玄疏 [Profound commentary on the Vimalakīrti-nirdeśa-sūtra], T1777.
48. Discussion of the Liao edition is based on Li Fuhua and He Mei, compiled
by Jiang Wu, "Appendix I: A Brief Survey of the Printed Editions of the
Chinese Buddhist Canon," in Wu and Chia, ed. *Spreading Buddha's Word*,
312; Chikusa Masaaki 竺沙雅章, *Sō Gen bukkyō* (Tokyo: Kyūko Shoin,
2000), 312–342; Chikusa Masaaki, "Keitan Daizōkyō shōkō" 契丹大藏経
小考 [Some thoughts on the Kitan Tripiṭaka], in *Tōyōshi ronshū* 東洋
史論集, ed. Uchida Ginpū Hakase Shōju Kinenkai 内田吟風博士頌寿
記念会 [Committee for the commemoration of Dr. Ginpū Uchida's sev-
entieth birthday] (Kyoto: Dōhōsha 同朋舎, 1978), 311–329; and Lothar
Ledderose, "Make Sutras, Not War: The Stele of 965/1005 A.D. at Cloud
Dwelling Monastery," Unpublished paper, *Perspectives on the Liao*, 2010,
157–216.
49. Chikusa, "Keitan Daizōkyō," 317–326.
50. Comparative analysis of end-times references in the Kaibao and Liao editions of the Canon is the obvious means to resolving this question, except
that both editions are known only in fragmentary form. Moreover, they
were collated for the second carving and publication of the Korean edition of the Chinese Buddhist Canon in the mid-thirteenth century, which
was later used as the basis for several Japanese editions of the Canon,
including the SAT Taishō Shinshū Daizōkyō Text Database (Taishō edition), whence most of the data in this study has been drawn. For the two
Korean editions of the Canon, see Jiang Wu and Ron Dziwenka, "Better

than the Original: The Creation of *Goryeo Canon* and the Formation of *Giyang Bulgyo*," in Wu and Chia, ed. *Spreading Buddha's Word*, 249–283.

51. Discussion of Yunjusi and the Liao sutra carving project at Yunjusi is based on Ledderose, "Make Sutras"; Sonya Lee, "Transmitting Buddhism to a Future Age: The Leiyin Cave at Fangshan and Cave-Temples with Stone Scriptures in Sixth-Century China," *Archives of Asian Art*, vol. 60 (2010), 43–78; Tanii Toshihito 谷井俊仁, "Keitan bukkyō seiji shiron" 契丹仏教政治史論 [Researches on the History of Kitan Buddhism and Government], in Kegasawa Yasunori 氣賀澤保規, ed. *Chūgoku bukkyō sekkyō no kenkyū* 中國佛教石經の研究 (Kyoto: Kyoto Daigaku Gaku-jutsu Shuppan Kai, 1996), 133–191; Hsueh-Man Shen, "Realizing the Buddha's 'Dharma' Body during the Mofa Period: A Study of Liao Buddhist Relic Deposits," *Artibus Asiae* 61, no. 2 (2001), 268; and Lewis R. Lancaster, "The Rock Cut Canon in China: Findings at Fang-Shan," in Tadeusz Skorupski, ed. *The Buddhist Heritage* (Tring, UK: Institute of Buddhist Studies, 1989), 143–156.

52. For two of Jingwan's four extant inscriptions expressing his desire to preserve the Dharma see "Jingwan Neipan jing tang diji" 静琬涅磐經堂題記 [Jingwan's inscription in the Mahāparinirvāṇa-sūtra hall] and "Zhenguan er nian Jingwan diji" 貞觀二年静琬題記 [Jingwan's inscription in the second year of the Zhenguan era, 628], in Chen Yanzhu 陳燕珠, ed. *Xinbian buzheng Fangshan shijing tiji huibian* 新編補正房山石經題記彙編 [Catalogue of the colophons on stone sutra carvings at Fangshan, revised) (henceforth *Fangshan shijing*; Taibei: Jueyuan Wen-jiao Jijin Hui, 1995), 1. For the stele inscriptions see "Zhongjuan Yunjusi beiji, Yingli shisi nian 重鐫雲居寺碑記, 應曆十四年 [Engraved stele inscription at Yunjusi, in the fourteenth year of the Yingli era, 964], and "Zhongxiu Fanyang Baidaishan Yunjusi bei, Tonghe ershisan nian" 重修范陽白帶山雲居寺碑, 統和二十三年 [Engraved inscription of restoration of Fanyang Baidaishan Yunjusi, in the twenty-third year of the Tonghe era, 1005], in *Fangshan shijing*, 11–12. For an English translation of the stele inscriptions see Ledderose, "Make Sutras," 184–195. The stele inscriptions are also found in Chen Shu 陳述, ed. *Quan Liao wen* (Beijing: Zhonghua Shuju, 1982), 79–81, 104–105.

53. For the inscription, by Zhao Zunren 趙遵仁 (?–?), see "Yunjusi Dongfeng Xujuan cheng Sidabujing ji, Qingning sinian" 雲居寺東峰續鐫成四大部經記, 清寧四年 [Record of continued carving of the four great Ssutras on the east peak at Yunjusi, in the fourth year of the

Qingning era, 1058] in *Fangshan shijing*, 13–14, and Shen, "Realizing the Buddha's 'Dharma' Body," 268n23; see also *Quan Liao wen*, 174–176.

54. Discussion of Chaoyang North Pagoda is based on Mizuno Saya 水野 さや, "Ryōdai chōyō hokutō ni kansuru kōsatsu" 遼代朝陽北塔に関す る考察 [Some thoughts on the Liao-period north pagoda at Chaoyang], *Kanazawa Bijutsu Kōgei Daigaku Kiyō* 金沢美術工芸大学紀要 [Bulletin of Kanazawa College of Art], 57 (2013), 91–110; Liaoning Sheng Wenwu Kaogu Yanjiusuo Chaoyangshi Beita Bowuguan 辽宁省文物考古研究 所朝阳市北塔博物馆, ed., *Chaoyang beita* 朝阳北塔 [Chaoyang north pagoda] (Beijing: Wenwu Chuban She, 2007), 26–61; and Youn-mi Kim, "The Hidden Link: Tracing Liao Buddhism in Shingon Ritual," *Journal of Song-Yuan Studies* 43 (2013), 117–170.

55. For the inscriptions *Chaoyang beita*, p. 72, pl. 62-1, and Chaoyang Beita Kaogu Kancha dui, "Liaoning Chaoyang Beita tiangong digong qingli jianbao" 辽宁省朝阳北塔天宫地宫清理简报 [Summary report on the excavation of the vault and upper chamber of the northern pagoda in Chaoyang, Liaoning Province], *Wenwu* 文物 7 (1992), 1–28, 97–103. Calculations are based on the lunisolar calendar including three intercalary months; see Furukawa Kiichirō, ed. *Nihon rekijitsu sōran Guchūreki hen Kodai kōki*, vol. 3, pp. 272–321, and vol. 4, p. 3, and Hong ed. *Liao Song Xia Jin Yuan wu chao ri li*, 145, 146.

56. See Heinz Bechert, ed. *The Dating of the Historical Buddha, Die Datierung des historischen Buddha, Parts 1-III* (Göttingen: Vandenhoeck & Ruprecht, 1991–1997), 3 vols.; Jan Nattier, *Once upon a Future Time: Studies in a Buddhist Prophecy of Decline* (Berkeley: Asian Humanities Press, 1991); Kusuyama Haruki, "Chūgoku bukkyō ni okeru Shaka shōmetsu no nendai" 中国仏教における釈迦生滅年代 [Chronology of the death date of Śākyamuni in Chinese Buddhism], in Hirakawa Akira Hakase Koki Kinenkai 平川彰博士古稀記念会, ed. *Bukkyō shisō no sho mondai* 仏教思想の問題 [Problems in Buddhist philosophy] (Tokyo: Shunjūsha, 1985), 665–678; Thomas Jülch, "The Buddhist Re-interpretation of the Legends Surrounding King Mu of Zhou," *Journal of the American Oriental Society*, 130: 4 (2010), 625–627; and Erik Zürcher, *The Buddhist Conquest of China* (Leiden: Brill, 2007 [1959]), 273–274, 286–287.

57. Kamens, *Three Jewels*, 92, 95.

58. Fei calculates by counting back from the seventeenth year of Kaihuang (597) with respect to any given hypothesis for Buddha's birth date. Various death dates can be calculated by adding seventy-nine years to the birth date. From the writings of Faxian (d. 418–423) Fei derives 1,681

years *bp*, which yields a birth date of 1084 BCE and death date of 1005 BCE (*Lidai sanbao ji*, T2034.49.23a16). From Fashang 法上 (495–580) he derives 1,486 years *bp*, or birth date 889 BCE and 810 BCE death date (23a17, 104c24-29); from the now-lost *Xiangzhengji* 像正記 [Chronicle of the correct and counterfeit), 1,323 *bp*, 727 BCE birth date, 648 BCE death date (23a18–19); from a stone inscription associated with Kumārajīva (344–413), 1,225 *bp*, 628 BCE birth date, 549 BCE death date (23a19–20); from the *Zhongsheng dianji* 眾聖點記 [Record of all sages] or "Dotted Record," 1,061 years *bp*, 464 BCE birth date, 485 BCE death date (23a20–21, 95c10–15); and from *Dehu Changjia jing* 德護長者經 (*Śrīgupta-sūtra*), translated by Fei's colleague Narêndrayaśas (517–589), death date at 1,196 *bp* or 598 BCE (107b07–15). For a discrepancy in the "Dotted Record" dating, see Hubert Durt, "La Date du Buddha," 488–489.

59. For Fei's preference see *Lidai sanbao ji*, T2034.49.23c1–2, 13–15; see also Durt, "La Date du Buddha," 487–488. Only one of these dates, 485 BCE, derived from the "Dotted Record" per Fei's citation (n. 56 *supra*), is within the range acceptable to modern scholars (i.e., 420–350 BCE); for a summary of current dating see D. Seyfort Ruegg, "A New Publication on the Date and Historiography of the Buddha's Decease ('nirvāṇa'): A Review Article," in *Bulletin of the School of Oriental and African Studies, University of London* 62, no. 1 (1999), 82–87.

60. *Kyōjijō*, T2395A.75.356b24–25.

61. *Nihon ryōiki*, "Preface by Kyōkai of Nara), in SNKBZ, vol. 10 (2008), part 3, p. 241.

62. The debate took place at the court of Wei Mingdi 魏明帝 (r. 516–528), with the Buddhists headed by Tanmozui 曇謨最 (fl. sixth century), and the Daoists by Jiang Bin 姜斌 (fl. sixth century); see *Poxielun*, T2109.52.41b–c, 485a7–12, and Thomas Jülch, "In Defense of the Saṃgha: The Buddhist Apologetic Mission of the Early Tang Monk Falin," in Thomas Jülch, ed. *The Middle Kingdom and the Dharma Wheel* (Leiden and Boston: Brill, 2016), 1, 60–61. Daoxuan 道宣 (596–667), writing in 644, gives the same date and sources in his *Guang hongming ji* 廣弘明集 [Expanded collection on the propagation and clarification of Buddhism], T2103.52.166b4–9.

63. *Lidai sanbao ji*, T2034.49.23a17–19.

64. Lewis Lancaster, "The Dating of the Buddha in Chinese Buddhism," in Heinz Bechert, ed. *The Dating of the Historical Buddha, Die Datierung des historischen Buddha, Part 1* (Göttingen: Vandenhoeck & Ruprecht, 1991), 454.

65. *Lidai sanbao ji*, T2034.49.120b2–3. As noted the tradition can be traced to the *Chunqiu*; see also Zürcher, *Buddhist Conquest*, 271–272, and Herbert Franke, "On Chinese Traditions concerning the Dates of the Buddha," in Heinz Bechert, ed. *The Dating of the Historical Buddha, Die Datierung des historischen Buddha, Part 1*, 444. The modern dating for King Zhuang is 696–682 BCE.

66. For the fifty-third year of King Mu see for example *Shijia fangzhi* 釋迦方志 [Reports on the spread of Buddhism], 695, by the Vinaya master Daoxuan 道宣 (596–667), T2088.51.970a18–21. Daoxuan gives the fifty-second year in *Guang honming ji* 廣弘明集; see, for example, T2103.52.100c10–12.

67. *Jōyuishikiron jukki joshaku* 成唯識論述記序釋 [Preface to explanatory notes on the *Cheng weishi lun* or *demonstration of consciousness only*], T2260.65.319c5–11, 321a17–b2. Han Mingdi dreamed of a divine golden man—Buddha—in the tenth year of Yongping, or 67 CE. Zenju counts back 1,020 years from that year to the fifty-second year of King Mu, which yields a death date of 953 BCE. Zenju probably knew Han Mingdi's dream from Daoxuan, who paraphrases the 5th-century Daoist text, *Huahu jing* 化胡經 [The scripture of Laozi converting the barbarians], whence the story originates; see *Guang hongming ji*, T2103.52.147c15–24.

68. *Jukkeshū*, T2367.74.297c27–29.

69. *Jingde chuandeng lu*, T2076.51.205c17–21. Daoyuan counts back 1,017 years from the tenth year of the Yongping era in the reign of Han Mingdi (i.e., 67 CE) to derive the 950 BCE date.

70. *Da Song seng shi lüe*, T2126.54.235b23–236a15, 236b7–9. For Zanning and his activities under Taizong see Albert Welter, "Confucian Monks and Buddhist *Junzi*: Zanning's *Topical Compendium of the Buddhist Clergy* (Da Song seng shi lüe) and the Politics of Buddhist Accommodation at the Song court," in Jülch, ed. *The Middle Kingdom*, 247–256.

71. *Weimojing lüeshou chuiyu ji* 維摩經略疏垂裕記 [Notes on the brief commentary on the Vimalakīrti-nirdeśa-sūtra], T1779.38.737a19–20. The modern reign dates for King Kuang are 612–697 BCE.

72. A search of the SAT or Taishō edition database, while generating multiple examples of *bp* scales, does not yield any countdowns of the sort in evidence at Chaoyang North Pagoda.

73. Jülch, "Legends Surrounding King Mu," 625; see also Edward L. Shaughnessy, *Sources of Western Zhou History* (Berkeley: University of California Press, 1991), 248–254.

74. For Shingō see *Yuishikigi shiki*, T2319.71.350a2–3; for Zhiyuan, *Weimo-jing lüeshou chuiyu ji*, T1779.38.716c17–18, 737a28–29; for Daocheng, *Shishi yaolan*, T2127.54.286a18ff.

75. *Fahua xuan lun*, T1720.34.449c29–450a1–10; for Falin see *Poxielun*, T2109.52.485a5–7; for Daoxuan see *Guang hongming ji*, T2103.52.166b2–5, and *Shijia fangzhi*, T2088.51.973c3–5.

76. For the *Candragarbha Sūtra* see *Yuezang fen* 月藏分 (*Candragarbha-parivarta*), in *Da fangdeng daji jing* 大方等大集經 [Great collection scripture], T397.13.379a5–9, and Nattier, *Once upon a Future Time*, 52–54. For Huisi see *Nanyue si dachanshi lishi yuanwen* 南嶽思大禪師立誓願文 [Tract on the vow made by the great master Huisi of the southern sacred peak, 558], T1933.46.787a3–4.

77. *Chūron soki*, T2255.65.22c14–17, 51a22–b16. Anchō is following Jizang, who also mentions the stele in *Fahua xuan lun*, T1720.34.450a2–3 but provides no other details about its provenance. According to Anchō the stele records Buddha's response when asked, on his deathbed, how long the Dharma would last. For Kūkai see *Himitsu mandara jūjishin ron* 祕密漫荼羅十住心論 [Ten abiding stages of the secret mind of the mandala, ca. 830], T2425.77.305c10–12; for Annen, *Kyōjijō*, T2395A.75.356a29–b1.

78. *Shōmangyō gisho* 勝鬘經義疏, T2185.56.9b9–11.

79. *Nihon ryōiki*, "Preface by Kyōkai of Nara," in SNKBZ, vol. 10 (2008), part 3, p. 241. There has been speculation that Kyōkai did not actually write this preface; see Marra, "Development of Mappō Thought I," 32–33.

80. *Mappō tōmyō ki*, in Eizan Gakuin, ed. *Dengyō Daishi zenshū*, 485.

81. "Everything is corrupted in the latter days of Buddha's Law" 浅くなりゆく世の末; see GM, "Umegae," in SNKBZ, vol. 22, p. 415, and Dennis Washburn, trans. *The Tale of Genji* (New York and London: W. W. Norton and Co., 2015), 615. Genji is speaking to the young Murasaki about the deterioration of taste and ability in calligraphy.

82. *Goryeosa*, fasc. 7, Munjong 文宗, pt. 1, in Kokusho Kankōkai, ed. *Kōraishi* (Tokyo: Kokusho Kankōkai, 1908–1909), 3 vols., vol. 1, p. 102b; and Yannick Bruneton, "Astrologues et devins du Koryŏ (918–1392): une analyse de l'histoire officielle," *Extrême-Orient Extrême-Occident*, no. 35 (2013), 45–46, 54.

83. Youn-mi Kim, "The Hidden Link," 120–121. For a list of the many dhāraṇīs inscribed on metal sheets and sutra containers deposited in the cella, see *Chaoyang beita*, 69.

84. *Zuisheng foding tuoluoni jingchu yezhang zhoujing* 最勝佛頂陀羅尼淨
除業障呪經 [Sutra of the dhāraṇī spell of the jubilant Buddha-Corona
which cleanses and abolishes karmic burdens], T970.19.361b19-23ff.
85. For a list of the dhāraṇīs see *Chaoyang beita*, 85. The version of the
Uṣṇīṣavijayā dhāraṇī on the pillar is the translation by Buddhapāli, T967;
see *Chaoyang beita*, fig. 71. The texts whose dhāraṇī offer solace during the Latter Dharma are *Pubian guangming qingjing chicheng ruy-
ibao yinxin wunengsheng damingwang dasuiqiu tuoluoni jing* 普遍光明
清淨熾盛如意寶印心無能勝大明王大隨求陀羅尼經 [Dhāraṇī of the
great protectress, queen of mantras], T1153.20.620c22-24; *Putichang
suoshuo Yizi ding lunwang jing* 菩提場所說一字頂輪王經 [Sutra of the
one-syllable wheel-turning ruler spoken at the seat of enlightenment],
T950.19.200c22, 205c17; and what appears to be a dhāraṇī prescribed
in Nāgārjuna's *Dazhi du lun* 大智度論 (Mahāprajñāpāramitā-śāstra),
T509.25.530b9-14ff.
86. For an iconographical and contextual analysis of the Phoenix Hall from
a cross-regional perspective see Mimi Yiengpruksawan, "A Pavilion for
Amitābha," in Victor H. Mair, ed. *Buddhist Transformations and Interactions* (Amherst: Cambria Press, 2017), 401-516.
87. At times the irascible Sanesuke even spoke of Yorimichi's governing
style as itself both product and exemplification of the end time; see
Shunki, Chōryaku 2/10/12 (Nov. 11, 1038), in ZST, vol. 7, pp. 5b-6a.
88. Washburn, *The Tale of Genji*, 935n5. For example see GM, "Agemaki 総
角," in SNKBZ, vol. 24, p. 296.
89. Franke, "On Chinese Traditions," 441.
90. For determination of calendrical epochs see Yamashita Katsuaki 山下
克明, "Senmyōreki ni tsuite—*Kōraishi* rekishi to Nihon no denbon" 宣
明暦について、「高麗史」暦志と日本の伝本 [On the Xuanmingli:
On the calendrical treatise in *Goryeosa* and Japanese versions], in Daitō
Bunka Daigaku Tōyō Kenkyūjo 大東文化大学東洋研究所, ed. *Kōraishi
rekishi Senmyōreki no kenkyū* 「高麗史」暦志宣明暦の研究 (Tokyo:
Daitō Bunka Daigaku Tōyō Kenkyūjo, 1998), 16. For the *Yingtian li*, see
Songshi 宋史 [History of Song; 1343], fasc. 68, Lülizhi 律曆志 [Treatises
on pitch-pipes and calendars], pt. 21, Lüli 律曆1, in *Ershisi shi* 二十四
史 [Standard histories or twenty-four histories) (henceforth *Ershisi shi*;
Taibei: Xin] Wenfeng Chuban Gufen Gongsi, 1975), vol. 30, p. 716a. For
the *Daming li* see *Liaoshi* 遼史 [History of Liao; 1344], fasc. 42, *Zhi* 志
[Treatises] 12, 歷象志上 [Treatise on calendars; pt. 1], in *Ershisi shi*,
vol. 37, p. 221b. For the *Xuanming li* see *Goryeosa* 高麗史, fasc. 50, Zhi

志 [Treatises], pt. 4, Li 曆 [Calendars], pt. 1, in *Kōraishi*, vol. 2, p. 64b. The start date for the Julian day number system is November 24, 4713 BCE (Gregorian) or January 1, 4713 (Julian); see Nachum Dershowitz and Edward M. Reingold, *Calendrical Calculations* (Cambridge: Cambridge University Press, 2008), 15.

91. *Suisaki*, Jōryaku 1/Intercalaris 12/14 *geng/shen* 庚申 (Jan. 30, 1078), in SZKT, vol. 8 (1965), p. 79a. For the NASA catalogue see https://eclipse.gsfc.nasa.gov/LEcat5/LEcatalog.html; see also Zhentao Xu, David W. Pankenier, and Yaotiao Jiang, *East Asian Archaeoastronomy: Historical Records of Astronomical Observations of China, Japan, and Korea* (Amsterdam: Gordon and Breach Science Publishers, 2000), 74.

92. *Shōyūki*, Chōwa 1 (Kankō 9)/7/25 (Aug. 15, 1012), in DNK, vol. 10, pt. 3, pp. 50–51. The event is mentioned in *Jiu Tangshu* 旧唐書 [History of Tang; fasc. 84, Liezhuan 列傳, pt. 30], which Sanesuke cites. When pheasants congregated at Taizong's palace in 643, the citation goes, he requested a prognostication from his advisors, most prominently Chu Suiliang 褚遂良 (597–658). Sanesuke's interest in the citation, which associates the pheasant cock with mandated rule and the hen with political collapse, may stem from tensions at the Heian court over the promotion to queen of a consort favored by Sanjō 三条天皇 (r. 1011–1016) but not by others, with the inevitable allusions to Yang Guifei; see *Shōyūki*, Chōwa 1 (Kankō 9)/4/27 (May 20, 1012), in DNK, pt. 10, vol. 3, pp. 11–16. The calendar consulted by Sanesuke was likely the *Wuyin li* 戊寅曆 [Fifteenth-year epoch], which was in use at the Tang court from 619 to 694.

93. *Shōyūki*, Chōwa 3/5/5 (June 5, 1014), in DNK, vol. 10, pt. 3, p. 220.

94. *Kaiyuan zhanjing*, fasc. 104, Suanfa 筭法 [Calculations], in Chang Bingyi, ed. *Kaiyuan zhanjing* (Beijing: Zhongyang Bianyi Chubanshe, 2006), 2 vols., vol. 2, p. 744; *Da Piluzhena chengfo jing shu* 大毘盧遮那成佛經疏 [Commentary on the Mahāvairocana-abhisaṃbodhi-tantra], T1796.39.618a17.

95. *Shōyūki*, Chōwa 3/10/23 (Nov. 18, 1014), in DNK, vol. 10, pt. 3, p. 244. The scholarly literature on the *Xiuyaojing* is extensive. For a recently updated classic on the topic, see Yano Michio 矢野道雄, *Mikkyō senseijutsu* 密教占星術 [Esoteric Buddhist astrology] (Tokyo: Tōyō Shoin, 2013); see also Marc Kalinowski, "The Use of the Twenty-eight Xiu as a Day-Count in Early China," *Chinese Science* 13 (1996), 64–66. For an exhaustive examination of Buddhist horoscopy and astrology see Niu Weixing 钮卫星, *Xiwang fantian* 西望梵天 [Gazing west at the Buddhist skies] (Shanghai: Shanghai Jiaotong Daxue Chubanshe, 2003).

96. Given the importance attached to the year 794 there is a remote possibility that *Fan li* was a shorthand name for *Qiyao rangzai jue*, a copy of which—according to the inscription at the end of the imprint utilized for the SAT Taishō edition—was in circulation in Kyoto by 999. See *Qiyao rangzai jue*, T1308.21.429c3, 452a29.

97. According to *Songshu* 宋書 (Book of Song, 493) the *Qiyao li* was promulgated in the twentieth year of Yuanjia, or 443, during the reign of Song Wendi of Liu-Song; see *Songshu*, fasc. 12, Zhi 志 [Treatises] 2, Lülizhi 律曆 [Treatises on pitch-pipes and calendars] 2, in *Ershisi shi* (Beijing: Zhonghua Shuju, 1997), vol. 5, p. 74a; see also Xin Yu, "Personal Fate and the Planets: A Documentary and Iconographical Study of Astrological Divination at Dunhuang, focusing on the 'Dhāraṇī Talisman for Offerings to Ketu and Mercury, Planetary Deity of the North,'" *Cahiers d'Extrême-Asie*, vol. 20, Buddhism, Daoism, and Chinese Religion (2011), 171. For Sanesuke's migraine-inducing technical concern with the degree of obscuration of a lunar eclipse crossing from the celestial lodge of Nü 女宿 (Albali, ε Aqr) all the way to Wei 危 (Sadalmelik, α Aqr), see *Shōyūki*, Chōgen 4/7/16 (Aug. 6, 1031), in DNK, vol. 10, pt. 9, p. 7.

98. The acquisition cost of the calendar and related texts was 80 *ryō* of gold particles (approximately 3 kilograms); see *Dazaifu jinja monjo* 大宰府神社文書 [Documents of the Dazaifu shrine], in Takeuchi Rizō 竹内理三, ed. *Heian ibun* 平安遺文 [Archives of the Heian period], 14 vols., vol. 9, no. 4623, pp. 3564–3565.

99. *Xin Wudai shi* 新五代史 [New History of the Five Dynasties; 1070], fasc. 58, Sitian kao 司天考 [Bureau of astronomy studies] 1, in *Ershisi shi* 13 (1997), 176a. Shigeru Nakayama, "Characteristics of Chinese Astrology, *Isis* 57, no. 4 (Winter 1966), 450–451. For "atypical canon" see Jean-Claude Martzloff, *Astronomy and Calendars—The Other Chinese Mathematics, 104BC – AD 1644* (Berlin and Heidelberg: Springer-Verlag, 2016), 109.

100. The calculation for "Sunday" in this dating is based on Furukawa et al. *Nihon rekijitsu sōran Guchūreki hen Kodai kōki* 3 (1994), 111, and the Fourmilab calendrical converter, which has February 9, 1018 as Sunday, Julian day 2092921.5. For a holograph see Kyoto National Museum, ed. *Fujiwara no Michinaga* 藤原道長 [Fujiwara no Michinaga] (Kyoto: Kyoto National Museum, 2007), pl. 2.

101. *Xiuyaojing*, T1299.21.398b05–18. A one-fascicle Qiyaoli from Dunhuang (Musée Guimet, P.2693) gives the Sogdian names with notes. These names have been variously transliterated in the literature as

Myr or *Mīr* 蜜, also 密 (Mi, Sunday, 日曜); M'x or Māq 莫, also 漠 (Mo, Monday, 月曜); Wnx'n or Wuqan 雲漢 (Yunhan, Tuesday, 火曜); Tyr or Tīr, 商 or 咥 (Shang or Die, Wednesday, 水曜); Wrmzt 鶻勿 斯 (Guwusi, Thursday, 木曜); N'xyo or Naqio 那歇 (Naxie, Friday, 金 曜; and Kyw'n or Kēwān 枳淙 (Zhicong, Saturday, 土曜). For Sogdian terms for the days of the week see Matsumoto Ikuyo, "Two Medieval Manuscripts on the Worship of the Stars from the Fujii Eikan Collection," *Culture and Cosmos* 10, no. 1–2 (Autumn/Winter and Spring/ Summer, 2006), 132–137; for the Sogdian calendar see B. I. Marshak, "The Historico-Cultural Significance of the Sogdian Calendar," *Iran* 30 (1992), 145–154. As the premier traders in the Silk Road regions for centuries, with a prominent enclave in Dunhuang as late as the tenth century, Sogdian merchants had a vested interest in the calendrical sciences, in keeping with their Zoroastrian faith and the Avestan calendar to be sure, but also for economic record keeping. Their influence was felt wherever Buddhist horoscopy was practiced. Indeed, the initial translator of the *Xiuyaojing*, Amoghavajra's disciple Shi Yao 史瑤 (fl. eighth century), famously said as much when he noted that, to learn about the days of the week, one asked a Sogdian 胡 (Hu); see *Xiuyaojing*, T1299.21.398b01. For the Sogdian enclave in Dunhuang see Frantz Grenet and Zhang Guangda, "The Last Refuge of the Sogdian Religion: Dunhuang in the Ninth and Tenth Centuries," *Bulletin of the Asia Institute*, New Series, vol. 10 (1996), 175–186, and Étienne de La Vaissière and Éric Trombert, "Des Chinois et des Hu: Migrations et integration des Iraniens orientaux en milieu chinois durant le haut Moyen Âge," *Annales: Histoire, Sciences Sociales*, 59e Année, No. 5/6 (2004), 965–969.

102. *Kōbō Daishi gyoden* 弘法大師御伝 [Biography of Kōbō Daishi; 1152], in Hanawa Hokinoichi, ed. *Zoku Gunsho ruijū* 続群書類聚 [Classified collection of Japanese texts, continued] (Tokyo: Kokusho Kankōkai, 1958), vol. 8, pt. 2, fasc. 209, p. 560. See also Yamashita Katsuaki, *Heian kizoku shakai to guchūreki* 平安貴族社会と具注暦 [Heian aristocratic society and the almanac] (Tokyo: Rinsen Shoten, 2017), 44–45.

103. *Nihonkoku genzaisho mokuroku* 日本国見在書目録 [Catalog of extant texts in the country of Japan; 891], in *Zoku Gunsho ruijū*, vol. 30, pt. 2, fasc. 884, p. 43b.

104. Kalinowski, "The Use of the Twenty-eight Xiu as a Day-Count," 64.

105. These were recent translations: *Mañjuśrīmūlakalpa*, by Tianxizai as noted, ca. 986, and *Grahamātṛkā* by Fatian 法天 (Dharmadeva, fl. tenth century), ca. 973–981. See Niu, *Xiwang fantian*, 192.

106. Kam-Wing Fung, "From Hellenistic Scientific Device to Islamic Astrolabe: Transmission of a Non-Chinese Scientific Instrument in Late Medieval China, in Dorothy C. Wong and Gustav Heldt, ed. *China and Beyond in the Medieval Period* (Amherst: Cambria Press, 2014), 196. See *Songshi*, fasc. 69, Lülizhi 律曆志 [Treatises on pitch-pipes and calendars], pt. 22, Lüli 律曆 2, in *Ershisi shi* 30, 726b. It should be noted that the citation here concerns the *Yitian li* 儀天曆, a corrected version of the *Yingtian li* issued under Song Zhenzong 真宗 (r. 997–1022) in 1001; see *infra*, n141.

107. The full title for S.95 is "Almanac for the Third Year Bing/Chen of the Xiande Era (956) 顯德三年丙辰歲具注曆日. For other similarly annotated calendars in the Dunhuang archive see British Museum S.2404 and British Museum S.276. The manuscript of the *Yingtian li* in the archive (British Library, S.612) does not show red-marked Sundays or other weekdays, but it is in fragmentary form.

108. *Xingming zongkuo zixu* 星命總括自序 [Preface to compendia of astrology and divination], in *Quan Liao wen*, 92–93. For the full text of the *Xingming zongkuo*, in three fascicles full of astronomical tables and calendrical lore, see *Wenyuange Siku quanshu dianziban* 文淵閣四庫全書电子版 [Wenyuange complete library of the four treasuries; electronic version].

109. Zürcher, *Buddhist Conquest of China*, 273.

110. *Lidai sanbao ji*, T2034.49.104c15–19. See also Lancaster, "Dating of the Buddha," 450, and *Haedong goseung jeon* 海東高僧傳 [Lives of eminent Korean monks; 1215], T2065.50.1016b16–c8.

111. Discussion of the Nanatsudera discovery is based on Makita Tairyō and Antonino Forte, ed., *The Manuscripts of Nanatsu-dera* (Kyoto: Istituto Italiano di Cultura, Scuola di Studi sull'Asia Orientale, 1991).

112. *Kaiyuan shijiao lu*, T2154.55.525b22, 699b20–25; *Zhenyuan xinding shijiao mulu*, T2157.55.822b6, 1046c24–29.

113. Ochiai Toshinori, "A Report on the Newly Found Texts of Nanatsudera," in Makita Tairyō and Antonino Forte, ed., *The Manuscripts of Nanatsu-dera*, 19–29. For the text of the *Piluo sanmei jing* see Makita Tairyō 牧田諦亮 and Ochiai Toshinori, ed., *Nanatsudera koitsu kyōten kenkyū sōsho* 七寺古逸經典研究叢書 [The long hidden scriptures of Nanatsudera; research series] (Kyoto: Daitō Shuppan, 1994–2000), 6 vols., vol. 1 (1994), 6–67.

114. For the text of the *Bi'an Sutra* see Makita and Ochiai, ed. *Nanatsudera koitsu kyōten* 4 (1999), 75–83, 84–86. Buddha Fragrant Sandalwood is

variously called Candana-puṣpa 栴檀花如来 and Candana-ghanda 栴檀香光明如來. It is one of a myriad of Buddhas preceding Śākyamuni. According to the list of Buddhas named in the translation of the Sanskrit version of the Sukhāvatīvyūha by Luis O. Gómez in *The Land of Bliss* (Honolulu: University of Hawaii Press, 1996), 65, Candana-ghanda is the 52nd Buddha predating Dīpaṃkara. Dīpaṃkara is the 24th predecessor of Śākyamuni.

115. Ochiai Toshinori, "A Report on the Newly Found Texts of Nanatsudera," 32.

116. Piero Corradini, "Notes on the Establishment of the Tuoba Power in North China and on the 'Tan Yao' Caves of Yungang," *Rivista degli studi orientali*, vol. 77, fasc. 1/4 (2003), 198–203.

117. Sofukawa Hiroshi 曽布川寛, "Unkō sekkutsu saikō" 雲岡石窟再考 [Yungang grottoes reconsidered], *Tōhō gakuhō* 東方學報 83 (2008), 121.

118. The inscription is entitled *Da Jin Wuzhoushan zhongxiu da shiku si bei* 大金西京武州山重修大石窟寺碑 [Stele inscription on restorations at the Great Rock Temple at Wuzhoushan at the western capital of Great Jin], or *Jin bei*; unfortunately, this document has not been digitized and is inaccessible. See Sofukawa, "Unkō sekkutsu," 4, 116–120; and Su Bai, "Yungang shiku fenqi shi lun 雲岡石窟分期試論 [Periodization of the Yungang Cave temples], in *Kaogu xuebao* 考古學報 *Acta archaeologia sinica* 1 (1978), 27n2.

119. Francois Louis, "Shaping Symbols of Privilege: Precious Metals and the Early Liao Aristocracy," *Journal of Song-Yuan Studies*, no. 33 (2003), 72, 89–91.

120. Chikusa, "Keitan Daizōkyō," 312–316. I am grateful to the anonymous reviewer of this essay for reminding me of the "southern" format utilized for the Kaibao imprint.

121. According to *Liaoshi*, there was direct contact in 1091 and 1092; see *Liaoshi*, fasc. 25, Benji 本紀 (Annals) 25, Daozong (道宗) 5, Da'an 7/1/2 (*ren/xu*) (Jan. 24, 1091) and Da'an 8/1/2 (*yi/you*) (Feb. 11, 1092), in *Ershisi shi* 37, 132b. By then it had been 167 years since a Japanese envoy appeared at the Kitan court; see also *Liaoshi*, fasc. 2, Benji 2, Taizu 太祖 2, Tianzan 4/10/10 (*xin/su*) (Oct. 29, 925), vol. 37, 23a.

122. Yiengpruksawan, "Pavilion for Amitābha," 447–452.

123. Ogawa Hiromitsu 小川裕充, "Ryō no kaiga" 遼の絵画 [Liao painting], in *Sekai bijutsu dai zenshū tōyōhen, dai go kan, Godai, Hokusō, Ryō, Seika* 世界美術全集東洋編, 第五卷, 五代-北宋-遼-西夏 [History of world

art, East Asia, vol. 5, Five Dynasties, Northern Song, Liao, Xi Xia], ed. Ogawa Hiromitsu and Yuba Tadanori 弓場紀知 (Tokyo: Shōgakkan, 1997), 132–135.

124. Tsunematsu Mikio, "Kawara no rūtsu o motomete" 瓦のルーツを求めて, in Kawazoe Shōji, Yomigaeru chūsei 1 Higashi Ajia no kokusai toshi Hakata よみがえる中世1東アジアの国際都市博多 (Tokyo: Heibonsha, 1988), 159.

125. Tsunematsu, "Kawara," 159–160. For early photographs of the roof tiles at Qingling see Tamura Jitsuzō and Kobayashi Yukio 小林行雄, Keiryō 慶陵 [Qingling] (Tokyo: Zauhō Kankōkai, 1952–1953), 2 vols., vol. 2, pl. 112, 116.

126. For an illustration of one of the tiles see Kyoto National Museum, Michinaga, pl. 134 (6). For Michinaga's building projects see Yiengpruksawan, "Pavilion for Amitābha," 446–447.

127. Midō Kanpaku ki, Chōwa 1 (Kankō 9)/9/21 (Oct. 9, 1012), in DNK, vol. 1, pt. 2, p. 167. Michinaga uses the term sakubun, "composition" or "writing," primarily for literary prose and poetry. For example, when he says there will be sakubun or "compositions" at his home in 1010, he means composition of classical Chinese poetry, in this case on the theme of a verse by Bai Juyi; see Midō Kanpaku ki, Kankō 7/9/6 (Oct. 15, 1010), in DNK, vol. 1, pt. 2, p. 74. For official communications Michinaga used the term chō 牒 "missive," as in the case of documents he sent to monks at Tiantaishan; see for example Midō Kanpaku ki, Chōwa 2/9/14 (Oct. 21, 1013), in DNK, vol. 1, pt. 2, p. 243.

128. Edmund H. Worthy, Jr. "Diplomacy for Survival: Domestic and Foreign Relations of Wu Yüeh, 907–978," in Morris Rossabi, ed. China among Equals: The Middle Kingdom and its Neighbors, 10th–14th Centuries (Berkeley, Los Angeles, London: University of California Press, 1983), 35–37.

129. Nihon kiryaku, Jōhei 5/9 hoc mense (Oct., 935), in SZKT, vol. 11, p. 35; Worthy, "Diplomacy for Survival," 35.

130. Nihon sandai jitsuroku 日本三代実録 [Record of three Japanese reigns], Jōgan 3/6/16 (July 27, 861), in Shintei zōho kokushi taikei fukyūban: Nihon sandai jitsuroku 新訂増補国史大系普及版：日本三代実録 [A Library of Japanese history, revised edition, popular edition: Record of three Japanese reigns] (Tokyo: Yoshikawa Kōbunkan, 1978), 2 vols., vol. 1, 76. For Balhae and the Balhae sea passage, see Kim Chang Seok, "Parhae's Maritime Routes to Japan in the Eighth Century," Seoul Journal of Korean Studies 23: 1 (June 2010), 1–22, and

Kojima Yoshitaka 小島芳孝, "Koguryō Bokkai to no kōryū" 高麗渤海
との交流 [Exchange with Goryeo and Parhae], in *Umi to rettō bunka 1
Nihonkai to hokkoku bunka* 海と列島文化 1 日本海と北国文化 [Cul-
ture of sea and archipelago: 1 culture of the Sea of Japan and Northern Provinces], ed. Amino Yoshihiko網野義彦 (Tokyo: Shōgakkan 小
学館, 1990), 208–209.

131. For Bae Gu as an envoy from Balhae, arriving in Wakasa then transfer-
ring to Echizen and finally Kyoto, see *Fusō ryakki*, Engi 延喜 19/11/25
(Dec. 20, 919), in SZKT, vol. 12, p. 192; and *Nihon kiryaku*, Engi 20/4/20
(May 11, 920) and 20/5/8 (May 28, 920), in SZKT, vol. 11 (2000), p. 23.
For Bae Gu as an envoy from Dong Qidan, see *Nihon kiryaku*, Enchō 延
長 7/12/24 (Jan. 26, 930), in SZKT, vol. 11, p. 29, and *Fusō ryakki*, Enchō
8/4/1 (May 1, 930), in SZKT, vol. 12, p. 204.

132. At his home Michinaga kept a library containing more than 2,000 fascicles of historical records and other writings, many of which were
Chinese dynastic histories. See *Midō Kanpaku ki*, Kankō 7/8/29 (Oct. 9,
1010), in DNK, vol. 1, pt. 2, p. 74.

133. Worthy, "Diplomacy for Survival," 35.

134. Murai Shōsuke 村井章介, *Kyōkai o matagu hitobito* 境界をまたぐ人
びと (People Astride Borders) (Tokyo: Yamakawa Shuppansha, 2016
[2006]), 27–31, 37.

135. Richard Pearson, "Japanese Medieval Trading Towns: Sakai and
Tosaminato," *Japanese Journal of Archaeology*, 3 (2016), 107–109.

136. *Shōyūki*, Chōwa 3/2/7 (Mar. 10, 1014), in DNK, vol. 10, pt. 3, p. 186.
Sanesuke had a poor opinion of the commanding officer, Taira no
Koreyoshi平惟良 (d. 1022), who bought his way to high office.

137. *Midō Kanpaku ki*, Chōwa 5/7/13 (Aug. 18, 1016), in DNK, vol. 1, pt. 3, p.
68. For Ōshū, Tosaminato, and the Eastern Sea trade see Kojima Yoshitaka, "Kodai Nihonkai sekai hokubu no kōryū" 古代日本海世界北部
の交流 (Exchange in the Northern Zone of the Ancient Sea of Japan
World), in Murai Shōsuke, Saitō Toshio 斉藤利男, and Oguchi Masashi
小口雅史, ed. *Kita no Kan Nihonkai sekai* 北の環日本海世界 (The
World of the Northern Circuit of the Sea of Japan) (Tokyo: Yamakawa
Shuppan, 2002), 36–56, and Murai Shōsuke, Kojima Yoshitaka, Sakak-
ibara Shigetaka 榊原滋高, Moriyama Kazō 森山嘉蔵, and Endō Iwao
遠藤巌, "Tōron: Kan Nihonkai Sekai Hokubu no shakai bunka to
kōryū" 討論：環日本海世界北部の社会・文化と交流 (Panel Dis-
cussion: Exchange and the Culture and Society of the Northern Zone

of the World of the Sea of Japan Circuit), in Murai et al., *Kita no Kan Nihonkai sekai*, 140–174.

138. David T. Bialock, *Eccentric Spaces, Hidden Histories: Narrative, Ritual, and Royal Authority from The Chronicles of Japan to The Tale of the Heike* (Stanford: Stanford University Press, 2007), 183. See also *Shōmonki* 将門記 (Account of Taira no Masakado), in *Gunsho ruijū*, vol. 20, fasc. 369, pp. 12a, 13b.

139. *Shunki*, Chōryaku 3/Intercalaris 12/28 (Feb. 13, 1040), in ZST, vol. 7, p. 92. Mistaken predictions were typically met with sarcasm. In 1014 an eclipse of the sun did not happen on the day predicted by the calendar makers, which prompted Michinaga to point out that the sun was perfectly round and could be seen clearly; see *Midō Kanpaku ki*, Chōwa 2/12/1 (Jan. 4, 1014), in DNK, vol. 1, pt. 2, p. 254. For Goryeo and Silla see Michael C. Rogers, "National Consciousness in Medieval Korea: The Impact of Liao and Chin on Koryŏ," in Rossabi, ed. *China among Equals*, 172n54.

140. *Shunki*, Chōryaku 4 (Chōkyū 1)/1/1 (February 15, 1040); for the citation see Kokusai Nihon Bunka Kenkyū Sentā 国際日本文化研究センター (International Research Center for Japanese Studies): Sekkanki kokiroku database 摂関期古記録データベース (Sekkan Period Documents Database) at http://rakusai.nichibun.ac.jp/kokiroku/list.php. Yorimichi was less sanguine, reminding everyone that Michihira had gotten the start time wrong, but agreed on the importance of having the correct end time.

141. For the holdings see *Songshi*, fasc. 206, Zhi 志 (Treatises) 159, 藝文 (Literature) 5, in *Ershisi shi*, vol. 32, p. 2395, and fasc. 207, Zhi 志 (Treatises) 160, 藝文 (Literature) 6, in *Ershisi shi*, vol. 32, p. 2405ff. For the *Qintian li*, *Yingtian li* and *Qianyuan li* see *Songshi*, fasc. 68, Lülizhi, pt. 21, Lüli 1, in *Ershisi shi*, vol. 30, pp. 712a, 715b. For the *Yitian li* see *Songshi*, fasc. 6, Benji 本紀 (Annals) 6, Zhenzong 1, in *Ershisi shi*, vol. 30, p. 53b7–10.

142. *Goryeosa* 高麗史, fasc. 50, Zhi 志 (Treatises), pt. 4, Li 曆 (Calendars), pt. 1, in *Kōraishi*, vol. 2, p. 64b.

143. For the *Chongxuan li* see Ji Zhigang, "The Development of Interpolation Methods in Ancient China: From Liu Zhuo to Hua Hengfang," in Alan K. L. Chan, Gregory K. Clancey, and Hui-Chieh Loy, ed. *Historical Perspectives on East Asian Science, Technology and Medicine* (Singapore: Singapore University Press, 2001), 261.

144. John M. Steele, On the Use of the Chinese "Hsuan-ming" Calendar to Predict the Times of Eclipses in Japan, *Bulletin of the School of Orien-*

tal and African Studies, University of London 61, no. 3 (1998), 528–532. For the Xuanmingli see also Shigeru Nakayama, *A History of Japanese Astronomy* (Cambridge, MA: Harvard University Press, 1969), 71. The coordinates for Kyoto are 35°0'45"N 135°46'6"E; those for Yangcheng are 34°27'19"N 113°1'31"E.

145. *Shōyūki*, Chōwa 1 (Kankō 9)/7/25 (Aug. 15, 1012), in DNK, vol. 10, pt. 3, pp. 50–51.

146. *Liaoshi*, fasc. 42, *Zhi* 志 (Treatises) 12, *Lixiang zhi Shang* 歷象志上 (Treatise on Calendars and Calendrical Representations, pt. 1), in *Ershisi shi*, vol. 37, pp. 221a–b.

147. Ye Mengde 葉夢得, *Shilin yanyu* 石林燕語 (Notes from Retirement in a Stone Forest, 1128), in Wang Yunwu 王雲五, *Cong shu ji cheng chu bian* 叢書集成初編 (Shanghai: Shangwu Yinshu Guan, 1935–1940), fasc. 3, pp. 30–31, and Joseph Needham, Wang Ling, and Derek J. Price, *Heavenly Clockwork* (Cambridge: Cambridge University Press, 1960), 6–7.

148. *Songshu*, fasc. 12, Zhi 2, Lülizhi 2, in *Ershisi shi* (1997), vol. 5, p. 73b.

149. *Liaoshi*, fasc. 44, *Zhi* (Treatises) 14, *Lixiang zhi Xia* 歷象志下 (Treatise on Calendars and Calendrical Representations, pt. 2), in *Ershisi shi*, vol. 37, p. 254b.

150. Toshifusa's calendar has the eclipse on the fourteenth day of the intercalary 12th month of year *ding/si* 丁巳—Jan. 30, 1078—whereas the Northern Song and Goryeo calendars, which did not utilize an intercalary month here—have the eclipse in the first month of the following year *wu/wu* 戊午. *Liaoshi* does not record the eclipse but does have an intercalary twelfth month for year *ding/si*. See Endō Mitsumasa 遠藤光正 and Ōtani Mitsuo 大谷光男, "Maegaki" まえがき (Preface), in Daitō Bunka Daigaku Tōyō Kenkyūjo, ed. *"Kōraishi" rekishi, Senmyōreki no kenkyū* 「高麗史」曆志、宣明曆の研究 (Calendrical Treatises of the *Goryeosa*: Studies in the Xuanming li) (Tokyo: Daitō Bunka Daigaku Tōyō Kenkyūjo, 1998), p. 1.

151. For example Sukefusa refers to some merchants as coming Guangzhou in "Great Song"; see *Shunki*, Chōryaku 4 [Chōkyū 1]/4/27 (June 9, 1040), in ZST, vol. 7, p. 149.

152. *Gonki*, Kankō 8/6/28 (July 31, 1011), in ZST, vol. 5, p. 169a.

About the Contributors

Mark Bender is Professor of Chinese literature and folklore at The Ohio State University. He did his undergraduate at The Ohio State University, then taught in China (Wuhan and Guangxi) during much of the 1980s, before returning to The Ohio State University for graduate school. Dr. Bender's publications include *The Borderlands of Asia: Culture, Place, Poetry*, *Plum and Bamboo: China's Suzhou Chantefable Tradition*; *Butterfly Mother: Miao (Hmong) Creation Epics from Guizhou, China*; and *The Columbia Anthology of Chinese Folk and Popular Literature*. He has published in journals such as *Asian Ethnology, Oral Tradition,* and *Chinese Literature Today.*

Nicola Di Cosmo is the Henry Luce Foundation Professor of East Asian Studies at the Institute for Advanced Study (Princeton, NJ). He holds a PhD from Indiana University in Uralic and Altaic Studies, and a BA from the University of Venice (Italy). His previous publications include *Ancient China and Its Enemies: The Rise of Nomadic Power in East Asian History,* and *Manchu-Mongol Relations on the Eve of the Qing Conquest.* He has published in several journals such as *Journal of Asian Studies, Journal of the American Oriental Society, Proceedings of the National Academy of Science,* and *Scientific Reports.* Among his edited books are *Military Culture in Imperial China* and *The Cambridge History of Inner Asia.*

Phyllis Granoff is the Lex Hixon Professor of Religious Studies at Yale University. She holds a PhD from Harvard University and a BA from Radcliffe College. Professor Granoff edits the *Journal of Indian Philosophy.* Her recent publications include *The Victorious Ones: Jain Images of Perfection,* an edited volume that accompanied the exhibition on Jain art that she curated at the Rubin Museum of Art. With Koichi Shinohara she has edited a number of volumes, including *Images in Asian Religions* and *Pilgrims, Patrons and Place.* She serves as senior advisor

to the Jain Heritage Preservation Project which is run by the Jiv Daya
Foundation in Dallas, Texas.

Wilt L. Idema is is Professor of Chinese literature at Harvard University
and a recipient of the prestigious Special Book Award of China. He holds
a PhD from Leiden University. His publications include *"The Immortal
Maiden Equal to Heaven" and Other Precious Scrolls from Western Gansu;
The Red Brush: Writing Women of Imperial China; Personal Salvation and
Filial Piety: Two Precious Scroll Narratives of Guanyin and Her Acolytes;
Meng Jiangnü Brings Down the Great Wall: Ten Versions of a Chinese
Legend; Heroines of Jiangyong: Chinese Narrative Ballads in Women's
Script; The White Snake and her Son; Judge Bao and the Rule of Law:
Eight Ballad-Stories from the Period 1250–1450; Monks, Bandits, Lovers and
Immortals: Eleven Early Chinese Plays; The Butterfly Lovers: The Legend
of Liang Shanbo and Zhu Yingtai; Escape from Blood Pond Hell: The Tales
of Mulian and Woman Huang; Battles, Betrayals, and Brotherhood: Early
Chinese Plays on the Three Kingdoms; The Generals of the Yang Family:
Four Early Plays;* and *The Resurrected Skeleton: From Zhuangzi to Lu Xun.*

Mabel Lee, PhD, FAHA, is currently an adjunct professor of Chinese
Studies at the University of Sydney where she taught twentieth-century
Chinese history and literature, 1966–2000. An honorary professor for
a number of years at the Open University of Hong Kong, Dr. Lee was
recently appointed a distinguished professor in their major research
project titled "Chinese Culture in the Global Context." She has published
numerous essays about Gao Xingjian, as well as translating English
editions of his works: two novels *Soul Mountain* and *One Man's Bible;*
a short-story collection *Buying a Fishing Rod for My Grandfather;* and
two collections of criticism *The Case for Literature* and his eponymous
book *Gao Xingjian: Aesthetics and Creation.* Her latest publications are *Gao
Xingjian and Transmedia Aesthetics* and Shen Jiawei's *Painting History:
China's Revolution in a Global Context.*

Perry Link is the Chancellorial Chair for Innovation in Teaching Across
Disciplines at the University of California, Riverside, and Emeritus

Professor of East Asian Studies at Princeton University. He received his PhD and BA from Harvard University. His books include *An Anatomy of Chinese: Rhythm, Metaphor, Politics*; a translation of the memoirs of the Chinese astrophysicist Fang Lizhi, entitled *The Most Wanted Man in China: My Journey from Scientist to Enemy of the State*; *The Uses of Literature: Life in the Socialist Chinese Literary System*; *Evening Chats in Beijing: Probing China's Predicament*; and *Mandarin Duck and the Butterflies: Popular Fiction in Early Twentieth-Century Chinese Cities*.

Haun Saussy is University Professor at the University of Chicago. He holds an MPhil and a PhD from Yale University and a BA from Duke University. His books include *The Problem of a Chinese Aesthetic*, *Great Walls of Discourse and Other Adventures in Cultural China*, *The Ethnography of Rhythm: Orality and its Technologies*, *Translation as Citation: Zhuangzi Inside Out*, and as editor or coeditor, *Comparative Literature in an Age of Globalization*, *Sinographies: Writing China*, *Fenollosa/Pound, The Chinese Written Character as a Medium for Poetry: A Critical Edition*, *Partner to the Poor: A Paul Farmer Reader*, and *A Book to Burn and a Book to Keep Hidden: Selected Writings of Li Zhi*.

Tansen Sen is Professor of History and the Director of the Center for Global Asia at NYU Shanghai, and Global Network Professor at NYU. He received his MA from Peking University and PhD from the University of Pennsylvania. His publications include *Buddhism, Diplomacy, and Trade: The Realignment of Sino-Indian Relations, 600–1400*; *India, China, and the World: A Connected History*; *Traditional China in Asian and World History*; and *Buddhism Across Asia: Networks of Material, Cultural and Intellectual Exchange*.

Koichi Shinohara is Senior Lecturer of Religious Studies and East Asian Languages & Literatures at Yale University. He holds a PhD from Columbia University and a Master of Letters and Bachelor of Letters from the University of Tokyo. Professor Shinohara is the coauthor of *Speaking of Monks: Religious Biography in India and China* and the coeditor of *Images in Asian Religions: Texts and Contexts* and *Sins and Sinners: Perspectives from Asian Religions.*

Jerome Silbergeld is the P. Y. and Kinmay W. Tang Professor of Chinese Art History, Emeritus, and founding director of the Tang Center for East Asian Art. He holds a PhD from Stanford University, an MA from the University of Oregon, and an MA and a BA from Stanford University. His publications include *Chinese Painting Style; Mind Landscapes: The Paintings of C. C. Wang; Contradictions: Artistic Life, the Socialist State, and the Chinese Painter Li Huasheng; China Into Film: Frames of Reference in Contemporary Chinese Cinema; Hitchcock with a Chinese Face; Body in Question: Image and Illusion in Two Chinese Films by Director Jiang Wen; Outside In: Chinese x American x Contemporary x Art; and Humanism in China: A Contemporary Record of Photography.*

Tanya Storch is Professor of Religious Studies at the University of the Pacific. She taught Asian religions at several universities, including the University of New Mexico, University of Pennsylvania, and University of Florida. She holds a PhD from the University of Pennsylvania and an MA from the University of St. Petersburg, Russia. her publications include *The History of Chinese Buddhist Bibliography: Censorship and Transformation of the Tripitaka; Chinese Scrolls; Religions and Missionaries in the Pacific, 1500–1800; Japan Under Snow;* and *Mastering the Five Elements,* in addition to thirty academic and artistic publications in the field of Asian religion and spirituality.

Emma J. Teng is the T.T. and Wei Fong Chao Professor of Asian Civilizations and the Head of Global Studies and Languages at MIT. She holds a PhD, AM, and AB from Harvard University. Her publications include *Taiwan's Imagined Geography: Chinese Colonial Travel Writing and Pictures, 1683–1895* and *Eurasian: Mixed Identities in the United States, China and Hong Kong, 1842–1943.* She has served on the Board of Directors of the Association for Asian Studies and currently serves on the Board of Directors for Mass Humanities and on the Faculty Advisory Committee of the Harvard-Yenching Institute.

David Der-wei Wang is the Edward C. Henderson Professor of Chinese Literature at Harvard University. He is Director of CCK Foundation Inter-University Center for Sinological Studies, and Academician, Academia Sinica. He holds a PhD and an MA from the University of Wisconsin at Madison and a BA from National Taiwan University. His publications include *A New Literary History of Modern China*; The *Lyrical in Epic Time: Modern Chinese Intellectuals and Artists Through the 1949 Crisis*; *The Monster That Is History: History, Violence, and Fictional Writing in Twentieth-Century China*; and *Fin-de-Siècle Splendor: Repressed Modernities of Late Qing Fiction, 1848–1911.*

Ellen Widmer is the Mayling Soong Professor of Chinese Studies and Professor of East Asian Studies at Wellesley College. She holds an MA and a PhD from Harvard University, an MA from the Fletcher School of Law and Diplomacy, and a BA from Wellesley College. Her publications include *Fiction's Family: Zhan Xi, Zhan Kai, and the Business of Women in Late-Qing China*; *The Beauty and the Book: Women and Fiction in Nineteenth-Century China*; and *The Margins of Utopia: Shui-hu hou-chuan and the Literature of Ming Loyalism.*

)

INDEX

CPSIA information can be obtained
at www.ICGtesting.com
Printed in the USA
FFOW02n1126180318
45698539-46534FF